Evidence-Based
Healthcare Chaplaincy

by the same author

Case Studies in Spiritual Care
Healthcare Chaplaincy Assessments, Interventions and Outcomes
Edited by George Fitchett and Steve Nolan
ISBN 978 1 78592 783 6
eISBN 978 1 78450 705 3

Spiritual Care in Practice
Case Studies in Healthcare Chaplaincy
Edited by George Fitchett and Steve Nolan
ISBN 978 1 84905 976 3
eISBN 978 0 85700 876 3

of related interest

Spiritual Care at the End of Life
The Chaplain as a 'Hopeful Presence'
Steve Nolan
ISBN 978 1 84905 199 6
eISBN 978 0 85700 513 7

Chaplaincy in Hospice and Palliative Care
Edited by Karen Murphy and Bob Whorton
Foreword by Baroness Finlay of Llandaff
ISBN 978 1 78592 068 4
eISBN 978 1 78450 329 1

Critical Care
Delivering Spiritual Care in Healthcare Contexts
Edited by Jonathan Pye, Peter Sedgwick and Andrew Todd
ISBN 978 1 84905 497 3
eISBN 978 0 85700 901 2

EVIDENCE-BASED HEALTHCARE CHAPLAINCY

A RESEARCH READER

Edited by George Fitchett,
Kelsey B. White and Kathryn Lyndes

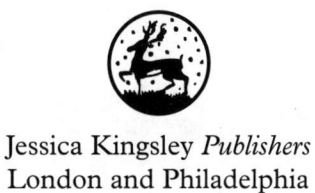

Jessica Kingsley *Publishers*
London and Philadelphia

[permissions granted]

First published in 2018
by Jessica Kingsley Publishers
73 Collier Street
London N1 9BE, UK
and
400 Market Street, Suite 400
Philadelphia, PA 19106, USA

www.jkp.com

Copyright © JKP 2018

Front cover image source: [iStockphoto®/Shutterstock®]. The cover image is for illustrative purposes only, and any person featuring is a model.

All rights reserved. No part of this publication may be reproduced in any material form (including photocopying, storing in any medium by electronic means or transmitting) without the written permission of the copyright owner except in accordance with the provisions of the law or under terms of a licence issued in the UK by the Copyright Licensing Agency Ltd. www.cla.co.uk or in overseas territories by the relevant reproduction rights organisation, for details see www.ifrro.org. Applications for the copyright owner's written permission to reproduce any part of this publication should be addressed to the publisher.

Warning: The doing of an unauthorised act in relation to a copyright work may result in both a civil claim for damages and criminal prosecution.

Library of Congress Cataloging in Publication Data
A CIP catalog record for this book is available from the Library of Congress

British Library Cataloguing in Publication Data
A CIP catalogue record for this book is available from the British Library

ISBN 978 1 78592 820 8
eISBN 978 1 78450 923 1

Printed and bound in the United States

Contents

Acknowledgments 9

Introduction: Advancing Evidence-Based Healthcare Chaplaincy 11

SECTION 1: HEALTHCARE CHAPLAINS: WHERE THEY WORK AND WHAT THEY DO

Introduction to Section 1 21

Article 1: The Provision of Hospital Chaplaincy in the
United States: A National Overview. 36
*Wendy Cadge, Jeremy Freese, and
Nicholas A. Christakis, 2008*

Article 2: "He Needs to Talk!": A Chaplain's Case Study of
Nonreligious Spiritual Care. 48
Steve Nolan, 2016

Article 3: What Do I Do? Developing a Taxonomy of
Chaplaincy Activities and Interventions for Spiritual Care in
Intensive Care Unit Palliative Care 66
*Kevin Massey, Marilyn JD Barnes, Dana Villines, Julie D Goldstein, Anna Lee
Hisey Pierson, Cheryl Scherer, Betty Vander Laan and Wm Thomas Summerfelt, 2015*

Article 4: Communicating Chaplains' Care: Narrative
Documentation in a Neuroscience–Spine Intensive Care Unit 82
*Rebecca Johnson, M. Jeanne Wirpsa, Lara Boyken, Matthew
Sakumoto, George Handzo, Abel Kho, Linda Emanuel, 2016*

Article 5: Determining Best Methods to Screen for
Religious/Spiritual Distress. 101
*Stephen D.W. King, George Fitchett, Patricia E. Murphy, Kenneth
I. Pargament, David A. Harrison, Elizabeth Trice Loggers, 2017*

Article 6: The Spiritual Distress Assessment Tool: An Instrument to
Assess Spiritual Distress in Hospitalised Elderly Persons 116
*Stefanie M Monod, Etienne Rochat, Christophe J Büla,
Guy Jobin, Estelle Martin, Brenda Spencer, 2010*

SECTION 2: PATIENT/FAMILY SPIRITUAL NEEDS AND SPIRITUAL CARE INTERESTS

Introduction to Section 2 135

Article 7: The Spiritual and Theological
Challenges of Stillbirth for Bereaved Parents 150
Daniel Nuzum, Sarah Meaney, Keelin O'Donoghue, 2017

Article 8: Identifying Religious and/or Spiritual Perspectives
of Adolescents and Young Adults Receiving Blood and
Marrow Transplants: A Prospective Qualitative Study 170
Judith R. Ragsdale, Mary Ann Hegner, Mark Mueller, Stella Davies, 2014

Article 9: Adolescents' Spirituality and Cystic Fibrosis Airway
Clearance Treatment Adherence: Examining Mediators 186
*Daniel H. Grossoehme, Rhonda D. Szczesniak, Sylvie Mrug,
Sophia M. Dimitriou, Alec Marshall, and Gary L. McPhail, 2016*

Article 10: Hospital Chaplains: Through the Eyes of
Parents of Hospitalized Children 207
*Pamela K. Donohue, Matt Norvell, Renee D. Boss, Jennifer Shepard,
Karen Frank, Christina Patron, and Thomas Y. Crowe, 2017*

Article 11: Service User Views of Spiritual and Pastoral Care
(Chaplaincy) in NHS Mental Health Services: A Co-Produced
Constructivist Grounded Theory Investigation 224
Julian Raffay, Emily Wood and Andrew Todd, 2016

Article 12: Cultural Differences in Spiritual Care:
Findings of an Israeli Oncologic Questionnaire
Examining Patient Interest in Spiritual Care 245
Michael Schultz, Doron Lulav-Grinwald and Gil Bar-Sela, 2014

Article 13: The Frequency and Correlates of Spiritual
Distress Among Patients with Advanced Cancer Admitted
to an Acute Palliative Care Unit 265
*David Hui, Maxine de la Cruz, Steve Thorney, Henrique A.
Parsons, Marvin Delgado-Guay, and Eduardo Bruera, 2011*

SECTION 3: CHAPLAINCY INTERVENTIONS AND THEIR IMPACT

Introduction to Section 3 281

Article 14: Relationship Between Chaplain Visits and
Patient Satisfaction 294
*Deborah B. Marin, Vanshdeep Sharma, Eugene Sosunov, Natalia
Egorova, Rafael Goldstein, and George F. Handzo, 2015*

Article 15: The Association of Spiritual Care Providers' Activities with Family Members' Satisfaction with Care after a Death in the ICU. . . . 306
Jeffrey R. Johnson, Ruth A. Engelberg, Elizabeth L. Nielsen, Erin K. Kross, Nicholas L. Smith, Julie C. Hanada, Sean K. Doll O'Mahoney, and J. Randall Curtis, 2014

Article 16: The Effect of Pastoral Care Services on Anxiety, Depression, Hope, Religious Coping, and Religious Problem Solving Styles: A Randomized Controlled Study 323
Paul S. Bay, Daniel Beckman, James Trippi, Richard Gunderman, and Colin Terry, 2008

Article 17: A Novel Picture Guide to Improve Spiritual Care and Reduce Anxiety in Mechanically Ventilated Adults in the Intensive Care Unit 340
Joel N. Berning, Armeen D. Poor, Sarah M. Buckley, Komal R. Patel, David J. Lederer, Nathan E. Goldstein, Daniel Brodie, and Matthew R. Baldwin, 2016

Article 18: The Impact of a Spiritual Legacy Intervention in Patients with Brain Cancers and Other Neurologic Illnesses and Their Support Persons 361
Katherine M. Piderman, Carmen Radecki Breitkopf, Sarah M. Jenkins, Maria I. Lapid, Gracia M. Kwete, Terin T. Sytsma, Laura A. Lovejoy, Timothy J. Yoder and Aminah Jatoi, 2017

Article 19: What Impact Do Chaplains Have? A Pilot Study of Spiritual AIM for Advanced Cancer Patients in Outpatient Palliative Care 379
Allison Kestenbaum, The Rev. Michele Shields, Jennifer James, The Rev. Will Hocker, Stefana Morgan, Shweta Karve, Michael W. Rabow, and Laura B. Dunn, 2017

Article 20: Patient Reported Outcome Measure of Spiritual Care as Delivered by Chaplains 393
Austyn Snowden and Iain Telfer, 2017

Article 21: A National Study of Chaplaincy Services and End-of-Life Outcomes 418
Kevin J Flannelly, Linda L Emanuel, George F Handzo, Kathleen Galek, Nava R Silton and Melissa Carlson, 2012

Full citations of the 21 articles 431

Acknowledgments

We wish to acknowledge that this *Reader* was produced with support from the Transforming Chaplaincy Project, which was funded by grants from the John Templeton Foundation. We also wish to thank Kristen Schenk for her help in preparing the manuscript.

Introduction: Advancing Evidence-Based Healthcare Chaplaincy

Around the world, a new evidence-based paradigm is informing the work of healthcare chaplains and spiritual care providers. We created this *Research Reader* to support this approach to chaplaincy and spiritual care. (We recognize that spiritual care and spiritual care provider are the preferred terms in some contexts. For simplicity, we will generally use the terms chaplain and chaplaincy.) One approach to the history of chaplaincy (Gleason 1998) describes the dominant model for spiritual care in the mid-20th century, shaped by the client-centered model of the psychologist Carl Rogers, as empathic presence and active listening. Gleason described a shift in the dominant paradigm for spiritual care at the beginning of the 21st century to spiritual care as a response to individual need. He pointed to the developing models of spiritual assessment as an indicator of the shift. As we will elaborate below, Gleason's 1998 observations about spiritual care in the 21st century were astute. However, now that we are well into the 21st century, it appears to us that the emerging paradigm for this period is an evidence-based approach to chaplaincy. Indicators of this are the inclusion of a standard about research in the Standards of Practice (SOP) of chaplaincy organizations, such as the US Association of Professional Chaplains (APC). (The first SOP was published in 2009. The Research Standard, Standard 12, reads in part, "The chaplain practices evidence-based care." For the current Standards see Association of Professional Chaplains 2015.) The Salzburg Statement of the European Network of Health Care Chaplaincy (2014) also reflects this paradigm, saying in part, "The European healthcare chaplaincy community actively promotes research as an integral part of chaplaincy activity… All chaplains must develop their ongoing practice in the light of current research." Surveys of chaplains both in the US and around the world suggest strong support for the paradigm (Fitchett et al. 2014; Snowden et al. 2017).

Two reasons are generally given for why healthcare chaplaincy needs to shift to an evidence-based paradigm. The reason which is often uppermost in chaplains' minds is that healthcare is an evidence-based activity, and, unless chaplains working in healthcare can provide evidence for the benefits associated with their work, they will be marginalized (Handzo et al. 2014). This is clearly important, but in our view it is the second reason for the profession to shift to an evidence-based paradigm. The first reason is that we need research to help us know if the care we are providing is having the effects we hope it will have. As Canadian chaplaincy researchers Thomas O'Connor and Elizabeth Meakes wrote in 1998 in the first paper to use the term "evidence-based pastoral care," "Evidence from research needs to inform our pastoral care. To remove the evidence from pastoral care can create a ministry that is ineffective or possibly even harmful" (p.367).

Fulfilling the potential of the evidence-based paradigm for healthcare chaplaincy requires that all chaplains become research *literate*. It is important to emphasize that it does not mean that all chaplains must do research; most will never be researchers, and that is fine. But all chaplains need to be research literate. There is a parallel in other healthcare professions (e.g., medicine, nutrition, physical therapy), where a relatively small proportion of the professionals are active researchers, but all members of the profession are research literate.

Being research literate means two things. First, it means having the ability to critically read and understand basic research and, if indicated, apply the findings of research studies to one's chaplaincy practice. Second, it means being generally familiar with the existing body of chaplaincy research, including topics that have been studied and important areas for future research.

The 21 research articles in this *Reader* were selected to help chaplains, chaplains in training, and their interested colleagues to develop both types of research literacy. Specifically, we selected articles that illustrate a variety of research methods, and we discuss how those different methods produce diverse findings that inform evidence-based practice for chaplaincy care. The articles were also selected to help readers develop awareness of some of the most important chaplaincy research that is currently being produced. This includes awareness of important contributors to chaplaincy research working in different national contexts.

We also made an effort to select articles that reflect the most recent chaplaincy research, that is, articles from the past five years. In some cases, however, important articles that are somewhat older were included. While the articles selected for the *Reader* provide a good introduction to chaplaincy research, there were many important articles that we could not include. Fortunately, there are a number of good reviews of the chaplaincy literature that will help chaplains develop a broad familiarity with the research in the field (Fitchett 2017; Jankowski, Handzo and Flannelly 2011; Kalish 2012; Mowat 2008; Pesut et al. 2016; Proserpio, Piccinelli and Clerici 2011; Spiritual Care Victoria 2015). There are also reviews of the quality of chaplaincy research, the latest by Galek and colleagues (2011).

The articles in the *Reader* are organized in three sections: Section 1, Healthcare Chaplains: Where They Work and What They Do; Section 2, Patient/Family Spiritual Needs and Spiritual Care Interest; and Section 3, Chaplaincy Interventions and Their Impact. These sections reflect three broad areas in which chaplaincy-related research is currently being conducted. Each of the sections begins with an introduction. These introductions start with an overview of the research in that section. This is then followed by a brief introduction to each article in that section. The article introductions provide background about the author(s) and the article. We also put each article in the context of the evidence-based paradigm for chaplaincy care and other chaplaincy research, including other articles in the *Reader*. Finally, we call attention to some of the research methods used in the article and invite chaplains to consider the implications of the article for their practice.

In addition to the themes that are mentioned in the section introductions, we want to call attention to several themes in chaplaincy-related research that are reflected in articles in different sections of the *Reader*. The first theme is about defining religion and spirituality. Most chaplains will be aware that there are many definitions of these terms and that the current perspective that views religion as one way of being spiritual is a switch from an earlier view (Oman 2013). Good research generally requires clarity about the constructs being investigated. However, the absence of a consensus about defining religion and spirituality is not preventing useful research about these constructs. Investigators just need to be clear about their definitions (e.g., Ragsdale et al. 2014 and Raffay, Wood, and Todd 2016) and any specific measures they are using (e.g., Grossoehme et al. 2016).

The second theme is about how chaplains are perceived by patients and their loved ones, the recipients of chaplaincy care. In an earlier view, chaplains saw themselves and were identified by others as representatives of faith traditions who mainly served members of that tradition who were ill and hospitalized. Now, many chaplains see themselves as healthcare professionals who address the religious, spiritual, and emotional needs of patients and their loved ones (Swift 2014; Swift, Handzo, and Cohen 2012). But how do patients and their loved ones view chaplains? Are they aware of this change? Several of the articles in the *Reader* address this question directly or indirectly. Donohue and her colleagues (2017) address it directly by asking parents of hospitalized children who had been seen by a chaplain if they viewed the chaplains as members of the healthcare team; 75 percent said they did. In Israel, where spiritual caregivers are still very new, Schultz, Lulav-Grinwald, and Bar-Sela (2014) asked 364 oncology patients how open they would be to a visit from a spiritual caregiver. Forty-one percent were definitely or possibly interested. Prior experience with a spiritual caregiver, or having an understanding of who a spiritual caregiver is, were strong predictors of interest in having a visit from one. Contrast this with the expectations family members of Den, a patient in a hospice in England, had of the hospice chaplain, Steve Nolan (2016). In many hospitals, nursing staff still ask new patients if they would like a visit from the chaplain. Further research about how patients and their families perceive chaplains may help us determine whether this practice should be continued.

The third theme that runs through a number of the articles in the *Reader* is religious/spiritual struggle, pain, and distress. It is the central focus of the research by King and colleagues (2017), who test the best methods to screen for spiritual pain. It is also central in the work by Monod and colleagues (2010) about developing a method to assess unmet spiritual needs in older patients and in the work by Hui and colleagues (2011) who report the prevalence and correlates of spiritual distress in a sample of patients receiving palliative care. It is also very evident in the quotes from bereaved parents in the report by Nuzum, Meaney, and O'Donoghue (2017) and in the adolescents and young adults interviewed by Ragsdale and colleagues (2014). In several of the articles, there are reports of the prevalence of spiritual pain (or need or struggle): it was noted to be present in 12 percent of the long-term survivors of stem cell transplants (King et al. 2017) and in 44 percent of the palliative care in-patients (Hui et al. 2011). These can be seen as measures of the acuity of unmet spiritual need in these clinical samples. Why is that information important for healthcare chaplains and their colleagues? Notice the different ways that these authors define and measure spiritual pain. What are the strengths and weaknesses of those definitions and measures?

The subject of spiritual pain leads us to the fourth theme that runs through a number of articles in different sections of the *Reader*. That theme is the changing paradigm for chaplaincy care that we discussed at the beginning of the Introduction. As we mentioned, Gleason (1998) described the dominant paradigm of the second half of the 20th century as empathic presence and active listening. The taxonomy of chaplain activities developed by Massey and colleagues (2015) reflects this paradigm; chaplains in that study reported "active listening" as both their most frequent and most important activity. Looking toward the 21st century, Gleason observed increased attention to models for spiritual assessment and described an emerging paradigm of identifying need and providing interventions. Accurately identifying patients in spiritual need or struggle so that chaplains can offer interventions to address that need is central to the research reported by King and colleagues (2017) and also Monod and colleagues (2010). In contrast to the ministry of presence paradigm, where the focus is on the process of the chaplains' care, the focus on addressing and ameliorating spiritual need fits well with an outcome-oriented, evidence-based approach to chaplaincy care (Handzo et al. 2014; Peery 2012). All the articles in Section 3 are about outcomes associated with chaplains' care. Which paradigm is reflected in the other articles in the *Reader*?

The aim of the *Reader* is to help chaplains develop research literacy, so they may function effectively in an evidence-based approach to chaplaincy care. Resources are available for chaplains who wish to continue learning about research. One resource is the reviews of chaplaincy research that were mentioned above. A very helpful book is *An Invitation to Chaplaincy Research: Entering the Process* (Myers and Roberts 2014). The book begins with brief accounts from several chaplain-researchers about how they got started on the path to research. Chapters include helpful introductory overviews of various steps in the research process (e.g., formulating a research question) and overviews of key research methods including statistics. Reading current chaplaincy research is an important way to develop and maintain research literacy. At present, the three main chaplaincy/spiritual care journals are *Journal of Health Care Chaplaincy*, *Journal of Pastoral Care & Counseling*, and *Health and Social Care Chaplaincy*.

The internet makes excellent resources easily available. The Joint Research Council is an organization made up of representatives of chaplaincy groups around the world. Its focus is advancing chaplaincy research and chaplaincy research literacy. With support from the Joint Research Council and the Association of Professional Chaplains, Transforming Chaplaincy has built and is maintaining a website to support chaplaincy research and research education (2015). It includes links to the sites of member organizations, many of whom have excellent research-related resources (e.g., European Research Institute for Chaplains in Healthcare 2017; Spiritual Care Victoria 2015). Another important website is the Association of Clinical Pastoral Education (ACPE) Research Network (2018). This site includes a monthly review of an article relevant to chaplaincy research by the Network's convener, Chaplain John Ehman. The archive contains over 15 years of very informative reviews.

The articles in the *Reader* illustrate the kind of chaplaincy-related research that has been conducted. What are the next steps in advancing the research for the profession? In our section and article introductions we have noted a number of areas for future research. In addition, a helpful overview of the priorities for chaplaincy research compares what chaplaincy leaders have written about priorities for chaplaincy research with the priorities of a convenience sample of 193 US chaplains (Damen, Delaney and Fitchett 2018). The team found considerable consistency in the priorities for research articulated by both groups. Specifically, both groups prioritize research on the outcomes of spiritual care, the development and testing of the effectiveness of chaplain interventions, and the development and evaluation of spiritual assessment and screening tools, as well as research about key subgroups of patients. The priorities of the surveyed chaplains also included research about chaplain competencies, education, and certification as well as research about the chaplain and the team.

The three sections of this *Reader* offer another way to think about priorities for future chaplaincy-related research. In line with the priorities identified by Damen and colleagues (2018), Section 3 focuses on chaplain interventions and the outcomes associated with chaplains' care. Section 1 focuses on what chaplains do, their methods for spiritual screening and assessment, and how they document their care, priorities that were also identified by Damen and colleagues (2018). Their work also found that chaplaincy leaders and practicing chaplains recognized that differences in those served by chaplains, including differences in age, gender, race/ethnicity, and religious/spiritual practice, would need to be addressed as research about chaplains' interventions, outcomes, screening, and assessment develops. As Jankowski and colleagues wrote in their review of chaplaincy research, future research needs to focus on "which practices are best for which kinds of patients in what patients' settings" (2011, p.117). The focus in Section 2 of the *Reader*, Patient/Family Spiritual Needs and Spiritual Case Interests, is mentioned as an area for future research by Damen and colleagues (2018), but we would put more emphasis on it. While a body of research has begun to examine the religious/spiritual resources, needs, and coping of people facing specific clinical situations (e.g., Ragsdale et al. 2014), there is a great need for additional research at this basic level. There are many conditions that have not been examined, and there is a similar need, as with research about interventions and assessment, for these studies to focus on key subgroups of people with those conditions. A high priority is for research that follows patients and their families over time to describe the trajectory of religious/spiritual coping with illness or loss. For example, Nuzum and colleagues (2017) describe the spiritual pain expressed by parents who experienced stillbirth. What would we learn if we could interview them again every year for the next five years? Examining trajectories such as these may disclose points of vulnerability or help identify those with prolonged intense spiritual anguish where chaplains' spiritual care may be especially important.

How will the research agenda we have described be accomplished? While we repeat the expectation that most chaplains will not be involved in research but will be research literate, we recognize that many chaplains may like to get involved in advancing the profession through research. For those colleagues, we suggest there are interesting and important opportunities to contribute to chaplaincy research at three different levels: small, medium, and large. Chaplains with a modest level of research literacy can partner with interested colleagues to replicate a small survey or other project in their local setting, to conduct a quality improvement project (e.g., Donohue et al. 2017), or to contribute to the growing body of chaplain case studies (e.g., Nolan 2016). Other chaplains may find the partners and resources to carry out a survey-based project (e.g., Schultz et al. 2014) or a series of qualitative interviews that shed light on how patients with a specific condition use religious/spiritual beliefs and practices to cope with their illness (e.g., Ragsdale et al. 2014). Finally, some chaplains will have the opportunity to partner with sophisticated major research efforts and address substantial questions about chaplaincy care and its impact (e.g., Johnson et al. 2014; Monod et al. 2010). The number of chaplains and collaborators who are interested in advancing this research is growing, and it is an exciting time to be involved in chaplaincy research.

In summary, we hope this *Research Reader* will further advance an evidence-based approach to healthcare chaplaincy by helping practicing chaplains and chaplains in training develop the ability to critically read and understand research so that, when indicated, they can apply the findings from research to their chaplaincy practice. In doing so, we trust that an evidence-based approach to chaplaincy practice will insure the highest quality spiritual care for the patients and families we serve. Further, we trust that an evidence-based approach to chaplaincy practice will enable us to better communicate what we do—and its value—to our healthcare colleagues and managers who need that information to make the best possible use of the services we provide.

References

Association of Clinical Pastoral Education (ACPE) Research Network (2018) website. Accessed on 2/12/18 at http://acperesearch.net.

Association of Professional Chaplains (2015) *Standards of Practice for Professional Chaplains*. Accessed on 2/12/18 at www.professionalchaplains.org/content.asp?pl=198&sl=198&contentid=200.

Damen, A., Delaney, A., and Fitchett, G. (2018) "Research priorities for healthcare chaplaincy: views of US chaplains." *Journal of Health Care Chaplaincy*, 24, 2:57–66.

Donohue, P.K., Norvell, M., Boss, R., Shepard, J., Frank, K., Patron, C., and Crowe, T. (2017) "Hospital chaplains: through the eyes of parents of hospitalized children." Journal of Palliative Medicine, 20, 2, 1352–1358.

European Network of Health Care Chaplaincy (2014) *Statement – Healthcare Chaplaincy in the Midst of Transition (aka The Salzburg Statement)*. Accessed on 2/12/18 at www.enhcc.eu.

European Research Institute for Chaplains in Healthcare (ERICH) (2017) Enhancing Spiritual Care through Chaplaincy Research. Accessed on 2/11/18 at www.pastoralezorg.be/page/erich.

Fitchett, G. (2017) "Recent progress in chaplaincy-related research." *Journal of Pastoral Care & Counseling*, 71, 3, 163–175.

Fitchett, G., Nieuwsma, J.A., Bates, M.J., Rhodes, J.E., Meador, K.G. (2014) "Evidence-based chaplaincy care: attitudes and practices in diverse healthcare chaplain samples." *Journal of Health Care Chaplaincy*, 20, 4, 144–160.

Galek, K., Flannelly, K.J., Jankowski, K.R.B., and Handzo, G.F. (2011) "A methodological analysis of chaplaincy research: 2000–2009." *Journal of Health Care Chaplaincy*, 17, 3–4, 126–145.

Gleason, J.J. (1998) "An emerging paradigm in professional chaplaincy." *Chaplaincy Today*, 14, 9–14.

Grossoehme, D.H., Szczesniak, R.D., Mrug, S., Dimitriou, S.M., Marshall, A.L., and McPhail, G.L. (2016) "Adolescents' spirituality and cystic fibrosis airway clearance treatment adherence: examining mediators." *Journal of Pediatric Psychology*, 41, 19, 1022–1032.

Handzo, G.F, Cobb, M., Holmes, C., Kelly, E., and Sinclair, S. (2014) "Outcomes for professional health care chaplaincy: an international call to action." *Journal of Health Care Chaplaincy*, 20, 2, 43–53.

Hui, D., de la Cruz, M., Thorney, S., Parsons, H.A., Delgado-Guay, M., and Bruera, E. (2011) "The frequency and correlates of spiritual distress among patients with advanced cancer admitted to an acute palliative care unit." *American Journal of Hospice and Palliative Medicine*, 28, 4, 264–270.

Jankowski, K.R., Handzo, G.F., and Flannelly, K.J. (2011) "Testing the efficacy of chaplaincy care." *Journal of Health Care Chaplaincy*, 17, 3-4, 100–125.

Johnson, J.R., Engelberg, R.A., Nielsen, E.L., Kross, E.K., et al. (2014) "The association of spiritual care providers' activities with family members' satisfaction with care after a death in the ICU." *Critical Care Medicine*, 42, 9, 1991–2000.

Kalish, N. (2012) "Evidence-based spiritual care: a literature review." *Current Opinion in Supportive and Palliative Care*, 6, 2, 242–246.

King, S.D.W., Fitchett, G., Murphy, P.E., Pargament, K.I., Harrison, D.A., and Loggers, E.T. (2017) "Determining best methods to screen for religious/spiritual distress." *Supportive Care in Cancer*, 25, 471–479.

Massey, K., Barnes, M.J.D., Villines, D., Goldstein, J.D., et al. (2015) "What do I do? Developing a taxonomy of chaplaincy activities and interventions for spiritual care in intensive care unit palliative care." *BMC Palliative Care*, 14, 10, 1–8.

Monod, S.M., Rochat, E., Büla, C.J., Jobin, G., Martin, E., and Spencer, B. (2010) "The Spiritual Distress Assessment Tool: an instrument to assess spiritual distress in hospitalized elderly persons." *BMC Geriatrics*, 10, 88–96.

Mowat, H. (2008) "The potential for efficacy of healthcare chaplaincy and spiritual care provision in the NHS (U.K.): a scoping review of recent research." Aberdeen, Scotland: Mowat Research Ltd. Accessed on 2/12/18 at www.ukbhc.org.uk/sites/default/files/The%20potential%20for%20effiicacy%20for%20healthcare%20chaplaincy.pdf.

Myers, G.E. and Roberts, S. (eds) (2014) *An Invitation to Chaplaincy Research: Entering the Process.* Accessed on 2/12/18 at www.healthcarechaplaincy.org/docs/publications/templeton_research/hcc_research_handbook_final.pdf.

Nolan, S. (2016) "'He needs to talk!': a chaplain's case study of nonreligious spiritual care." *Journal of Health Care Chaplaincy*, 22, 1, 1–16.

Nuzum, D., Meaney, S., and O'Donoghue, K. (2017) "The spiritual and theological challenges of stillbirth for bereaved parents." *The Journal of Religion & Health*, 56, 1081–1095.

O'Connor, T.S. and Meakes, E. (1998) "Hope in the midst of challenge: evidence-based pastoral care." *Journal of Pastoral Care*, 52, 4, 359–367.

Oman, D. (2013) "Defining Religion and Spirituality." In R.F. Paloutzian and C.L. Park (eds) *Handbook of the Psychology of Religion and Spirituality* (2nd ed.). New York: Guilford.

Peery, B. (2012) "Outcome Oriented Chaplaincy: Intentional Caring." In S.B. Roberts (ed.) *Professional Spiritual and Pastoral Care: A Practical Clergy and Chaplain's Handbook.* Woodstock, Vermont: Skylight Paths Publishing.

Pesut, B., Sinclair, S., Fitchett, G., Greig, M., and Koss, S.E. (2016) "Health care chaplaincy: a scoping review of the evidence 2009–2014." *Journal of Health Care Chaplaincy*, 22, 2, 67–84.

Proserpio, T., Piccinelli, C., and Clerici, CA. (2011) "Pastoral care in hospitals: a literature review." *Tumori*, 97, 5, 666–671.

Raffay, J., Wood, E., and Todd, A. (2016) "Service user views of spiritual and pastoral care (chaplaincy) in NHS mental health services: a co-produced constructivist grounded theory investigation." *BMC Psychiatry*, 16, 200.

Ragsdale, J.R., Hegner, M.A., Mueller, M., and Davies, S. (2014) "Identifying religious and/or spiritual perspectives of adolescents and young adults receiving blood and marrow transplants: a prospective qualitative study." *Biological Blood Marrow Transplantation*, 20, 8, 1242–1257.

Schultz, M., Lulav-Grinwald, D., and Bar-Sela, G. (2014) "Cultural differences in spiritual care: findings of an Israeli oncologic questionnaire examining patient interest in spiritual care." *BMC Palliative Care*, 13, 1, 19–29.

Snowden, A., Fitchett, G., Grossoehme, D.H., Handzo, G., et al. (2017) "International study of chaplains' attitudes about research." *Journal of Health Care Chaplaincy*, 23, 1, 34–43.

Spiritual Care Victoria (2015) *Review of Literature.* Accessed on 2/12/18 at www.spiritualhealthvictoria.org.au/research.

Swift, C. (2014) *Hospital Chaplaincy in the Twenty-First Century: The Crisis of Spiritual Care on the NHS* (2nd ed.). Farnham: Ashgate Publishing.

Swift, C., Handzo, G., and Cohen, J. (2012) "Healthcare Chaplaincy." In M. Cobb, C. Puchalski, and B. Rumbold (eds) *Oxford Textbook of Spirituality in Healthcare.* Oxford: Oxford University Press.

Transforming Chaplaincy website (2015) Joint Research Council. Accessed on 1/25/18 at www.transformchaplaincy.org.

SECTION 1

HEALTHCARE CHAPLAINS: WHERE THEY WORK AND WHAT THEY DO

Introduction

Research has provided snapshots of what healthcare chaplains do and where they practice. Section 1 begins with an overview of where chaplains work and moves more specifically into the components of their care. We encourage you to consider a multidisciplinary conversation as you work through the *Reader*; a rich variety of perspectives will inform the conversation. For example, the implication of the chaplain taxonomy (Massey et al. 2015) may be different for a physician than for a chaplain. The perspectives of non-chaplain colleagues will strengthen chaplain practice and research, and the insights of chaplains will strengthen the holistic care provided by other clinicians to patients and families.

The first article by Cadge, Freese, and Christakis (2008) provides an overview of the proportion of hospitals in the US with chaplaincy departments. Then, a case study by Nolan (2016) takes an in-depth look at chaplaincy care for those who identify as non-religious. Articles 3 and 4 offer different perspectives on the language we use to describe chaplain activities. One perspective arises out of the work of chaplain-researchers (Massey et al. 2015), while the other comes from a multidisciplinary team reviewing chart notes (Johnson et al. 2016). Finally, the section concludes with two articles focused on spiritual screening and assessment. King et al. (2017) and Monod et al. (2010a) will help you think through the differences between these activities and initiate conversation about their clinical application. As the profession shifts from a paradigm focused on presence to a paradigm focused on interventions and outcomes, the work of chaplains will need to move past the simple identification of spiritual distress to a more nuanced assessment of the type and degree of spiritual distress.

As you read, also pay attention to the study designs and the amount of evidence each article offers. The design type of each study determines the amount of evidence or generalizations one can take from the results. Cross-sectional studies (measuring one point in time) can help you identify relationships between variables while randomized control trials (see Article 16) permit stronger causal inferences. Within Section 1, King et al. (2017) used a study design that provides some of the most substantial evidence. When a study provides stronger evidence, one can then begin to consider its wider application and generalization.

Several themes emerge throughout the articles in Section 1. First, consider the theme of spiritual pain and how chaplains identify unmet spiritual need. Section 1 articles that attend to spiritual pain focus on its prevalence and how best to identify it. For example, King et al. (2017) sought the best method for screening for distress, and Monod et al. (2010a) created a validated assessment of spiritual distress for use with elderly rehabilitation patients. When studying the articles by Massey et al. (2015) and Johnson et al. (2016), consider not only what their results say about the specific work chaplains do but also about the intensity of chaplaincy treatment in specific patient populations. People receiving care from chaplains are often in the midst of significant life events, and these articles in Section 1 help us better understand how to identify the spiritual needs associated with those events.

A second theme in the articles is refining the language of chaplaincy care. The profession, through research and practice, is still working to identify the best way to describe its role. For example, Cadge et al. (2008) indirectly explore the language of chaplaincy organizational structures, and Nolan (2016) begins to delve theologically into the mystical connection that can occur in relationship with another. Some chaplains refer to this connection as a ministry of presence. Through different avenues, each of these articles attempts to bridge a gap between the practice of routine chaplain care and the language used to communicate routine chaplain care. As you will see, and as discussed in the Introduction, the articles look at routine care in different ways, and research helps us refine that language. We are clarifying what we do and how we communicate about it in a multidisciplinary environment.

The articles in Section 1 also highlight the paradigm shift within the profession. The model of intentional care that includes a plan focused on changing an outcome is quite different from chaplaincy care informed by a paradigm focused on pastoral presence (Cadge 2012, see especially Chapter 4). Research will need to continue to address how the structures (e.g., departmental organization, clinical assignments, on-call coverage) of chaplaincy work impact patients, families, and staff. If these structural details influence factors such as patient/family satisfaction, then they could help improve the case for the value of chaplaincy departments.

Think of the content of Section 1, Healthcare Chaplains: Where They Work and What They Do, as a beginning for chaplaincy's intentional engagement with—and your own shift toward—practice informed by evidence. Professional chaplaincy research will continue to refine study designs, increase the number of evidence-based practices, and help the profession make sure our care is the best it can be. We hope this section adds a unique dynamic as you improve your research literacy and energize the development of your own research ideas.

Article 1: Cadge, W., Freese, J., and Christakis, N. (2008) The Provision of Hospital Chaplaincy in the United States: A National Overview

In the US, informal conversations among chaplains often include stories of hospitals downsizing or eliminating chaplaincy programs. These stories evoke concern, even among chaplaincy departments that consider themselves part of a supportive healthcare system. The concern is felt in multiple national contexts. Christopher Swift (2014) wrote about an effort to eliminate the chaplaincy program in the Worcestershire Acute Hospitals NHS Trust. The prospects for chaplains sometimes feel daunting. To begin piecing together a realistic picture of the extent of chaplaincy programs, Cadge et al. (2008) analyzed the American Hospital Association's (AHA) annual survey of hospitals between 1980 and 2003. They were interested in where chaplains work and what influences the existence of their services. The article starts the *Reader* as one example of the chaplaincy landscape in the US context. As you read, consider how the existence of chaplaincy services follows similar patterns as the existence of (and gaps within) other healthcare services.

Wendy Cadge is a professor of sociology from Brandeis University near Boston with over ten years of experience in studying chaplaincy. Cadge's observations, such as those in her 2012 book *Paging God: Religion in the Halls of Medicine*, often challenge healthcare chaplains to re-examine what they do and how they think about what they do. With George Fitchett, she is a Co-Director of the Transforming Chaplaincy Project (2015), which is advancing an evidence-based approach to the profession.

US chaplains have often believed that chaplaincy would become universal and more secure if professional chaplaincy were required in the hospital accreditation guidelines of our major accrediting body, the Joint Commission. Cadge and colleagues (2008) take this into account in their study and observe whether changes in those guidelines in the 1990s had any impact on the provision of chaplaincy. Note that the AHA Survey does not set guidelines for what constitutes a chaplaincy department.

Cadge and colleagues address chaplains' hopes about the effects of Joint Commission requirements by noting that their results showed a consistent proportion of hospitals with chaplaincy programs throughout the period of changing regulations. Questions to consider as you read this study include: what constitutes or defines a chaplaincy department? What specific regulations influence the prevalence of chaplaincy programs in your context? When considering healthcare disparities between rural and urban settings, what do those disparities mean for the prevalence of chaplaincy services?

Interestingly, the proportion of hospitals reporting chaplaincy services and the predictors of those services reported by Cadge and colleagues (2008) were similar to those reported in a 2004 study that used a different approach to gather their information (Flannelly, Handzo, and Weaver 2004). When it comes to research, finding consistency in results, especially from studies that take somewhat different approaches, adds to the confidence we place in them. As you read this article, also think about the results that may surprise you – for example, the results about the existence and demise of chaplaincy programs within faith-based systems.

To examine possible predictors of a hospital reporting chaplaincy services, the investigators used a statistical technique called logistic regression. Logistic regression is used with a dichotomous dependent variable (e.g., have chaplaincy services: yes/no). Generally, results of logistic regression are reported as odds ratios (ORs); for example, the odds of faith-based hospitals having chaplaincy services compared to for-profit hospitals. Cadge and colleagues (2008) reported their results as regression coefficients – a little less clear, but still permitting the reader to identify which predictor variables are significant. For an example of reporting ORs for logistic regression, see Hui et al. (2011) in Section 2.

Article 2: Nolan, S. (2016) "He Needs to Talk!": A Chaplain's Case Study of Non-Religious Spiritual Care

In many places around the world, an increasing number of people identify as non-religious or with an emerging spiritual orientation. For European countries, this has meant a shift towards what Nolan calls the "secularist narrative." These changes raise the question of how chaplains care for people with diverse spiritual-but-not-religious orientations. Nolan's article invites chaplains to examine whether their current approaches are adequate to care for people who consider themselves non-religious. The article will also help non-chaplain colleagues see that chaplains care for all people, not just those who identify as religious.

Steve Nolan is a leading chaplaincy researcher and hospice chaplain in the UK. His book, *Spiritual Care at the End of Life: The Chaplain as a*

'Hopeful Presence' (2012), is an important contribution to the literature of our profession. His case study in the *Reader* was published about a year after the publication of a book of case studies that he co-edited with George Fitchett (Fitchett and Nolan 2015). The introduction to that book describes the important contributions of case studies to the development of evidence-based chaplaincy.

Research via case study provides an avenue for documenting and investigating the detail of chaplaincy craft. We cannot generalize the findings of case studies, but they provide rich descriptions of chaplaincy care and a foundation for future research. Two responses to Nolan's case study were published with it: one by a chaplain (Hess 2016) and the other by a nurse-researcher (Pesut 2016). These responses provide a model for the critical conversation about case studies that will enrich chaplaincy care.

In this case, Nolan claims that part of what makes chaplaincy important is that all individuals, whether religious or not, have religious/spiritual instincts. Those instincts come from an individual's innate being. Chaplain care attends to that instinct, which may be expressed in the religious/spiritual projections evoked by the chaplain. Nolan argues that only a professional chaplain can address the religious and spiritual aspects of an individual's identity. The diverse and changing religious and spiritual dynamics within cultures require a professional who can evoke that innate religious/spiritual framework as well as someone who has the training to directly address it. Interestingly, the family members in this case study do not appear to be struggling with finding or making meaning, a frequently named component of chaplaincy care. Nolan's case study may ignite strong conversation regarding the content of the care he provided. Could he be offering a theological interpretation of "presence?" What do you think of his approach to using research to explain chaplain care?

An outcome-based paradigm will require further study of chaplain encounters with the spiritual, non-religious, or those of emerging spiritual orientations. Perhaps as a profession, we will be able to figure out if care for individuals like Den will differ from individuals who identify in more traditional ways.

How would you evaluate this encounter? Nolan claims a non-chaplain could not have provided effective care in this situation. What do you think? Rituals are a prominent feature of this case. What do the rituals appear to mean to each individual? What impact do they appear to have? What are the challenges of spiritual care for the non-religious? Do mystical moments, as described by Nolan, qualify as mystical moments for Den, the patient at the center of this case? Why or why not?

Article 3: Massey, K., Barnes, M.J.D., Villines, D., Goldstein, J.D., Pierson, A.L.H., Scherer, C., Vander Laan, B., and Summerfelt, W.T. (2015) What Do I Do? Developing a Taxonomy of Chaplaincy Activities and Interventions for Spiritual Care in Intensive Care Unit Palliative Care

Chaplaincy documentation and communication about the care provided in an encounter varies from hospital to hospital and sometimes from one chaplain to the next. Recognizing the need for consistency, Kevin Massey and colleagues (2015) undertook a mixed-methods approach to develop an evidence-based, consistent taxonomy of chaplain activities. The taxonomy has been adopted by a number of chaplaincy departments. The taxonomy website invites feedback; as research using it emerges, the team intends to publish updated versions (Massey and Barnes 2014). Massey, the leader of the team that developed this taxonomy, is a chaplaincy manager for several Chicago-area hospitals in Advocate Health Care. He has a strong interest in using research to strengthen chaplaincy practice and chaplaincy education.

This study used a number of research methods to develop the taxonomy. The work included generating a list of chaplain activities using a literature review, retrospective chart reviews, and focus groups and interviews with chaplains.

Several concepts that are important for developing research literacy are illustrated in this article. First, the authors describe important background literature for their project. Massey et al. (2015) write that this study is not the first publication about chaplain activities (see their references numbers 2–6; also see Gibbons, Retsas, and Pinikahaha 1999, a study that was not included in their review of literature). Second, the study introduces the concepts of validity and reliability, which are important in research when developing measures (see Article 20). Reliability refers to the consistency of a measure (e.g., can the measure repeatedly get the same results from different users?), and validity indicates the ability of an instrument to measure what it aims to measure. An instrument can be reliable but not valid, but it cannot be valid without being reliable. This team examined the reliability of the taxonomy and several different types of validity.

Categorizing items into intended effects, methods, and interventions gave the taxonomy structure; however, it lacks directly naming spiritual assessment as an activity. The team suggested using multiple items from each of the categories to create "pathways" that constitute a spiritual care plan.

Other studies (Cadge, Calle, and Dillinger 2011; Lyndes et al. 2012) have highlighted how chaplains focus on the process of chaplaincy care while our healthcare colleagues have begun to describe the outcomes associated with our care. Additionally, healthcare chaplaincy leaders have urged a shift toward outcomes and evidence in clinical practice (Handzo et al. 2014). However, the content of the taxonomy shows us that descriptors of chaplain activities developed by chaplains are still very focused on the process of their care. Even many of the items about the "intended effects" of chaplain care focus on the process of care (e.g., "build relationship of care and support").

The taxonomy authors intended this work to create a consistent language within the profession and to guide future research efforts. Do you think they succeeded? In multidisciplinary conversation, what are clinician-specific perceptions of the activities in the taxonomy? What are the implications of those perceptions? Does the taxonomy continue to use chaplaincy jargon to describe what chaplains do, or does it paint a clearer picture of spiritual care? How do the activities rated by the chaplains as most important and most frequently performed (see Table 2) compare with your care? What do these items say about chaplaincy? How could a chaplaincy program implement the taxonomy? What do we need to do to improve it?

Article 4: Johnson, R., Wirpsa, M.J., Boyken, L., Sakumoto, M., Handzo, G., Kho, A., and Emanuel, L. (2016) Communicating Chaplains' Care: Narrative Documentation in a Neuroscience-Spine Intensive Care Unit

Little is known about how chaplains document their care in patient records. Given the absence of a professional consensus, it is likely that the content of chaplains' documentation and how they document varies widely across chaplains and systems. A multidisciplinary team at Northwestern University conducted one of the first examinations of the free-text portions of chaplains' notes. The team framed the study within the American College of Critical Care Medicine 2004–05 Clinical Practice Guidelines for support of the family in the patient-centered intensive care unit. (For the current version, see Davidson et al. 2017.) The guidelines specifically address the documentation of spiritual care within intensive care unit (ICU) care plans and emphasize the role of spirituality within family- and patient-centered treatment.

Johnson's team collected over 400 chaplain notes from an intensive care setting for a qualitative analysis. Using inductive content analysis, the team thematically coded the free-text portion of the notes written by staff and resident chaplains. After coding these notes, a chaplain on the team categorized the codes within the chaplaincy-specific activities of assessment, intervention, and outcome. Coding is often a subjective process that requires assessing its reliability. Inter-rater reliability refers to the consistency of the coding and reports how consistently multiple coders assigned the same codes. (Details of their process is found in their methods section.)

The authors of this study thought that the chaplains thoroughly documented important content related to religious practices relevant to care. In contrast, the study team noted the colloquial use of diagnosis/medical terminology (e.g., anxiety) as well as the suggestion that chaplains have the ability to assess for decisional capacity. Notes about assessment appeared descriptive in nature, and notes about interventions were more concrete; assessments were documented more frequently than interventions or outcomes. On occasion, the chaplains were able to link an intervention with an outcome, but at times the outcome seemed unclear. Johnson et al. (2016) identify that chaplains may need collaboration with other healthcare professionals to identify important documentation strategies and develop standardized language for their care. What do you think?

Since Johnson et al.'s efforts in 2016, three other papers have continued the discussion of chaplain documentation (Lee, Curlin, and Choi 2017; Stang 2017; Tartaglia et al. 2017). Future chaplaincy research on documentation could identify how other clinicians use chaplain notes for patient care. For example, what beliefs, background, family dynamics, and so on are most important to document? Would the patient's medical diagnosis impact the content of documentation? How could you imagine a conversation between Massey et al. (2015) and Johnson et al. (2016)? Where do you think they would agree or disagree? Could the pathways created by the taxonomy improve chaplaincy documentation?

Article 5: King, S.D.W., Fitchett, G., Murphy, P.E., Pargament, K.I., Harrison, D.A., and Loggers, E.T. (2017) Determining Best Methods to Screen for Religious/Spiritual Distress

How do busy chaplains determine whom to visit? There appears to be considerable variation in practices and protocols that inform these decisions. Some hospitals ask new patients if they want to see a chaplain, while chaplains at other hospitals visit patients only based on referral. Research suggests those who request chaplain care may not be those with the greatest need for it (Fitchett, Meyer, and Burton 2000). Screenings for spiritual need conducted by non-chaplain healthcare colleagues allow chaplains to function as the spiritual care specialists who follow up on these screening-based referrals to provide further assessment and spiritual care as indicated (see also Handzo and Koenig 2004).

Fitchett (2012) has described the differences in depth of spiritual inquiry between spiritual screening, spiritual history taking, and spiritual assessment. Spiritual assessment, the process conducted by a spiritual care professional, takes an in-depth look at an individual's religious/spiritual identity and resources to identify areas of spiritual need. Spiritual history taking, often conducted by a clinician other than a chaplain, identifies spiritual dynamics intertwined with treatment and potential decision-making. Finally, all clinicians can spiritually screen with one or two questions that probe for symptoms of or risks for spiritual distress.

Stephen King, a chaplain-researcher and spiritual care manager at the Seattle Cancer Care Alliance, has extensive experience studying screening for religious/spiritual struggle. He and his colleagues (including Kenneth Pargament, whose work on religious/spiritual coping and struggle continues to inform the work of practicing chaplains) published this first attempt to assess the validity of several religious/spiritual distress screening tools.

The evaluation of the screening tools was based on their sensitivity and specificity. Think about these concepts in terms of a two by two table; each participant will fall into either A, B, C, or D:

	Distressed	No Distress	Totals
+ Screening Result	A (True Positive)	B (False Positive)	A + B
− Screening Result	C (False Negative)	D (True Negative)	C + D
Totals	A + C	B + D	A + B + C + D

Figure 1. Calculating sensitivity and specificity of a screening protocol

Everyone screened will have either a positive (spiritually distressed) or negative (no spiritual distress) result based on a reference protocol. In this study, the team used a participant's result from the Negative Religious Coping Scale of the Brief RCOPE (Pargament, Feuille, and Burdzy 2011) as the reference standard and compared that result with six screening measures. Sensitivity is the percentage of individuals who had a positive screening result and who are actually distressed (A/A+C). Specificity is the percentage of individuals with a negative screening result who are not distressed (D/B+D). Ideally, researchers want both numbers as high as possible, but increasing one decreases the other (see Table 4). King et al. (2017) set their pre-specified (ideal) sensitivity at 85 percent.

None of the six screening items met the pre-specified sensitivity, but further analysis identified a combination of two items with net sensitivity of 82 percent. King et al. (2017) recommend these two items as the strongest approach to screening for spiritual struggle for practicing chaplains within oncology. The evidence supporting the use of these two items may also give non-chaplain healthcare colleagues greater confidence about using them to identify patients who should be referred to a spiritual care professional. Additionally, by surveying an oncology population, the results help to identify the best method for spiritual screening and complement the requirement for spiritual screening by the American College of Surgeons' Commission on Cancer (2016 mandate). Future research includes similar testing of spiritual screening tools in other clinical populations.

Before you read the results in this paper, read the screening protocols. Which of the selected protocols would you have thought would work best? Why or why not? Why do you think none of the items independently met the targeted sensitivity? Which screening tools do you think would work within your patient population?

Article 6: Monod, S.M., Rochat, E., Büla, C.J., Jobin, G., Martin, E., and Spencer, B. (2010a) The Spiritual Distress Assessment Tool: An Instrument to Assess Spiritual Distress in Hospitalised Elderly Persons

One of the biggest challenges for healthcare chaplains is advancing an evidence-based approach to spiritual assessment. Existing published models for spiritual assessment can be said to be evidence-based only insofar as expert opinion is considered evidence. It is important to remember that expert opinion is the least rigorous form of evidence. The Spiritual Distress Assessment Tool (SDAT), described in this article, is based on more rigorous research than previous models for assessment and thus provides a unique new resource for spiritual assessment for chaplains.

Stefanie Monod, a physician with interests in geriatrics and spirituality, and her multidisciplinary colleagues based at the Lausanne Medical Center in Switzerland, published the next paper in the *Reader* along with several other articles that describe the development of SDAT model (Monod et al. 2010a; Monod et al. 2010b; Monod et al. 2012). Monod et al. (2012) is the paper in which the team reports further evidence of the validity and reliability of their SDAT model. It is a unique and important contribution to evidence-based chaplaincy research. Monod et al. (2010a) is the paper in which the team describes the skills needed by those implementing the SDAT, including the ability to develop a relationship prior to conducting a semi-structured interview.

The research team examined other spiritual assessment tools and noticed that some tools capture spiritual well-being while others capture spiritual distress. To their knowledge, no assessment tool captured both. Instead of assessing a person's spiritual state on a spectrum from spiritually well to spiritually distressed, they developed a model that measures a person's overall spiritual state within the individual's own religious/spiritual framework.

The SDAT is built on a model of four spiritual dimensions of older medical rehabilitation patients (meaning, transcendence, values, and psycho-social identity; Monod et al. 2010b). The team identified five spiritual needs associated with these dimensions. After an interview with the patient, the chaplain rates the severity of unmet spiritual needs for each of the five spiritual needs. In the article included in the *Reader*, the team describes its assessment of the face validity (subjective assessment of its validity) of the instrument among chaplains previously exposed to the SDAT and chaplains with no previous exposure. The team reported that the chaplains thought identifying the presence of unmet need was not difficult, but assessing its severity was challenging. Do you think the authors provided enough information to help chaplains determine the difference between the ratings?

What do you think it would take to implement this model in your setting? Do you think the SDAT allows the chaplain to address the needs of patients as they arise? How does the numeric component strengthen or weaken the communication of an individual's distress? Can the SDAT bridge the gap between those favoring evidence-based practices and those hesitant to quantify spiritual assessment? Where do you see religious practices fitting into this model? The authors also identify this as a tool that will improve communication between disciplines. What is your opinion of that claim? The SDAT is based on the team's Spiritual Needs Model. What are the strengths and limitations of that model?

References

American College of Surgeons' Commission on Cancer (2016) *Cancer Program Standards: Ensuring Patient-Centered Care.* Accessed on 1/25/18 at www.facs.org/quality-programs/cancer/coc/standards.

Cadge, W. (2012) *Paging God: Religion in the Halls of Medicine.* Chicago: The University of Chicago Press.

Cadge, W., Calle, K., and Dillinger, J. (2011) "What do chaplains contribute to large academic hospitals? The perspectives of pediatric physicians and chaplains." *Journal of Religion & Health*, 50, 2, 300–312.

Cadge, W., Freese, J., and Christakis, N.A. (2008) "The provision of hospital chaplaincy in the United States: a national overview." *Southern Medical Journal*, 101, 6, 626–630.

Davidson, J.E., Aslakson, R.A., Long, A.C., Puntillo, K.A., et al. (2017) "Guidelines for family-centered care in the neonatal, pediatric, and adult ICU." *Critical Care Medicine*, 45, 1, 103–128.

Fitchett, G. (2012) "Next Steps for Spiritual Assessment in Healthcare." In M. Cobb, C. Puchalski, and B. Rumbold (eds) *Oxford Textbook of Spirituality in Healthcare.* Oxford: Oxford University Press.

Fitchett, G., Meyer, P., and Burton, L.A. (2000) "Spiritual care: Who requests it? Who needs it?" *Journal of Pastoral Care*, 54, 2, 173–186.

Fitchett, G. and Nolan, S. (eds) (2015) *Spiritual Care in Practice: Case Studies in Healthcare Chaplaincy.* London: Jessica Kingsley Publishers.

Flannelly, K.J., Handzo, G.F., and Weaver, A.J. (2004) "Factors affecting healthcare chaplaincy and the provision of pastoral care in the United States." *Journal of Pastoral Care & Counseling*, 58, 1–2, 127–130.

Gibbons, G., Retsas A., and Pinikahaha, J. (1999) "Describing what chaplains do in hospitals." *Journal of Pastoral Care*, 53, 2, 201–207.

Handzo, G.F, Cobb, M., Holmes, C., Kelly, E., and Sinclair, S. (2014) "Outcomes for professional health care chaplaincy: an international call to action." *Journal of Health Care Chaplaincy*, 20, 2, 43–53.

Handzo, G. and Koenig, H.G. (2004) "Spiritual care: whose job is it anyway?" *Southern Medical Journal*, 97, 1242–1244.

Hess, D. (2016) "Myths and systems: a response to '"He needs to talk!"': a chaplain's case study of nonreligious spiritual care'." *Journal of Health Care Chaplaincy*, 22, 1, 17–27.

Hui, D., de la Cruz, M., Thorney, S., Parsons, H.A., Delgado-Guay, M., and Bruera, E. (2011) "The frequency and correlates of spiritual distress among patients with advanced cancer admitted to an acute palliative care unit." *American Journal of Hospice and Palliative Medicine*, 28, 4, 264–270.

Johnson, R., Wirpsa, M.J., Boyken, L., Sakumoto, M., Handzo, G., Kho, A., and Emanuel, L. (2016) "Communicating chaplains' care: narrative documentation in a neuroscience-spine intensive care unit." *Journal of Health Care Chaplaincy*, 22, 4, 133–150.

King, S.D.W., Fitchett, G., Murphy, P.E., Pargament, K.I., Harrison, D.A., and Loggers, E.T. (2017) "Determining best methods to screen for religious/spiritual distress." *Supportive Care in Cancer*, 25, 471–479.

Lee, B.M., Curlin, F.A., and Choi, P.J. (2017) "Documenting presence: a descriptive study of chaplain notes in the intensive care unit." *Palliative Supportive Care*, 15, 2, 190–196.

Lyndes, K.A., Fitchett, G., Berlinger, N., Cadge, W., Misasi, J., and Flanagan, E. (2012) "A survey of chaplains' roles in pediatric palliative care: integral members of the team." *Journal of Health Care Chaplaincy*, 18, 1–2, 74–93.

Massey, K. and Barnes, M. (2014) *The Advocate Health Care Chaplain Taxonomy.* Advocate Health Care. Accessed on 1/25/18 at www.advocatehealth.com/chaplaincyresearch.

Massey, K., Barnes, M.J.D., Villines, D., Goldstein, J.D., et al. (2015) "What do I do? Developing a taxonomy of chaplaincy activities and interventions for spiritual care in intensive care unit palliative care." *BMC Palliative Care*, 14, 10, 1–8.

Monod, S., Martin, E., Spencer, B., Rochat, E., and Bula, C. (2012) "Validation of the Spiritual Distress Assessment Tool in older hospitalized patients." *BMC Geriatrics*, 12, 13.

Monod, S.M., Rochat, E., Büla, C.J., Jobin, G., Martin, E., and Spencer, B. (2010a) "The Spiritual Distress Assessment Tool: an instrument to assess spiritual distress in hospitalized elderly persons." *BMC Geriatrics*, 10, 88–96.

Monod, S., Rochat, E., Büla, C., and Spencer, B. (2010b) "The spiritual needs model: spirituality assessment in the geriatric hospital setting." *Journal of Religion, Spirituality & Aging*, 22, 271–282.

Nolan, S. (2012) *Spiritual Care at the End of Life*. London: Jessica Kingsley Publishers.

Nolan, S. (2016) "'He needs to talk!': a chaplain's case study of nonreligious spiritual care." *Journal of Health Care Chaplaincy*, 22, 1, 1–16.

Pargament, K.I., Feuille, M., and Burdzy, D. (2011) "The Brief RCOPE: current psychometric status of a short measure of religious coping." *Religions*, 2, 51–76.

Pesut, B. (2016) "Recovering religious voice and imagination: a response to Nolan's case study 'He needs to talk!'" *Journal of Health Care Chaplaincy*, 22, 1, 28–39.

Stang, V.B. (2017) "An e-chart review of chaplains' interventions and outcomes: a quality improvement and documentation practice enhancement project." *Journal of Pastoral Care & Counseling*, 71, 3, 183–191.

Swift, C. (2014) *Hospital Chaplaincy in the Twenty-First Century: The Crisis of Spiritual Care on the NHS* (2nd ed.). Farnham: Ashgate Publishing.

Tartaglia, A., Ford, T., Dodd-McCue, D., Reid, C., Hawley, C., and Hassell, A. (2017) "Charting our course: chaplain documentation as a performance improvement project." *Journal of Health Care Chaplaincy*, 2, 1–11. [Epub ahead of print]

Transforming Chaplaincy Project website (2015) Joint Research Council. Accessed on 1/25/18 at www.transformchaplaincy.org.

ARTICLE 1

The Provision of Hospital Chaplaincy in the United States: A National Overview

Wendy Cadge, PhD, Jeremy Freese, PhD, and Nicholas A. Christakis, MD, PhD, MPH

From the Department of Sociology, Brandeis University, Waltham, MA; the Department of Sociology, Northwestern University, Evanston, IL; and the Department of Health Care Policy, Harvard Medical School, Boston, MA.

Reprint requests to Wendy Cadge, Assistant Professor of Sociology, Brandeis University, MS 071, Waltham, MA 02454-9110. Email: wcadge@brandeis.edu

Supported by the Robert Wood Johnson Foundation Scholars in Health Policy Research Program at Harvard University.

Accepted November 29, 2007.

Copyright © 2008 by The Southern Medical Association

0038-4348/0 – 2000/10100-0626

Abstract

Over the past 25 years, the Joint Commission for the Accreditation of Healthcare Organizations has changed its guidelines regarding religious/spiritual care of hospitalized patients to increase attention concerning this aspect of hospital-based care. Little empirical evidence assesses the extent to which hospitals relied on hospital chaplains as care providers during these years. This study investigates 1) the extent of chaplaincy service availability in US hospitals between 1980 and 2003; 2) the predictors of having chaplaincy services in 1993 and 2003; and 3) the change in the magnitude of these predictors between years. This study examines the presence or absence of chaplaincy or pastoral care services in hospitals using the American Hospital Association Annual Survey of Hospitals (ranging from 4,946–6,353 hospitals) in 1980–1985, 1992–1993, and 2002–2003. Between 54% and 64% of hospitals had chaplaincy services between 1980 and 2003, with no systematic trend over this period. In 1993 and 2003, hospital size, location, and church affiliation were central factors influencing the presence of chaplaincy services. Smaller hospitals and those in rural areas were less likely to have chaplaincy services.

Cadge, W., Freese, J., and Christakis, N.A. (2008) "The provision of hospital chaplaincy in the United States: a national overview." *Southern Medical Journal*, 101, 6, 626–630.

Church-operated hospitals were much more likely to have chaplaincy services; but between 1993 and 2003, church-operated hospitals were more likely to drop chaplaincy services than to add them. Not-for-profit hospitals were more likely than investor-owned hospitals to add chaplaincy services. Changes to Joint Commission for the Accreditation of Healthcare Organizations policies about the religious/spiritual care of hospitalized patients between 1980 and 2003 seem to have had no discernible effect on the fraction of US hospitals that had chaplaincy services. Rather, characteristics of hospitals, their surroundings, and their religious affiliations influenced whether they provided chaplaincy services to patients.

Key words: hospital chaplaincy, provision of healthcare services, religion, spirituality

---

KEY POINTS

- Between 54% and 64% of hospitals had chaplaincy services between 1980 and 2003, with no systematic trend over this period.

- Smaller hospitals and those in rural areas were less likely to have chaplaincy services.

- Church-operated hospitals were much more likely to have chaplaincy services.

- Between 1993 and 2003, church-operated hospitals were more likely to drop chaplaincy services than to add them.

- Not-for-profit hospitals were more likely than investor-owned hospitals to add chaplaincy services.

The Joint Commission for the Accreditation of Healthcare Organizations (JCAHO) guidelines regarding religion and spirituality have evolved since 1969, when the Commission first addressed the topic. In 2003, JCAHO stated that "patients have a fundamental right to considerate care that safeguards their personal dignity and respects their cultural, psychosocial, and spiritual values." Hospitals were to "demonstrate respect" for patient needs, including the need for "pastoral care and other spiritual services." Additional language about religion and spirituality was included in the guidelines about dietary options, pain concerns, resolving dilemmas about patient care issues, end-of-life issues, and the treatment and responsibilities of staff. JCAHO Associate Director of Standards Interpretation explained that the Commission "expects you to conduct a spiritual assessment of every patient in every healthcare setting […] to determine how a patient's religion or spiritual outlook might affect the care he or she receives […] At minimum the spiritual assessment should determine the patient's religious denomination, beliefs, and what spiritual practices are important to the patient."[1]

Little prior research has evaluated whether the Joint Commission's recommendations have had an appreciable impact and, more importantly, whether and how hospitals have met patients' religious and spiritual needs as outlined in these guidelines. Many hospitals have done so through the use of voluntary and employed hospital chaplains supported financially by the hospital or local religious organizations. Knowing which hospitals have chaplains is the first step in understanding whether they work collaboratively with nurses, physicians, and other healthcare professionals.[2, 3, 4, 5, 6, 7, 8]

Limited empirical data exist describing these hospital chaplains, and existing studies[9, 10, 11, 12] (Sakurai, Unpublished Dissertation, 2005) have used nonrepresentative samples and/or surveys with low response rates. To our knowledge, this study provides the first systematic national overview of hospital chaplaincy based on a well-regarded survey, the American Hospital Association's Annual Survey of Hospitals. A question about the presence of a hospital chaplaincy service was asked in this survey intermittently from 1980 through 2003. We evaluated the overall percentage of hospitals providing chaplaincy services between 1980 and 2003. We also provide a more detailed examination of predictors of chaplaincy services in 1993, when JCAHO guidelines began to change, and in 2003, after guideline changes had been made.

Materials and methods

This study analyzes survey data about the presence of hospital chaplaincy services collected in the American Hospital Association's Annual Survey of Hospitals in 1980–1985, 1992–1993, and 2002–2003; the included years are the only ones to date in which the survey has asked about chaplaincy services. This survey is regularly administered to a full sample of hospital facilities in the United States, and there was a consistently high response rate over the studied period. The number of hospitals surveyed in these years varied from 4,946 to 6,353.

In 1981, the survey distinguished between hospital-based/staffed and hospital-based/contracted services, but the two categories are combined here for consistency with other years. The 2003 survey distinguished between hospital-based/staffed chaplaincy/pastoral care and care provided through the hospital's health system affiliation, integrated delivery network affiliation, or joint venture arrangement; these categories are also combined in the analysis. Other analyses that disaggregated these categories did not yield different results (data not shown).

Hypotheses

Independent variables used in this study are summarized in Table 1. Based on the existing literature and 10 interviews we conducted with professional chaplaincy leaders, we had six hypotheses about the relationship between these variables and the presence of chaplaincy services:

1. We expected that larger hospitals (as measured by adjusted average daily census) would be more likely to have hospital chaplains.

2. We expected that hospitals in larger metropolitan areas would be more likely to have chaplains.

3–4. In addition to expecting that church-operated hospitals would be much more likely to have chaplains than other hospitals, we hypothesized that—as chaplains do not directly contribute to hospital revenues—investor-owned hospitals would be less likely to have chaplains than either government (nonfederal) or (nongovernment and non-church-operated) not-for-profit hospitals. In our analyses, we exclude hospitals in the Veterans Administration, as they have all had chaplains since the Veterans Administration Chaplaincy was established in 1945.

5. We expected that teaching hospitals would be more likely to have chaplains, which we measured by whether they belonged to the Council of Teaching Hospitals.

6. Several chaplaincy leaders we interviewed discussed the special value of chaplains in providing religious/spiritual care for oncology patients. Therefore, we hypothesized that hospitals with oncology services would be more likely to have chaplains. Because we worried that the observed effects of having an oncology service could merely reflect the hospital size, we also

included in our model whether hospitals had an occupational health service; we did this because such a presence was roughly as common as that of an oncology service in the American Hospital Association data, and there would be no reason to expect a special relationship between occupational health services and the presence of chaplaincy services.

As additional covariates, we included the mean number of patients on Medicare and Medicaid to avoid confounding by these aspects of a hospital's client population.

We first present descriptive statistics about hospital chaplaincy between 1980 and 2003 and then examine logistic regression models predicting the presence of chaplaincy in 1993 and 2003. We also compare results from these models to assess changes in the predictors of chaplaincy services between these 2 years. Additional analyses of change between 1993 and 2003 as a single model did not yield substantially different results (data not shown).

Table 1: Percentages and means for selected variables, 1993 and 2003 American Hospital Association Annual Survey

	1993	2003
Region		
Northeast	15.8	13.5
South	38.7	39.3
Midwest	28.9	29.2
West	16.6	18.1
Metropolitan statistical area		
Rural—nonmetro areas	39.5	42.0
Small (0–250,000)	9.5	9.2
Medium (250,001–1,000,000)	18.4	18.5
Large (larger than 1,000,000)	32.7	30.3
Average daily census (adjusted)		
0–50	30.2	26.3
51–100	20.8	20.1
101–150	12.9	11.6
151–200	8.7	10.2
200+	27.5	31.8

Control		
Church-operated	10.8	10.7
Nongovernment, not-for-profit	45.3	47.7
Government, nonfederal	28.1	24.4
Investor-owned	15.8	17.3
Other operating characteristics		
Member, council of teaching hospitals	5.6	6.2
Church-operated	10.8	10.7
Patient characteristics		
Mean % of patients on Medicare (SD)	43.3 (21.9)	46.8 (23.6)
Mean % of patients on Medicaid (SD)	18.4 (18.0)	19.5 (19.7)
Services and technologies		
Oncology specialists at hospital or subsidiary	40.8	52.2
Occupational health services	44.7	61.7
N	5587	4793

Cases excluded are missing values for the dependent variable or membership in the Council of Teaching Hospitals and/or have their regions coded as other (i.e, "associated areas").

Results

As described in Table 2, between 54% and 64% of hospitals had chaplaincy services between 1980 and 2003. No trends are evident in the fraction of hospitals that had chaplaincy services during these years. Approximately 59% of hospitals had chaplains in both 1993 and 2003.

Table 3 presents logistic regression results for 1993 and 2003. A comparison of the models for the 2 years shows that the factors that led hospitals to have chaplaincy services were relatively consistent in 1993 and 2003. As predicted, hospital size was strongly associated with having a chaplain; hospitals with a smaller average daily census were less likely than those with more patients to have chaplains. Holding other variables constant at their mean, the predicted probability of having a chaplaincy service in 2003 was 0.48 for hospitals with an average daily census of 50 or less, compared with 0.79 for hospitals of 200 or more. The largest hospitals were more likely to be teaching hospitals, and our results show that, consistent with our predictions, teaching hospitals were more likely to have chaplains, which is not surprising, given that even net of size that teaching hospitals typically have larger than average nonmedical staffs.

Church-operated hospitals were much more likely to have chaplains than other kinds of (non-Veterans Administration) hospitals. Holding other variables at their mean, church-owned hospitals had a 0.86 predicted probability of having a chaplain in 2003, compared with only 0.48 for government-owned hospitals. In comparison with investor-owned hospitals, nongovernment or church-operated not-for-profit hospitals were also more likely to have chaplains. There was no significant difference between government-owned and investor-owned hospitals.

Hospitals in rural areas were much less likely than those in large urban areas to have hospital chaplaincy in both 1993 and 2003. The difference in 2003 corresponds to a change in predicted probabilities from 0.58 for rural hospitals to 0.71 for hospitals in large urban areas. We observed no other effect of locality other than this difference.

We did find a positive relationship between having an oncology service and chaplains, which might otherwise support the suggestion from the chaplains interviewed that the provision of chaplaincy services was particularly responsive to the needs of cancer patients. However, we can see that when an occupational health service is also included, it has effects as large or larger than having an oncology service.

Given the lack of change in the overall percentage of chaplains between 1993 and 2003, comparisons in coefficients between 1993 and 2003 also provided an analysis of whether the variables were associated with any changes in which hospitals had chaplains. To confirm, we also conducted a multinominal logistic regression analysis of the four-category outcome implied by the absence of chaplaincy services in 1993 and 2003 (results not shown) and obtained results consistent with those discussed here. The only significant differences were for types of hospitals. The coefficient for church-operated hospitals was larger in 1993 than 2003, suggesting that, compared with other types of hospitals, church-operated hospitals were relatively more likely to have dropped chaplains in the intervening period than to have added them. Not-for-profit hospitals were more likely than investor-owned hospitals to have added hospitals in the intervening period than to have dropped them.

Table 2: Chaplaincy service in US hospitals

Year	Total hospitals	Reporting hospitals	Hospitals reporting chaplaincy service	Percentage of reporting hospitals with chaplaincy
1980	6,965	6,277	3,643	58.0
1981[a]	6,933	6,276	3,371	53.7

1982	6,915	6,277	3,499	55.7
1983	6,888	6,353	3,670	57.8
1984	6,872	6,302	3,817	60.6
1985	6,872	6,304	4,000	63.5
1992	6,539	5,916	3,175	53.7
1993	–	5,789	3,398	58.7
2002	5,794	4,876	2,581	52.9
2003[a]	–	4,946	2,934	59.3

Data sources: AHA Annual Survey, Health Forum, LLC, a subsidiary of the American Hospital Association. Fiscal years 1980–1985, 1992 and 2002; and AHA Hospital Statistics, 1993 and 2003.

[a] See Discussion in text of differences in the survey item for these two years.

Table 3: Coefficient for logistic regressions of presence of chaplaincy, 1993 and 2003. American Hospital Association Annual Survey of Hospitals

	1993		2003	
	Model 1	Model 2	Model 1	Model 2
Northeast	0.03 (0.12)	0.12 (0.12)	-0.02 (0.14)	-0.09 (0.14)
South	0.06 (0.09)	0.17 (0.10)	0.19 (0.10)	0.27[b] (0.10)
Midwest	0.23 (0.10)[b]	0.24[b] (0.10)	0.28[d] (0.11)	0.13 (0.11)
Rural	-0.43 (0.08)[c]	-0.33[c] (0.10)	-0.47[c] (0.10)	-0.61[c] (0.10)
Small MSA	-0.13 (0.12)	-0.12 (0.13)	0.04 (0.14)	-0.08 (0.15)
Medium MSA	-0.05 (0.01)	-0.02 (0.10)	-0.13 (0.11)	-0.13 (0.11)
Average census 1–50	-2.26 (0.11)[c]	-1.88[c] (0.12)	-2.18[c] (0.12)	-1.40[c] (0.13)
Average census 51–100	-1.43 (0.11)[c]	-1.19[c] (0.12)	-1.35[c] (0.11)	-0.88[c] (0.12)
Average census 101–150	-1.23 (0.12)[c]	-1.08[c] (0.12)	-1.01[c] (0.13)	-0.73[c] (0.13)
Average census 151–200	-0.75 (0.14)[c]	-0.71[c] (0.14)	-0.74[c] (0.13)	-0.62[c] (0.14)
Teaching hospital	1.53 (0.31)[c]	1.42[c] (0.31)	1.58[c] (0.31)	1.23[c] (0.31)
Church-operated	2.56 (0.21)[c]	2.57[c] (0.21)	2.00[c] (0.16)	1.91[c] (0.17)
Other not-for-profit	0.36 (0.10)[c]	0.34[c] (0.10)	0.97[c] (0.10)	0.89[c] (0.10)
Government, nonfederal	0.18 (0.10)	0.24[b] (0.10)	0.41[c] (0.11)	0.40[c] (0.12)
% Medicaid	-0.007 (0.002)[c]	-0.008[c] (0.002)	-0.01[c] (0.002)	-0.01[c] (0.002)
% Medicare	0.011 (0.002)[c]	0.007[c] (0.002)	0.01[c] (0.002)	0.01[c] (0.002)
Oncology service		0.18[b] (0.09)		0.76[c] (0.08)
Occupational health		0.64[c] (0.07)		0.75[c] (0.08)
Intercept	1.18 (0.16)	0.69 (0.18)	0.58 (0.17)	-0.13 (0.18)

cont.

	1993		2003	
	Model 1	Model 2	Model 1	Model 2
-2 Log likelihood	5912.2	5824.3	5009.93	4777.99
N	5587	5587	4793	4793

[a]MSA, Metropolitan Statistical Area; [b]$P < 0.010$; [c]$P < 0.05$; [d]$P < 0.01$.

Standard errors are given in parentheses. Reference categories are west (region), large MSA (area size), average census 201+ (hospital size), and investor-owner (institutional type).

Discussion and conclusion

Our findings suggest three main conclusions: first, these results show that whether hospitals had chaplains in 1993 and 2003 was strongly predicted by general demographic and institutional characteristics of the hospitals. As in previous analyses[10] of smaller datasets, hospital size, location, and church affiliation were the central factors influencing the presence of chaplaincy services. Smaller hospitals and those in rural areas were less likely to have chaplaincy services than larger hospitals and those in more urban areas in 1993 and 2003, likely reflecting differences in financial and religious leadership resources in these areas. Smaller and/or rural hospitals might not have resources available to hire chaplains and/ or there may be less need because local religious leaders are more readily available.

Church-affiliated hospitals were also much more likely than others to have chaplaincy services, potentially indicating different value commitments around religious/spiritual care and/or greater ease of finding and financially supporting chaplains. Additional information about the religious affiliations of hospitals and their chaplains would enable further consideration. In comparison with investor-owned hospitals, nongovernment, or church-operated not-for-profit hospitals were also more likely to have chaplains, perhaps indicating different value commitments or financial management priorities.

Second, although positive changes in JCAHO guidelines concerning religion and spirituality occurred between the early 1980s and early 2000s, there is not yet evidence that they had any effect on the fraction of hospitals with hospital chaplaincy services between 1993 and 2003. Though the Joint Commission first considered religion and spirituality in 1969, the guidelines were significantly revised in the 1990s when the religious/spiritual care of patients was framed as a "right," addressed under the heading of "Patient Rights." In the 1990s, there was also a transition in the standards about what the religious/spiritual care of patients should be called and who specifically might provide it. In 1996, the Joint Commission stated that hospitals were to demonstrate respect for "pastoral counseling," a phrase replaced with "pastoral care and other spiritual services" in 1999 after chaplaincy leaders argued that this phrase better reflected their jobs. Although the Joint Commission has not established specific guidelines or licensing requirements that mandate who can provide religious/spiritual care, in their 1999 guidelines they mentioned pastoral services departments and pastoral personnel from outside of the facility as possibilities.

Leaders in hospital chaplaincy described the changes the Commission has made as overwhelmingly positive. "Ten years ago the Joint Commission didn't ask about spiritual care," one chaplain explained. "Today it's one of the first things they ask about." Another leader explained, "Anytime you get standards like that, whether it's JCAHO or HIPAA [Health Insurance Portability and Accountability Act] or anything else, you know it certainly becomes a powerful tool for advocating for pastoral care." Although changes in JCAHO policies in the 1990s may have influenced the number and visibility of chaplains at individual hospitals, they have not increased the fraction of hospitals that have chaplains.

Third, the only changes evident in the fraction of hospitals that had chaplains in 1993 and 2003 were related to whether the hospital was church-operated or not-for-profit. Compared with other types of hospitals, church-operated hospitals were relatively more likely to have dropped chaplains between 1993 and 2003 than to have added them. This could reflect greater financial pressures on church-operated hospitals in these years. If so, however, these pressures did not extend to not-for-profit hospitals, as these hospitals were actually more likely than investor-owned hospitals to have added chaplains in the intervening period than dropped them. These findings require additional study. Not only did the percentage of hospitals with chaplaincy services not change between 1993 and 2003, but the magnitude of different predictors of chaplaincy services changed little.

This study presents the first national overview of hospital chaplaincy, but it is limited in several ways. Primarily, it examines only the presence or absence of hospital chaplaincy services, a very broad measure of the presence and work of hospital chaplains. It is certainly possible that the structure and functioning of chaplaincy departments changed based on changes in healthcare financing, the professionalization of hospital chaplaincy, the strategic work of professional chaplaincy organizations, etc. Additional, more detailed data collection is needed to assess variations, specifically in how hospitals have and continue to provide chaplaincy services, what impact JCAHO policy changes may have had on that provision, and what influence (if any) chaplaincy services have on patient satisfaction and other relevant outcomes.

Rather than being an impetus for change in hospital chaplaincy services, our findings begin to suggest that changes to JCAHO guidelines around religion/spirituality may be largely symbolic, reflecting changes already being made in hospitals. These findings[2,13] suggest that the increased attention to religion/spirituality in JCAHO guidelines, some hospitals, and the medical literature, may not be related to the changing presence of hospital chaplains but to increased attention to religion and spirituality among other healthcare providers. Physicians and nurses currently occupy some of the most prominent places in related medical and societal discourse about religion/spirituality and are contributing to broader trends in medicine around spiritual and ethical concerns.[14]

Acknowledgments

Programming assistance was provided by Laurie Meneades.

References

1. Staten P. Spiritual assessment required in all settings. *Hosp Peer Rev* 2003;28:55–56.
2. Weaver AJ, Koenig HK, Flannelly KJ, et al. A review of research on chaplains and community-based clergy in the Journal of the American Medical Association, Lancet, and the New England Journal of Medicine: 1998–2000. *J Pastoral Care Counsel* 2004;58:343–350.
3. Hall C. *Head and Heart: The Story of the Clinical Pastoral Education Movement.* Journal of Pastoral Care Publications, 1992.
4. Holst L. The hospital chaplain between worlds, in Marty ME, Vaux KL (eds): *Health/Medicine and the Faith Traditions.* Philadelphia, Fortress, 1982, pp. 293–309.
5. Norwood F. The ambivalent chaplain: negotiating structural and ideological difference on the margins of modern-day hospital medicine. *Med Anthropol* 2006;25:1–29.
6. Lee SJC. In a secular spirit: strategies of clinical pastoral education. *Health Care Anal* 2002; 10:339–356.
7. VandeCreek L. *Contract Pastoral Care and Education: The Trend of the Future?* New York, Haworth Pastoral Press, 1999.
8. Flannelly KJ, Weaver AJ, Smith WJ, et al. Psychologists and health care chaplains doing research together. *J Psychol* 2003;22:327–332.
9. VandeCreek L. Professional Chaplaincy: What is Happening to it During Health Care Reform? Binghamton, NY, Haworth Press, 2000.
10. Flannelly KJ, Handzo GF, Weaver AJ. Factors affecting healthcare chaplaincy and the provision of pastoral care in the United States. *J Pastoral Care Counsel* 2004;5:1–2.
11. VandeCreek L. How has health care reform affected professional chaplaincy programs and how are department directors responding? in VandeCreek L. (ed): *Professional Chaplaincy: What Is Happening to It During Health Care Reform?* Binghamton, NY, Haworth Press, 2000.

12. VandeCreek L, Siegel K, Gorey E, et al. How many chaplains per 100 inpatients? Benchmarks of health care chaplaincy departments. *J Pastoral Care Counsel* 2001;55:289–301.
13. Weaver AJ, Flannelly KJ, Oppenheimer JE. Religion, spirituality, and chaplains in the biomedical literature: 1965–2000. *Int J Psychiatry Med* 2003;33:155–161.
14. Curlin FA, Lawrence RE, Chin MH, et al. Religion, conscience, and controversial clinical practices. *N Engl J Med* 2007;356:593–600.

ARTICLE 2

"He Needs to Talk!": A Chaplain's Case Study of Nonreligious Spiritual Care

Steve Nolan

Princess Alice Hospice, Esher, Surrey, UK; University of Winchester, Hampshire, UK
Address correspondence to Steve Nolan, MA, MSc, PhD, Princess Alice Hospice, West End Lane, Esher KT10 8NA, UK. E-mail: stevenolan@PAH.org.uk
Copyright © 2016 Taylor & Francis Group, LLC
ISSN: 0885-4726 print/1528-6916 online
DOI: 10.1080/08854726.2015.1113805

Abstract

Chaplains have always worked with nonreligious people, but it is not always clear what is distinctive about their contribution. This case describes an episode of nonreligious spiritual care in order to explore the value of chaplaincy work with people who regard themselves as nonreligious. This case reports on work with a dying man and his family—wife, daughter, sister, and son-in-law—whose religion is secularized, but whose secularism is touched by the sacred.

Key words: case study, chaplain, nonreligious, presence, spiritual care

"Religion in Britain is not what it used to be" (Woodhead, 2012, p.1). This unremarkable statement sums up the changing nature of religions in Britain. *Religions* in the plural because, to whatever extent the nations of Britain may have once been Christian, they are now a multifaith mix of European, Asian, and African religions. The success of this mix is perhaps surprising given that the secularist narrative has long described the inevitable privatization and decline of religion. On the face of it, the secularist narrative has validity. According to the United Kingdom Office of National Statistics:

> Between 2001 and 2011 there has been a decrease in people who identify as Christian (from 71.7% to 59.3%) and an increase in those reporting no religion (from 14.8% to 25.1%). (Office for National Statistics [ONS], 2012)

Nolan, S. (2016) "'He needs to talk!': a chaplain's case study of nonreligious spiritual care." Journal of Health Care Chaplaincy, 22, 1, 1–16.

These figures for England and Wales compare with those for Scotland, where over the same period the number identifying as Christian (54%) decreased by 11%, while those stating that they had no religion increased by 9% (to 37%) (National Records of Scotland [NRS], 2013).

However, based on research for the Adults' Spirituality Project at the University of Nottingham, David Hay identified an upward trend in the number of people who admitted to having had some kind of spiritual experience, from 48%, in 1987, to 75%, in 2000, an increase of around 60% (Hay, 2002, p.4). It is possible that the decline in traditional religion may be confounded by a rise in "spirituality." In consequence, Linda Woodhead (2012), Director of the Religion and Society Programme, Lancaster University, argues that post-war Britain is both religious *and* secular. With her colleague, Paul Heelas, she coined the term "subjectivization" to name a set of processes they argue account for the secularizing *decline* of religion and the simultaneous sacralizing *growth* of spirituality (Heelas & Woodhead, 2005).

This is not the place to discuss the complexities of the religious/spiritual context, or to debate definitions of *religion* and *spirituality* (Hill et al., 2000; Nolan, 2011). I simply note here that chaplains are challenged by working in this highly subjectivized environment, where the religious is secularized and the secular is sacralized. Authorized by their faith community, chaplains are paid by and accountable to secular healthcare managers; their services are valued by those they serve, but they minister to people who are beyond the borders of religious communities and who may have little to no understanding of theology or religious polity. Working in the liminality of this context, Mowat and Swinton (2005, 2007) ask, "What do chaplains do?" and conclude that healthcare chaplaincy involves "an active process of finding people who need spiritual care, identifying the nature of the need and responding to the need through theological reflection and the sharing of spiritual practices" (Mowat & Swinton, 2007, p.8). It is of interest that their qualitative study emphasizes *spiritual* care and *spiritual* practices (however they may be defined), rather than *religious* care and *religious* practices.

The situation in the United States differs from that of the United Kingdom, in that in the United States, researchers tend to treat spirituality and religion as interchangeable terms. However, a report by Handzo et al. (2008) hints at the possible re-evaluation of spirituality as a nonreligious phenomenon of the kind that has been taking place in the United Kingdom over at least the last decade. Analyzing data about the nature of spiritual care, the researchers classified certain interventions as nonreligious, which some chaplains regarded as spiritual (Handzo et al., 2008, p.50).

The case I have chosen exemplifies work in this context. The case involved a range of chaplaincy interventions and practices, most of which would not be considered *religious* and some of which could have been delivered by another healthcare professional. However, all the work reported is pastoral care of the kind delivered by a religious pastor, and I would argue that, because it attends to that "natural extension of the conscious self" that some regard as "transcendent" (Elkins, Hedstrom, Hughes, Leaf, & Saunders, 1988, p.10), it is spiritual care of the kind best delivered by a chaplain (Nolan, 2011).

Formal permission from an ethics committee is not necessary for a case study; however, the article was submitted to, and approved for publication by, Princess Alice Hospice, on condition that identities and identifying details are disguised. All the verbatim accounts were written up within 24 hours of the intervention.

Background

Den was clerked into hospice suffering from small cell carcinoma of the lung, with liver and bone metastases. Now in his 80s, Den began his career as a manual worker before re-training in mid-life in a professional role. In the late 1950s, he met Connie. The couple married and set up home in a rented flat. A few years later, Elaine, their daughter, was born.

Den was an intelligent and grounded man, with wide interests. He enjoyed practical hobbies, classical and jazz music, and collecting; he followed south London football teams and was a lifelong camper. Generous with his time and energies, Den had been financial and emotional provider to Connie, who with his sister, Millie, showed conspicuous devotion. Connie and Millie visited from late morning every day, staying with him until taken home by a friend or by Elaine, who visited several times a week. While Den had not been religious, Connie brought Elaine up within the Roman Catholic tradition that she had known from childhood. However, Elaine had become alienated from the Church following her divorce. Now, with her teenaged child, she lived with her long-term partner, Alan, who was very close to Den. Elaine and Alan were planning to marry, but had not yet "got around to it."

In 2013 Den was admitted to Princess Alice Hospice, an independent 28-bedded in-patient hospice, in the south of England. This independent charity provides palliative care, free at the point of need, to adults with cancer and other life-limiting illnesses. The hospice supports families and carers during the illness and provides bereavement care afterward. The hospice catchment area takes in over one million people across a large part of Surrey, southwest London, and Middlesex.

I began work as a chaplain in this hospice in June 2004. My spiritual formation began within Roman Catholicism, but, after exploring the possibility of the priesthood and engaging with the Charismatic Renewal, I left to join an independent evangelical church, whose style was Pentecostal. In my early 20s, I spent two years in an evangelical Bible college and then worked in churches in Kent and the Midlands. My theological understanding began to change and, following a short break working in advertising, I trained for Baptist ministry in a liberal theological college in my home city, Manchester. Following ordination, I served seven years in a small church in northwest London, where I began to engage in interfaith work. I consider myself fluent in several dialects of Christian spirituality, but I have found wisdom and spiritual nurture in eastern faiths, particularly Buddhism. I am dual qualified, with British Association for Counselling and Psychotherapy accreditation as a counsellor/psychotherapist. At the time of writing, I am 56.

Case study

Initial encounters

I visited Den and his family shortly after his admission, because his nurses felt he needed to talk. When I arrived he was asleep, so I introduced myself to his wife, Connie, and his sister, Millie. They seemed pleased that I had called, but seemed not to want any support. Indeed, our chaplaincy volunteers, who visited four times over the next ten days, found no obvious desire to engage, certainly not from Den, although one volunteer recorded that Den had "seemed to be quite stressed emotionally." During these initial encounters, I was asked to contact Den's daughter, who had enquired about the possibility of arranging her wedding in the hospice, and I arranged a meeting to discuss what was possible.

Den

Two weeks after admission, Den was referred to me again. Connie had expressed concern that Den had something on his mind, but would not talk to her about it. Could I help? When I visited, he was alone in his room.

Chaplain: How's it going Den?

Den: (*Pause*) About the same as yesterday.

Chaplain: And how was that?

Den: (*Pause*) Muddled and confused.

Chaplain: (*Pause*) Do you have anything on your mind, Den?

Den: (*Pause*) Connie and I haven't really spoken about... (*His voice trailed off*).

Chaplain: Is that something you like to speak about? (*Long pause suggesting Den didn't want to respond*) You and Connie have been together a long time, Den. (*Nods*) She seems a lovely lady.

Den: The best!

Chaplain: I met your daughter, Elaine, yesterday. She seems very nice.

Den: (*Pause*) My sister's here and you say you've met my daughter.

Chaplain: Yes.

Den: It's not the best time.

Chaplain: It's not the best time?

Den: I find when they're here... It's not the best time to make decisions.

Chaplain: (*Pause. Den's whole demeanor seemed to say that he was too weary to talk and wanted to be left alone*) Would you like me to come back tomorrow? (*Nods*) Okay, Den. I'll wish you well.

Den extended his hand to shake mine and engaged me with a look that felt very purposeful. We held each other's gaze as I walked around his bed and toward the door. Later, I summarized our meeting in Den's medical records:

> Den indicated he has things to speak about, but didn't want to talk today. I offered to see him again tomorrow.

Connie

I found Connie and Millie in the hospice coffee lounge and joined them at their table.

Connie: Did he speak to you?

Chaplain: (*I was protective of Den's confidentiality*) He was tired today and said I could come back tomorrow.

Connie:	But did you say anything to him?
Chaplain:	No, but he said I could come back tomorrow.
Connie:	That's a shame.
Chaplain:	I'll see him tomorrow. (*Connie looked worried*) Is there something you think he needs to talk about?
Connie:	Not really. He doesn't talk to me about how things are, only about how he's feeling.
Chaplain:	(*I wanted to understand Den*) Has Den always been a private man?
Connie:	(*Nods*) He has. He's done it to protect me. He's always been the one... I'm the stupid one, the one who doesn't text, or email, or set the programme on the TV.
Chaplain:	But Den's looked after things and been the provider.
Connie:	Hasn't he just. Well, we'll go back now.

Den

I visited Den the following day.

Chaplain:	How's it going, Den?
Den:	About the same as yesterday.
Chaplain:	So a bit muddled and confused then. (*Nods*)
Chaplain:	(*Pause*) Connie told me you've always been very protective and looked after her. (*He sighed*) Do you worry about Connie?
Den:	Not as much as I used to.
Chaplain:	Not as much.
Den:	She's hard.
Chaplain:	(*I was puzzled by his use of "hard"*) She's become tougher?
Den:	More than she was. (*Den looked very tired*)
Chaplain:	Is there something you'd like to talk about?
Den:	Not really.
Chaplain:	Okay, Den. Shall I let you rest?

Den: Yes, please.

I summarized our meeting in Den's notes:

Tried to give Den the opportunity to talk, but he declined.

Connie

That afternoon, I had a call from Den's health care assistant (HCA): Connie would like me to come and talk with Den. Before going to his room, I checked with his HCA. Connie had received bad news: she had been expecting Den would return home, but he was deteriorating. With his health carers, we agreed to try to help Connie manage her anxieties. I found Connie walking alone in the garden.

Chaplain: You've seen the doctors today.

Connie: Yes. It wasn't good.

Chaplain: Would you like to have a cup of tea and sit and talk about it?

Connie: I won't have a cup of tea, but I will sit down.

We found seats in the coffee lounge.

Connie: We were told by the cancer hospital that he might have about two years, but it doesn't look that way now. Den's happy to stay here. I don't think I'll tell Elaine. She has such a long drive home, and she's so tired. I think I'll tell Alan (*Elaine's partner*).

Chaplain: That's a good idea.

Connie: We always said we would go together. Elaine doesn't agree with that. She says what about her, but she has Alan. We didn't have many friends. (*She began to cry*) We were always enough for each other. But it wouldn't be difficult.

Chaplain: (*This sounded like suicidal ideation, but I wanted Connie to be more explicit*) How do you mean?

Connie: A few sleeping tablets. A few *more* tablets.

I felt Connie had taken me into her confidence, and I was cautious about challenging her immediately; nonetheless, I felt I should say something about the implications of her possible action. I expressed how difficult it would be for those close to her. On reflection, I should probably have tried to explore Connie's suicidal ideation with her, to check how serious she was, and what she felt life would be like without Den. In Den's notes, I summarized my meeting with Connie:

> Spent time with Connie. She expressed she had suicidal thoughts and spoke about not wanting to "go on" after Den's death. I discussed this with my line manager.

Elaine

Accompanying Connie to Den's room, I found Elaine with her dad. I had news about her wedding plans and we agreed to talk. Elaine had been with Alan for over 20 years. They had always intended to marry, but they "just hadn't got around to it." She wanted Den to "give her away" and was eager to make the arrangements. I was advised that a registrar would not attend the hospice, because it was not a patient who wanted to marry. The next best option was for Elaine and Alan to marry at a convenient register office and then have a blessing in Den's hospice room. However, because it was felt that time was short, I agreed to conduct the blessing first, and we set a date. I wrote a personalized service of blessing on their intention to marry that specifically included within it a question for Den:

> Chaplain: Who gives Elaine's hand to Alan?
>
> Den: I do.

Connie and Millie

A week after the blessing, Den's condition had begun to improve, to the point where there was talk of discharging him. I found Connie and Millie in the hospice dining room. Connie said they were waiting for the social worker to talk to Den about nursing homes, and she expressed her anxieties about having Den home.

> Connie: He'd prefer to stay here. He likes it here. He doesn't want to go to a nursing home. I understand why they're saying that, but...

Millie sat quietly, her facial expressions reflecting Connie's anxiety. I felt compromised. I had a strong urge to explain the hospice policy, but held back to allow Connie to express her feelings. In any case, Connie's sense of helplessness silenced us all. I wanted to reach out and hold her hands, which she rested on the table. I regret that I did not.

Later, I saw Millie sitting alone in the corridor. I sat down next to her. Her eyes instantly watered and she blinked back tears. I asked about Connie, and Millie told me how heavily the decision weighed on her. Millie said that the family had offered to help Connie to have Den at home.

> Millie: I'm a widow, so I could be there to help during the day, and Elaine and Alan could be there at the weekend!

I learned from Millie that her husband had died under the hospice's care. At the time, she had been offered bereavement support, but declined to have it. I reminded her that the offer remained available to her and that she may find it helpful now. She said she would consider it.

Den and Connie

The following day, I visited Den in his room. Wide-eyed, he looked like a rabbit caught in the headlights. I squeezed his hand, but with little response. Plaintively, Connie voiced, "He doesn't speak now."

Den stared at the wall behind my head. Connie was pouring a tot of whisky. Millie was in search of ice. We distilled opinions about malts, and Den nodded his preference was for Irish. Connie was again awaiting the social worker to talk about nursing homes. Rehearsing the previous day's conversation, I moved to sit beside Den. Taking his hand, I squeezed it and he responded in kind. He closed his eyes and seemed to drift off to sleep. Connie dabbed her eyes with a tissue. Still holding Den's hand I stood and reached out to Connie. Millie returned without ice. I offered to get some from the kitchen. Den was asleep when I returned.

Later, I found my social worker colleague. Like me, he felt Den's condition had deteriorated, and rather than prematurely burden Den and Connie with talk about discharge, he felt it wise to wait until after Ward Round, when the doctors had been able to assess Den.

Den, Connie, and Millie

Three days later, Den was unresponsive. Geraldine, a Chaplaincy volunteer, visited and sat a while with him. As she left the room, Den died. It was Friday morning. Geraldine and a young trainee nurse waited with Den, and left him when Connie and Millie arrived. I joined them a few minutes later. Den had not been religious and religion had not been part of my involvement with his family. They did not ask for prayers, and it felt inappropriate to offer any. Therefore, I watched quietly with them, and witnessed Den's womenfolk anxiously caress him, their pink-warm hands in salient contrast to the paling ochre of his now-cold fingers. I listened to the words they whispered to each other:

Connie: I just want to be with him.

Millie: You can't do that to Elaine.

Connie: But she has a husband now.

Millie: But she needs you.

Since our earlier conversation, I had looked for an opportunity to speak again with Connie about her suicidal ideation. I had discussed the situation with colleagues and agreed that, while we could not prevent Connie taking her own life, I should nevertheless try to speak further with her and also alert her general practitioner (GP). Later that morning, after Elaine had arrived, I asked to speak privately with Connie.

Chaplain: I remember a conversation we had some time ago, and you said that you didn't want to go on without Den. (*Nods*) You mentioned in the room, just now, that you didn't want to be without him. (*Nods*) Connie, I'm very concerned about you. Have you thought about what you might do?

Connie: No.

Chaplain: But you're thinking about it. (*Nods*) Connie, Elaine would be devastated.

Connie: But she has Alan.

Chaplain: But she loves you and needs you now. It would be devastating if you did anything.

Connie: It's devastating for me.

Chaplain: I know. (*Pause*) Connie, I want to speak to your doctor.

Connie: And tell him about Den.

Chaplain: And tell him what you've said to me.

Connie agreed I could contact her GP. I documented what I had done:

Spent time supporting Connie and Millie after Den's death. Connie mentioned again that she doesn't want to go on without Den. Millie's reaction indicated she was expressing suicidal thinking and I later asked to speak with Connie alone. I wanted to check with her about her thoughts and she acknowledged that she was thinking how to end things. I told her I would speak to her GP and she agreed I should. I spoke to Dr [Name], who said he would like someone to bring Connie to see him. I wanted to discuss this with Elaine, but she left before I had chance. I will try to contact Elaine.

Connie, Elaine, Millie, and Alan

After the weekend, I met Connie, Elaine, and Millie in the Sanctuary, the hospice quiet room. They were tearful and I sat with them for a short while. Elaine asked if I would take the service for her dad, and we arranged a time to meet later in the week. When they arrived, I spent over an hour with them, listening to and writing up their memories and anecdotes about Den, which I used to construct a eulogy. As we ended the appointment, Alan voiced: "It's good to talk like this. Actually, it's quite therapeutic." I conducted Den's funeral a week later.

Assessments, interventions, and outcomes

Assessment: Den

Initial concerns were raised about Den's spiritual needs by his nurses, who felt that he "needed to talk." This informal observation, in which nurses responded to visual cues, probably informed by their assumptions about his wellbeing, was an intuitive form of the kind of spiritual screening described by Fitchett and Risk (2009) (the formal protocol was unknown to the hospice at the time of the case). The feeling that Den needed to talk was underlined by Connie, who expressed her husband had something on his mind but was not talking to her about it. Yet, she was ambivalent when I asked if there was something he needed to talk about. Several colleagues, including chaplaincy volunteers, had tried to engage Den, but while he had hinted that he wanted to talk, he declined every opportunity. It seemed that Den had always kept things to himself, probably because he wanted to "protect" those closest to him. Den's resistance to talk freely made his spiritual needs difficult to assess.

Assessment: Connie

A core value of palliative care is extending care to family and carers. Connie's spiritual needs involved her anxieties around losing Den, which implied her loss of security and anxiety about her own mortality. She appeared to cope by externalizing her need on to Den: *he* needed to talk.

When Connie was told Den's condition was deteriorating and that he was unlikely to return home, she responded by requesting that I come and talk with him, even though she had no idea what he might want to talk about, nor any basis for expecting that he would talk. Connie's dependency on Den was such that she was unable to imagine a life without him—she presented as being helpless and unable to cope—and it is tempting to speculate that Connie may have an ambivalent style of attachment (Parks, 2009). At Den's bedside, Connie articulated the desperation of the clinging nature of her loss: "I just want to be with him." Suicide might enact the extremity of Connie's anxiety and the overwhelming existential threat to her sense of self.

Assessment: Elaine

Elaine's spiritual needs were less obvious than those of her parents, but she expressed them clearly in wanting her dad to "give her away." He had done this when Elaine first married, but that marriage had long since ended. Now Elaine was with her soul-partner she wanted to show her dad that this was a relationship that was solid, permanent, and dependable (like him). On the other hand, Elaine's identity seemed closely associated with her role as a carer. She worked in a caring profession and was literally going the extra mile(s) in caring for her parents. To that extent, it is possible Elaine's caring was meeting one of her significant spiritual needs: the need to actualize her identity as she had constructed it. However, taking the form of "selfless" caring for her parents, partner, and daughter, while holding down a full-time job and driving in excess of three hours several times each week after work, this actualization was very likely damaging her health. Elaine's desire that her dad should "give her away" was one more expression of her caring.

Assessment: Millie

Millie's spiritual needs were the least conspicuous because she was so undemanding, faithfully accompanying her sister-in-law. Yet, despite her unassertive demeanor, there were layers to Millie's psychospiritual pain that needed attention. Accepting bereavement support after the death of her own husband may have proved helpful in dealing with the dying of her brother, perhaps recognizing this prompted her to urge Connie to make use of the service. As it was, Den's protracted decline was reopening Millie's emotional wounds.

Intervention: Den

Den defied our attempts to address his perceived need to talk. Perhaps I should have been more persistent in inviting him to speak, but the signals Den gave seemed consistent and strong: he did not want to talk, to his wife or his care team, and no one was going to cajole him otherwise. This not only proscribed our talking interventions, it made redundant any rational assessment of his needs, spiritual or otherwise. However, spiritual care transcends objective, rational communication and speaks without words at the level of the subjective and immediate, in a form of relating Martin Buber characterizes as "I–Thou" (Buber, 1958). Although unable to evidence this objectively, it is my sense that, on two occasions, Den and I communicated in this subjective, immediate way. The first occasion was when we shook hands and he engaged me with what I experienced as a very purposeful gaze. This felt to me to be more than the look that typically passes between two people in regular social interaction. It disquieted but did not unsettle me; it searched me and seemed to hang on to me, inviting me to return the gaze as a recognition that in that moment we were present to each other. On reflection, maybe I should have stayed longer with his gaze; but then maybe more would have been less; in the same way that those rare moments of unexpected encounter with the sacred dissipate in the recognition, maybe overstaying would have stolen presence from the moment and left us only embarrassment. Months later, the moment retains its resonance for me.

The other occasion was when I sat beside him shortly before he died, and Den responded to my gentle squeeze of his hand, before drifting off to sleep. The communication went unnoticed, but it both gave and received quiet recognition. In contrast with my reaching out to Connie, who was lost in her grief, Den's gesture seemed to express his content with the moment, and he drifted off to sleep. My interpretation is that Den and I subtly communicated that we were present to each other. We did this without words, I would say beyond words, and on both occasions we did it in a passing, yet enduring, moment. Because our communication was beyond words, it was also beyond rational analysis. Nevertheless, my sense is that it was meaningful and not untypical of the communication many chaplains experience.

Intervention: Connie

The direct cause of Connie's spiritual need was Den's dying. My work with Connie was first to build a relationship of trust. This seemed to develop naturally as I was able to spend time with her on the ward and in the coffee lounge; but I also deliberately sought out Connie to speak with her in private. This allowed her to talk candidly, and to say she did not want to "go on" without Den. This was significant information, and, while I respected Connie's right to determine her own future, my duty of care nonetheless required me to take what she said at face value and treat it seriously. After speaking with my line manager, I decided to speak again with Connie and (with her consent) with her GP. Den's unexpected death almost robbed me of a suitable opportunity. Connie's GP took my call and asked to see her as soon as practicable. My relationship with Connie and her family was such that they asked me to take Den's funeral. When I have had a sustained relationship with a family it can feel important to me, at a personal level, to provide aftercare in the form of a funeral; however, the services take time to prepare and conduct, and I therefore refrain from offering. Clearly, it was important to Connie and her family, and, as Alan observed, it was at some level therapeutic—for us all.

Intervention: Elaine

Addressing Elaine's need to care for her parents, I focused on helping her plan a service analogous to a wedding that would bless her intention to marry, but which would also allow Den to play his part as father of the bride (-to-be). The short service, conducted around Den's bed, included a pre-amble about their relationship, it highlighted their intention to marry, and it acknowledged that their family had gathered to anticipate their wedding. I ended with:

> Today as we gladly and with real joy anticipate your wedding we stand together with you, and ask a blessing upon you as you join hands to anticipate your wedding.

Then, to allow Den to participate, I asked: "Who will give Elaine's hand to Alan?" To which he replied: "I do." Den passed Elaine's hand to Alan. I followed this with an edited version of the wedding promises and concluded with a specially written blessing.

Intervention: Millie

Regrettably, it was not possible to address any of Millie's psychospiritual pain around the loss of her husband. I had been mindful of her needs and looked for opportunities to give her time to talk. However, the only occasion that arose naturally was when I found her sitting alone in the corridor. I tried, then, to encourage her to talk, but she was too overcome to speak about herself. I was able, later, to tell Millie about the hospice's bereavement support aftercare, and I subsequently referred her to the service.

Outcomes: Den

It is tempting to assert that the presence of those who sat with Den made a difference to how he experienced his dying. This was the view of one nurse who said that, in being there with him where he was, Geraldine had been "a real presence for him" and that this was "just what she [the nurse] felt he needed." My instinct is that the nurse was right; however, it is not possible to know the state of a dying person's subjectivity, and such assertions risk a form of self-indulgence that is unwarranted. The uncomfortable reality is that it is impossible to know what Den's end-of-life experience was.

Outcomes: Connie

Connie's faith had not been to the fore in her adult life, although she retained a respect for religion, and perhaps an expectation that clergy could be trusted. She seemed, at least, to regard me as able to contain her anxiety, such that she always appeared pleased to see me and to trust me. She was certainly open to me referring her to other professionals. Den died on Friday and Connie saw her GP the following Monday. He spent time with her and prescribed antidepressants. When I met Connie the following day at the hospice, she was heartbroken. When we met to plan Den's funeral, she was less emotionally labile; however, on the day of the funeral, she was inconsolable, and I referred her to the hospice bereavement support service. Within about a week, Connie had been contacted by the service and began seeing an experienced support worker.

Outcomes: Elaine

Elaine had one outcome she wanted. Estranged from her Roman Catholicism, she wanted her union with Alan to be blessed. I tried to respond in a pastorally sensitive and creative way to Elaine's spiritual needs, which I interpreted as being accepted by God, as represented by a minister of the Church. However, in my view, Elaine had another need that remained unaddressed. I regard actualizing the identity one has constructed as a spiritual need, and that, for Elaine, this need had developed a deleterious quality that was potentially, if not actually, harming her, physically and emotionally. It was disappointing that there was no opportunity to address it with her.

Discussion

My work with Den and his family represents an episode of nonreligious spiritual care. Nonetheless, I would argue the work responded to their religious/spiritual instincts. Such instincts are often expressed in non-rational, "I–Thou" communication (Buber, 1958), the unconscious connection that transcends objective rationality and communicates without words in the subjective and immediate (Frankl, 2000, pp.31, 37). Some chaplains call this *presence* and regard it as a key and distinctive aspect of their spiritual care.

For me, the idea of being present, or being-*with*, is core to spiritual care (Nolan, 2012). In every encounter, I aim to communicate that my attention is focused fully on the person I am with and that, for those few moments, I am entirely with them. In part, this approach is informed by training in integrative psychotherapy; in part by learning from eastern spiritual practices; and in part by formation as a Christian minister; but I try also to be sensitive to the possibilities that open by virtue of what I *represent*, or evoke as a chaplain. For example, with some I evoke benign indifference, while with others I evoke confidence that I can be trusted with personal issues, private fears, or troubling questions about life and death. Again, I remind some that there is that which is mysterious and other (however that is understood), and others that important life events can be marked by rites or rituals.

Critics misunderstand and misrepresent the purpose of healthcare chaplaincy when they present it as a relic of its religious heritage, and argue that healthcare chaplains provide care that could be provided equally well, and at less cost, by community faith leaders (Christian, 2011; Paley, 2008a, 2008b). Yet, in working with those whose religion is secularized and whose secularism is touched by the sacred, chaplains do much more. Chaplains care for the religious/spiritual instinct, which, while often expressed religiously, is never fully contained within a religious tradition, nor fully represented by a nonreligious philosophy or psychology. The religious/spiritual instinct is fundamental to being human, regardless of religion, and should be met with an ethic of respect and dignity, in other words, with love. Therefore, I approached Den and his family with the aim of supporting them, religiously or otherwise. Such an approach did not reduce my chaplaincy care to a form of humanistic psychotherapy, nor did it induce tension in me as one who is both a chaplain and a psychotherapist. Rather it acknowledged the genius of the human spirit.

Certainly, aspects of my work in this case could have been delivered by another healthcare professional. However, another healthcare professional would be unlikely to open the particular possibilities for engaging the religious/spiritual instinct that were evoked by me as a chaplain. Arguably, Den would have preferred a humanist funeral, but that would not have answered the religious/spiritual instinct of his family. This instinct was apparent in Elaine's desire to ritualize her major life event in a way that allowed her father to enact his approval of their relationship. The instinct was less obvious in working with Connie. However, faith had been significant in her early life and informed a respect for the clergy. She confided in me some of her personal issues, private fears and troubling questions about life and death (suicide). She also trusted me to refer her to her GP. Den's expression of the religious/spiritual instinct was perhaps least obvious, but I identify it in a desire for connection beyond words. I suggest the religious/spiritual instinct was expressed and met in the holding of a gaze and the squeezing of hands.

It remains important to make the case for the relevance and impact of religious interventions, but the evolving healthcare context demands chaplains demonstrate the value of spiritual care to people who regard themselves as nonreligious. I chose this case to describe an episode of nonreligious spiritual care and demonstrate the value of chaplaincy work with people who regard themselves as nonreligious, in this case people whose religion is being secularized, but whose secularism is touched by the sacred.

References

Buber, M. (1958). *I and thou*. Edinburgh, Scotland: T&T Clark.
Christian, R. (2011). *Costing the heavens: Chaplaincy services in English NHS provider trusts 2009/10*. London, UK: National Secular Society.
Elkins, D. N., Hedstrom, L. J., Hughes, L. L., Leaf, J. A., & Saunders, C. L. (1988). Toward a humanistic–phenomenological spirituality: Definition, description and measurement. *Journal of Humanistic Psychology, 28*(4), 5–18. doi:10.1177/ 0022167888284002
Fitchett, G., & Risk, J. L. (2009). Screening for spiritual struggle. *Journal of Pastoral Care and Counseling, 63*(1–2), 1–12. doi:10.1177/154230500906300104
Frankl, V. E. (2000). *Man's search for ultimate meaning*. New York, NY: Basic Books.
Handzo, G. F., Flannelly, K. J., Kudler, T., Fogg, S. L., Harding, S. R., Hasan, Y. ... Taylor, B. E. (2008). What do chaplains really do? II. Interventions in the New York chaplaincy study. *Journal of Health Care Chaplaincy, 14*(1), 39–56. doi:10.1080/08854720802053853
Hay, D. (2002). The spirituality of adults in Britain – Recent research. *Scottish Journal of Healthcare Chaplaincy, 5*(1), 4–9. doi:10.1558/hscc.v5i1.4

Heelas, P., & Woodhead, L. (2005). *The spiritual revolution: Why religion is giving way to spirituality.* Oxford, UK: Blackwell.

Hill, P. C., Pargament, K. I., Hood, R. W., McCullough, M. E., Jr, Swyers, J. P., Larson, D. B. & Zinnbauer, B. J. (2000). Conceptualizing religion and spirituality: Points of commonality, points of departure. *Journal for the Theory of Social Behaviour, 30*(1), 51–77. doi: 10.1111/1468-5914.00119

Mowat, H., & Swinton, J. (2005). *What do chaplains do? A report on a two year investigation into the nature of chaplaincy in the NHS in Scotland.* Edinburgh, Scotland: Scottish Executive.

Mowat, H., & Swinton, J. (2007). *What do chaplains do? The role of the chaplain in meeting the spiritual needs of patients* (2nd ed.). Aberdeen, Scotland: Mowat Research.

National Records of Scotland (NRS). (2013). *Census 2011: Key results on population, ethnicity, identity, language, religion, health, housing and accommodation in Scotland – Release 2A.* Retrieved November 9, 2014, from www.scotlandscensus.gov.uk/documents/censusresults/release2a/StatsBulletin2A.pdf.

Nolan, S. (2011). Psychospiritual care: New content for old concepts—Towards a new paradigm for non-religious spiritual care. *Journal for the Study of Spirituality, 1*(1), 50–64. doi:10.1558/jss.v1i1.50

Nolan, S. (2012). *Spiritual care at the end of life: The chaplain as a "hopeful presence."* London, UK: Jessica Kingsley.

Office for National Statistics (ONS). (2012). *Religion in England and Wales 2011.* Retrieved November 9, 2014, from www.ons.gov.uk/ons/rel/census/2011-census/key-statistics-for-local-authorities-in-england-and-wales/rpt-religion.html.

Paley, J. (2008a). Spirituality and nursing: A reductionist approach. *Nursing Philosophy, 9,* 3–18. doi:10.1111/j.1466-769x.2007.00330.x

Paley, J. (2008b). The concept of spirituality in palliative care: An alternative view. *International Journal of Palliative Nursing, 14,* 448–452. doi: 10.12968/ijpn.2008.14.9.31125

Parks, C. M. (2009). *Love and Loss: The Roots of Grief and its Complications.* Hove, UK: Routledge.

Woodhead, L. (2012). Introduction. In L. Woodhead & R. Catto (Eds). *Religion and Change in Modern Britain* (pp. 1–33). New York, NY/Abingdon, UK: Routledge.

ARTICLE 3

What Do I Do? Developing a Taxonomy of Chaplaincy Activities and Interventions for Spiritual Care in Intensive Care Unit Palliative Care

Kevin Massey, Marilyn JD Barnes, Dana Villines, Julie D Goldstein, Anna Lee Hisey Pierson, Cheryl Scherer, Betty Vander Laan and Wm Thomas Summerfelt

Correspondence: kevin.massey@advocatehealth.com

Advocate Health Care, 3075 Highland Parkway, Downers Grove, IL 60515, USA

Copyright © 2015 Massey et al.; licensee BioMed Central. This is an Open Access article distributed under the terms of the Creative Commons Attribution License (http://creativecommons.org/licenses/by/4.0), which permits unrestricted use, distribution, and reproduction in any medium, provided the original work is properly credited. The Creative Commons Public Domain Dedication waiver (http://creativecommons.org/publicdomain/zero/1.0/) applies to the data made available in this article, unless otherwise stated.

Abstract

Background: Chaplains are increasingly seen as key members of interdisciplinary palliative care teams, yet the specific interventions and hoped for outcomes of their work are poorly understood. This project served to develop a standard terminology inventory for the chaplaincy field, to be called the chaplaincy taxonomy.

Methods: The research team used a mixed methods approach to generate, evaluate and validate items for the taxonomy. We conducted a literature review, retrospective chart review, focus groups, self-observation, experience sampling, concept mapping, and reliability testing. Chaplaincy activities focused primarily on palliative care in an intensive care unit setting in order to capture a broad cross-section of chaplaincy activities.

Results: Literature and chart review resulted in 438 taxonomy items for testing. Chaplain focus groups generated an additional 100 items and removed 421 items as duplications. Self-observation, Experience Sampling and Concept Mapping provided validity that the taxonomy items were

---

Massey, K., Barnes, M.J.D., Villines, D., Goldstein, J.D., Hisey Pierson, A.L., Scherer, C., Vander Laan, B., and Summerfelt, W.T. (2015) "What do I do? Developing a taxonomy of chaplaincy activities and interventions for spiritual care in intensive care unit palliative care." *BMC Palliative Care*, 14, 10, 1–8.

actual activities that chaplains perform in their spiritual care. Inter-rater reliability for chaplains to identify taxonomy items from vignettes was 0.903.

Conclusions: The 100 item chaplaincy taxonomy provides a strong foundation for a normative inventory of chaplaincy activities and outcomes. A deliberative process is proposed to further expand and refine the taxonomy to create a standard terminological inventory for the field of chaplaincy. A standard terminology could improve the ways interdisciplinary palliative care teams communicate about chaplaincy activities and outcomes.

Keywords: taxonomy, spiritual care, chaplaincy, palliative care, standard terminology

Background

Chaplains are increasingly seen as key members of interdisciplinary palliative care teams, yet what chaplains specifically do in terms of assessments, hoped for outcomes, and interventions remains poorly understood.[1] Chaplains lack a consistent way to describe their activities. Attempts have been made to develop inventories of chaplain activities and propose standard terminologies, yet none of these attempts were empirically based and none of these attempts has emerged as normative.[2,3,4,5,6] Chaplains perform a variety of interventions with therapeutic intent yet lack a unified and consistent naming set for these interventions which would better portray to the inter-disciplinary medical team what goals and results they strive to achieve.

Our study undertook to meet this identified[7] gap in the field of chaplaincy by building an inventory of chaplain activities through a series of mixed methods in which chaplains provided and refined their own terms and verbal preferences for their practice. This was executed in both patient care contexts and through qualitative steps involving groups of chaplains.

Methods

A qualitative and quantitative approach was used to execute three phases of the study: item generation, validity, and reliability. The Advocate Health Care Institutional Review Board of our organization approved this study.

Item generation

LITERATURE AND RETROSPECTIVE CHART REVIEW

Four published inventories[2, 3, 4, 5] of chaplain activities were reviewed by team members. The review criteria for inclusion included being published and employing research methodology. These inventories were judged by the team members to be the best previous efforts preceding this project. The team incorporated these inventories into a collective initial inventory. As the initial items were emerging from the literature review and the retrospective chart review, the chaplain researchers perceived three categories of "granularity." Some items were very specific concrete actions. Some items were more like goals or outcomes. Some items seemed like something in between concrete items and goals. As the study progressed and as is seen in the results, we began grouping the items into these three categories, which we named "interventions" for concrete items, "intended effects" for goals and outcomes, and "methods." These categories were later validated by the concept mapping phase described below. In the retrospective chart review phase, chaplain care data was taken from patient records (n = 1126 patient encounters) that had at least one interaction with a hospital chaplain and were also seen in the Intensive Care Unit (ICU). Patients who had the following Diagnosis Related Groups (DRG) were included: Intracranial Hemorrhage/Cerebral Infarction (DRG 65), Intracranial Hemorrhage Malignancy of Hepatobiliary System or Pancreas with Morbidity (DRG 435), Respiratory System Diagnosis with Ventilator Support (DRG 207–208), Septicemia or Severe Sepsis with or without Mechanical Ventilation 96+ Hours (DRG 870–711), and Simple Pneumonia and Pleurisy with Complication or Comorbidity (DRG 193). These DRGs were used in this step at the suggestion of the palliative care physician on our team to encompass patients mirroring the palliative care and ICU context that would follow in later steps.

External validity

FOCUS GROUP/KEY INFORMANT INTERVIEWS

Board Certified Chaplains (BCCs) and Board Certified-Eligible Chaplains (BCC-Es), who contributed to the care of patients, (n = 27) participated in one of five focus groups conducted at five hospitals within our system. The chaplains were asked to complete four tasks based on their experiences within patient care to determine: which items could be categorized together, which items did not apply to their activities, which items were redundant and which new items should be included. Additionally, eight key informant interviews[8] approximating the focus group experience were conducted with chaplains in administrative positions.

Construct validity

Self-observation and experience sampling methodology[9, 10, 11] was used to determine that we were creating a taxonomy that accurately reflected chaplain activities. Three chaplains at different sites made daily observations of their activities with palliative care patients, their family member(s) and the intensive care unit (ICU) care team using the activity list that was generated by the previous item generation phase. Electronic data collection was used by the three chaplains to record their activities.

SELF-OBSERVATION

Three Board Certified chaplains operating at three different though comparable acute care hospitals made daily observations of their activities with ICU palliative care patients, their family member(s), and the ICU care team using the activity list generated in the previous steps. Each chaplain self-selected activities to be recorded in an electronic collection tool (one to five per day). For each activity, they were asked to select the intervention performed, the intended effect and method corresponding to the intervention, and with whom the intervention was performed.

EXPERIENCE SAMPLING

Chaplains were paged at random intervals during each shift for 28 days to record their current activity, similar to the method pioneered by Larson & Csikszentmihalyi.[9, 10, 11] The chaplains were asked to record their activities within 15 minutes after receiving the page and were alerted by pager six times per shift to identify on the electronic tracking tool if they were engaged in spiritual care or another activity such as administrative duties or on personal time. If a spiritual care intervention was selected, they also recorded the intended effect from the inventory.

CONCEPT MAPPING

Concept mapping is a group-oriented, decision-making process to develop a framework of stakeholders' views for a specific topic.[12] BCCs were recruited from focus group participants and from other institutions participating in the grant opportunity that supported this project. Participants (n = 30) were asked to group the activities into three categories (intended effect, method, and intervention) after receiving training on the data collection tool. Participants were then given a list of activity items and asked to rate each item on a five point Likert-type scale for frequency of use and importance.

Reliability

INTER-RATER RELIABILITY SESSIONS

Vignettes of chaplain activities portraying the care of patients, family member(s), and care team were created from real-life chaplain examples. All vignettes were voice-acted and audio recorded by members of the research team so participants in each session would respond to a standardized vignette presentation. Participants were provided with a list of the taxonomy items divided into intended effect, method, and intervention, as well as a transcript of the vignettes. For each vignette, participants listened to the audio recording of the vignette while reading the transcript, if desired, and identified a Spiritual Care Plan (SCP). An SCP is an assembly of an intended effect, method, and intervention encompassing spiritual care provided.

Figure 1 provides a high level view of the methods process.

Data analyses and statistics

Counts and percentages were used for the patient chart review, chaplain focus group, self-observation and experience sampling data, and the concept map Likert-type ratings of frequency of use and importance are displayed as means with standard deviations. Inter-rater reliability was assessed using the intra-class correlation (ICC).[13] The ICC is an advanced correlation that allows for a random-effects model and estimates agreement among raters. Analysis was performed using SPSS®18 with the exception of analysis for concept clusters. The concept mapping software organized and displayed data using multidimensional scaling and cluster analysis displayed as maps which show the relationship between clusters created by the participants.

Results

The research engaged 67 religiously, ethnically, and geographically diverse chaplains; with 24% of the chaplains participating in three or more research methods.

Item generation

LITERATURE AND RETROSPECTIVE CHART REVIEW

The first version of the taxonomy was generated from the 348 items abstracted from the literature review and clinical experience, with 122 items identified in the previously published inventories and 226 additional items generated by the primary research team, reflecting on their own chaplain experiences. Apparent redundancies were purposely retained in the literature review and retrospective chart review stages to allow later stages to express chaplain preferences. Each additional step would result in a new version built upon the previous steps.

From the population of 1126 cases that met selection criteria for chart abstraction, a random sample of 50 cases from each of three hospitals (n = 150) was selected for review to abstract free text from the progress notes in the charts in search of unique chaplaincy activities for the inventory. Review of the charts resulted in 261 activities recorded. This step generated 90 additional items for placement within the taxonomy, bringing the total number of items to 438.

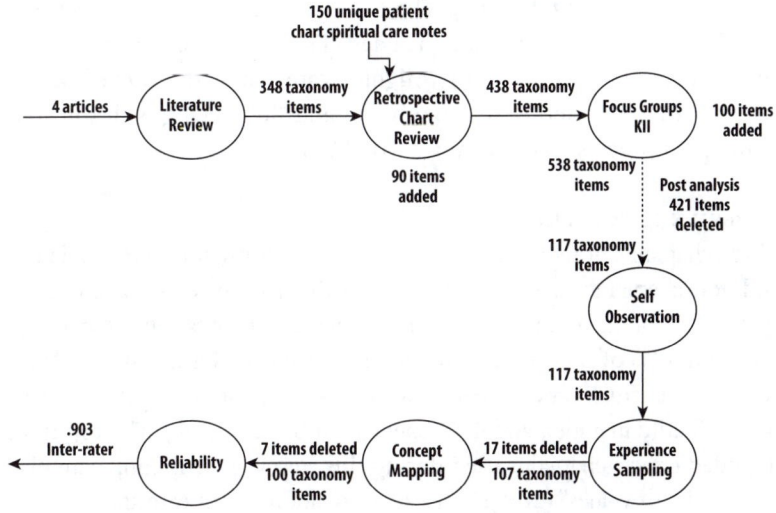

Figure 1: Summary of methods used and taxonomy development

External validity

Focus groups/key informant interviews

The focus groups and key informant interviews generated, deleted, added and revised numerous items of the taxonomy. Session four of the focus groups added the most items (n = 57). Session one identified the most items as duplicates (n = 278), and session two identified the most items as chaplain specific interventions (n = 245). Table 1 provides all session data. The key informant interviews generated similar items to the focus group sessions. After data analysis, the focus groups and key informant interviews generated an additional 100 items and deleted 421 items as duplicate or similar items leaving 117 chaplaincy taxonomy items.

SELF-OBSERVATION

Each chaplain self-selected activities (n = 646 chaplain activities) performed throughout their work shift. For the interventions, 79% of the items were used and 100% of the items were used for methods and intended effects.

The top five interventions accounting for 28% of the responses included "Active listening" (n = 46, 7.1%), "Prayer for healing" (n = 36, 5.6%) and "Silent prayer at bedside", "Facilitate story-telling", and "Facilitate communication between patient and/or family member and care team" each with n = 33, 5.1%. The top three methods accounting for 36% of the responses were "Demonstrate caring and concern" (n = 89, 13.8%), "Provide emotional support" (n = 79, 12.2%), and "Collaborate with care team member" (n = 64, 9.9%). The top four intended effects accounted for 58.1% of the responses and included "Establish a relationship of care and support" (n = 142, 22.0%), "Aligning care plan with patient's values" (n = 134, 20.7%), and "Exploring hope" and "Journeying with someone in the grief process" each with n = 50, 7.7%.

EXPERIENCE SAMPLING

Three chaplains provided 244 data points accounting for their chaplaincy and non-chaplaincy activities. Analysis of the data showed that chaplains spent 56% of their time on administrative, documentation, or personal time and 44% of their time providing spiritual care. Of this 44% of time spent on spiritual care, 42% of the time was spent with patients, 36% with a family member, and 43% spent with the care team. The top three intended effects chaplains used during this step were "Aligning care plan with patient's values" (26%); "Establish a relationship of care and support" (21%); and "Journeying with someone in the grief process" (19%).

Table 1: Focus group results

Session #	# of items added to taxonomy	# of items identified as duplicates	# of items identified as chaplain interventions
1	13	278	173
2	10	219	245
3	7	235	210
4	57	125	198
5	13	271	180

CONCEPT MAPPING

There were a total of 30 BCC and BCC-E participants, from nine health care systems. Other demographic information of the participants included:

23% non-Christian, 67% Christian, 57% female, 73% Caucasian, and 80% of the chaplains identified hospitals as their work setting. The average years of chaplain experience across the participants was 15 years. The top ten frequency and importance rated items are provided in Table 2.

Content Validity

Participant categorizations were compared to the categories established for the experience sampling data collection. Categorizations were compared between the data collection steps and each item was coded as congruent (same categorization in experience sampling and concept mapping) and/or incongruent (different categorization in experience sampling and concept mapping). Of the 107 activities, 72 were congruent (67%) and 35 activities were incongruent (33%). A thorough review of all data collected and group discussion was used to resolve incongruent results and 19 (54%) of the 35 incongruent activities retained the concept mapping categorization with two activities (6%) removed from the activity list.

Reliability

Twenty-seven BCCs, BCC-Es and chaplain residents (student chaplains engaged in a year-long training program) participated in five inter-rater reliability sessions at four hospitals within our system, plus one hospital within the region from a different health care system to increase sample diversity. Fifty different vignettes from actual chaplaincy encounters with an associated correct response were used during each session. Fifteen practice vignettes were used to familiarize participants with intended effects, methods and interventions used to describe why and how a chaplain performed an activity. Thirty-five different vignettes were used for the inter-rater reliability assessment.

Upon completion of the data gathering and analysis, an inter-rater reliability of 0.903 was achieved based on an inter-rater reliability testing process. This was achieved without the elimination of any participant responses or testing questions. We note that there was one participant who scored 66%, four participants who scored 97% and two questions had less than a 50% correct response rate.

Table 2: Concept mapping results

Top 10 frequency rated items	Frequency rating	Top 10 importance rated items	Importance rating
Active listening	5	Active listening	5
Provide a pastoral presence	5	Demonstrate caring and concern	4.9

cont.

Top 10 frequency rated items	Frequency rating	Top 10 importance rated items	Importance rating
Demonstrate caring and concern	4.9	Provide a pastoral presence	4.8
Preserve dignity and respect	4.9	Preserve dignity and respect	4.8
Remain open to patient's beliefs	4.9	Collaborate with care team member	4.8
Collaborate with care team member	4.8	Build rapport and connectedness	4.8
Demonstrate acceptance	4.8	Establish a relationship of care and support	4.8
Build rapport and connectedness	4.8	Demonstrate acceptance	4.7
Provide emotional support	4.8	Provide emotional support	4.7
Establish a relationship of care and support	4.8	Provide support	4.7

Discussion

Taxonomy description

Following the completion of all the generation, evaluation, and validation steps, the resulting taxonomy consisted of 100 items, presented in Table 3. The resulting inventory is practical, robust, and yet economical. While additional efforts are required to address remaining gaps and limitations, this taxonomy of chaplaincy activities provides a strong foundation for the sorely needed normative inventory of chaplaincy activities and a starting place for a standardized chaplaincy language.

The taxonomy

As the taxonomy emerged, we tried out a variety of patterns of how to group and assemble items to represent spiritual care interactions. A pattern that emerged was one in which items can be assembled to represent a plan of progression, including specific actions and the effects of those actions. The taxonomy items can be grouped and associated together in nearly infinite combinations to develop a grouping we have come to call a "pathway;" which is the assemblage of an intended Effect—Method—Intervention. A pathway or pathways make up a Spiritual Care Plan which is developed in response to the identified spiritual care needs surfaced in a Spiritual Assessment. A variety of methods of Spiritual Assessment are current,[14] which were out of the scope of our study. Spiritual Care Plans

can be comprised of many different combinations ranging from a s
intervention with numerous intended effects to numerous interven
with a single intended effect. Additionally, Intended Effect, Methods, and
Interventions are provisional categories, and a case could be made for
grouping the items into two categories such as Actions and Outcomes or
Means and Ends.

Chaplains in our organization have found it more natural to assemble
items and create pathways than to think about individual items in isolation.
Chaplains in our organization have discussed assembling care plans of
intended effects, methods, and interventions to match the spiritual care
needs of particular patient populations. Some of these pathways common
to palliative care of interest to readers of this journal include:

- Aligning care plan with patient's values—Ask guided questions about cultural and religious values—Explore cultural values.

- Preserve dignity and respect—Communicate patient's needs/concerns to others—Collaborate with care team member.

- Demonstrate caring and concern—Provide compassionate touch—Offer emotional support.

- Faith affirmation—Perform a religious rite or ritual—Assist with spiritual/religious practices.

- Meaning making—Invite someone to reminisce—Encourage self-reflection.

- Establish rapport and connectedness—Provide hospitality—Offer support.

- Sense of peace—Pray for healing—Exploring hope.

The taxonomy and palliative care

Previous studies in spirituality and palliative care have foreshadowed many of the themes that emerged in the intended effects list of the chaplaincy taxonomy. The item "Preserve dignity and respect" mirrors the important work on Dignity Therapy by Chochinov.[15] The item "Align care plan with patient's values" mirrors a recent study showing connection between chaplains and hospice and palliative care use.[16] The emphasis on relationship; such as "Lessen someone's feelings of isolation," "Build rapport and connectedness," and "Mending broken relationships" is important.[17] The multidimensional elements uplifted in the Special Report—Improving the Quality of Spiritual Care as a

Dimension of Palliative Care: The Report of the Consensus Conference,[18] which was a contributing inventory in the literature review for the chaplaincy taxonomy, are also well represented by the items that emerged. The taxonomy then is a recognizable inventory of chaplaincy activities known among palliative care teams.

The taxonomy could be used in a number of ways to enhance interdisciplinary team understanding of chaplaincy work. The taxonomy could form the basis of a clinical documentation set to standardize the descriptions chaplains share about their Spiritual Care Plan.

Table 3: The chaplaincy taxonomy

Intended effects	Methods	Interventions	
Aligning care plan with patient's values	Accompany someone in their spiritual/religious practice outside your faith tradition	Acknowledge current situation	Facilitate closure
Build relationship of care and support	Assist with finding purpose	Acknowledge response to difficult experience	Facilitate communication
Convey a calming presence	Assist with spiritual/religious practices	Active listening	Facilitate communication between patient and/or family member and care team
De-escalate emotionally charged situations	Collaborate with care team member	Ask guided questions	Facilitate communication between patient/family member(s)
Demonstrate caring and concern	Demonstrate acceptance	Ask guided questions about cultural and religious values	Facilitate decision making
Establish rapport and connectedness	Educate care team about cultural and religious values	Ask guided questions about faith	Facilitate grief recovery groups
Faith affirmation	Encourage end of life review	Ask guided questions about purpose	Facilitate life review
Helping someone feel comforted	Encourage self care	Ask guided questions about the nature and presence of God	Facilitate preparing for end of life
Journeying with someone in the grief process	Encourage self reflection	Ask questions to bring forth feelings	Facilitate spirituality groups

Lessen anxiety	Encourage sharing of feelings	Assist patient with documenting choices	Facilitate understanding of limitations
Lessen someone's feelings of isolation	Encourage someone to recognize their strengths	Assist patient with documenting values	Identify supportive relationship(s)
Meaning-Making	Encourage story-telling	Assist someone with Advance Directives	Incorporate cultural and religious needs in plan of care
Mending broken relationships	Encouraging spiritual/religious practices	Assist with determining decision maker	Invite someone to reminisce
Preserve dignity and respect	Explore cultural values	Assist with identifying strengths	Perform a blessing
Promote a sense of peace	Explore ethical dilemmas	Bless religious item(s)	Perform a religious rite or ritual
	Explore faith and values	Blessing for care team member(s)	Pray
	Explore nature of God	Communicate patient's needs/concerns to others	Prayer for healing
	Explore presence of God	Conduct a memorial service	Provide a religious item(s)
	Explore quality of life	Conduct a religious service	Provide access to a quiet place
	Explore spiritual/religious beliefs	Connect someone with their faith community/clergy	Provide compassionate touch
	Explore values conflict	Crisis intervention	Provide Grief Processing Session
	Exploring hope	Discuss concerns	Provide grief resources
	Offer emotional support	Discuss coping mechanism with someone	Provide hospitality

cont.

Intended effects	Methods	Interventions	
	Offer spiritual/ religious support	Discuss frustrations with someone	Provide religious music
	Offer support	Discuss plan of care	Provide sacred reading(s)
	Setting boundaries	Discuss spirituality/ religion with someone	Provide spiritual/ religious resources
		Ethical consultation	Respond as chaplain to a defined crisis event
		Explain chaplain role	Share words of hope and inspiration
		Facilitate advance care planning	Share written prayer
			Silent prayer

Further resources and structuring of the taxonomy

We have completed a User's Guide to the Taxonomy[19] that will assist chaplains and other palliative care members in using the taxonomy more reliably and consistently. The User's Guide includes definitions of the specific taxonomy intended effects, methods, and interventions. The User's Guide includes both the alphabetical listing of the taxonomy items found in Table 3 of this piece and another listing of the taxonomy items grouped into categories of similarity to assist a user in selecting items. For example, categories such as "Grief," "Relationships" and "Spiritual/ Religious Practice" group together items that pertain to each other on these themes.

Limitations

While the taxonomy project involved chaplains from outside our health care system and outside the Chicagoland area, the majority of chaplains were from our system and area. Some questions of generalizability are raised by this fact. Further generalizability questions arise in that the taxonomy was developed mostly in a specific clinical context, namely ICU and palliative care. Inevitably there are gaps concerning interventions, methods, and intended effects perhaps unique to other contexts. For example, there may be items particular to pediatric contexts that are missing from this initial taxonomy. These generalizability concerns may have been addressed by the two steps, Focus Groups and Concept Mapping which included chaplains from other practice settings. Continued practice and use of the taxonomy in diverse geographic and organizational contexts can address these issues and may identify additional improvements to the taxonomy.

Some apparent redundancies and contradictions have survived the taxonomy formation process. For example, one intervention, "Ask guided questions about the nature and presence of God," might be paired with two different methods, "Explore presence of God" and "Explore nature of God." Either these two methods should be merged, or if it were judged that the two concepts are very distinct, then "Ask guided questions about the nature and presence of God" should be split into two different interventions. As the taxonomy is used, questions such as this should be re-evaluated and, if need be, the taxonomy should be updated.

Conclusion

The adoption of a normative language among chaplains working on palliative care teams would be a welcome development in helping interdisciplinary teams better describe chaplaincy actions and goals. This taxonomy provides a firm foundation upon which such a normative language could be built. Further practice of this inventory by chaplains working on palliative care teams would continue to identify gaps and eliminate redundancy and refine and improve the inventory.

We propose testing this taxonomy in practice with all members of the palliative care team in order to facilitate communication and assessing outcomes. We encourage chaplains and other members of the palliative care team to identify redundancies and gaps and to further enrich the taxonomy for future use.

Abbreviations

BCC: Board Certified Chaplain; BCC–E: Board Certified Chaplain-Eligible; DRG: Diagnosis Related Group; ICC: Intra-Class Correlation; ICU: Intensive Care Unit; KII: Key Informant Interviews.

Competing interests
The authors declare that they have no competing interests.

Authors' contributions
KM, MJDB, DV, and WTS contributed to project conception and design, project management, data acquisition, data analysis and manuscript authoring. JDG contributed to project conception and design and data analysis. ALHP, CS, and BV contributed to project conceptions and design, data acquisition, and data analysis. All authors read and approved the final manuscript.

Acknowledgements
This project and the preparation of this article were funded by a generous grant from the New York based Health Care Chaplaincy provided by the John Templeton Foundation. In addition to our generous grantors the authors gratefully acknowledge the assistance of Barbara E. Giloth, DrPH for her invaluable guidance during every step of this project and other members of the project's Research Council: Rev. Bonnie Condon, MA, MTS, Rev. David McCurdy, DMin, BCC, Sr. Patricia Murphy, PhD, BCC, and Michael Ries, MD, MBA, FCCM, FCCP, FACP. We thank Kathy Dobbs for her diligent service and Rev. Kathie Bender Schwich, MDiv for her support and encouragement.

Finally, we dedicate this paper to our late colleague, The Rev. Brenda S. Jackson, MDiv, BCC whose wit and wisdom inspired many, and by her insights left a personal mark on the taxonomy.

Received: 2 June 2014
Accepted: 4 March 2015
Published online: 15 April 2015

References
1. Fitchett G. Screening for Spiritual Risk. Chaplaincy Today. 1999;15(1):2–12.
2. Handzo G, Flannelly KJ, Murphy KM, Mauman JP, Oettenger, M, et al. What do chaplains really do? II. Interventions in the New York chaplaincy study. J Health Care Chaplain. 2008;14(1):39–56.
3. Hummel L, Galek K, Murphy KM, Tannenbaum HP, Flannelly KJ, Goodell, E. Defining spiritual care: an exploratory study. J Health Care Chaplain. 2008;15:40–51.
4. Puchalski C, Ferrell B, Virani R, Otis-Green S, Baird P, Bull J, et al. Special report – improving the quality of spiritual care as a dimension of palliative care: the report of the consensus conference. J Palliat Med. 2009;12(10):885–904.

5. Aldridge A, Fraser DJ, Morrison K. What do people talk to chaplains about? Scottish Journal of Healthcare Chaplaincy. 2009;12(2):3–9.
6. Lyndes KA, Fitchett G, Berlinger N, Cadge W, Misasi J, Flanagan E. A survey of chaplains' roles in pediatric palliative care: integral members of the team. J Health Care Chaplain. 2012; 18(1–2):74–93.
7. Jankowski K, Handzo G, Flannelly K. Testing the efficacy of chaplaincy care. J Health Care Chaplain. 2011; 17(3–4):100–25.
8. USAID Center for Development Information and Evaluation, Cfr. Performance Monitoring and Evaluation TIPS: Conducting key information interviews. Report No. 2. PN ABS 541.
9. Csikszentmihalyi M, Larson R. Validity and reliability of the Experience-Sampling Method. J Nervous and Mental Disease. 1987;175(9):526–536.
10. Larson R, Csikszentmihalyi M. The Experience Sampling Method. New Directions for Methodology of Social and Behavioral Science. 1983;15:41–56.
11. Hektner JM, Schmidt JA, Csikszentmihalyi M. Experience Sampling Method: Measuring the quality of everyday life. Thousand Oaks, CA: Sage; 2006.
12. Trochim W. Pattern matching, validity and conceptualization in program evaluation. Eval Rev. 1985;9(5):575–604.
13. Shrout PE and Fleiss JL. Intraclass Correlation: Uses in assessing rater reliability. Psychol Bull. 1979;86(2):420–428.
14. Massey K, Fitchett G, Roberts P. Assessment and diagnosis in spiritual care. In: Mauk KL, Shmidt NK, editors. *Spiritual care in nursing practice.* Philadelphia, PA: Lippincott, Williams and Wilkins; 2004. pp.209–242.
15. Chochinov HM, Hack T, Hassard T, Kristjanson LJ, McClement S, Harlos M. Dignity Therapy: A Novel Psychotherapeutic Intervention for Patients Near the End of Life. J Clin Oncol. 2005; 23(24):5520–25.
16. Flannelly KJ, Emanuel LL, Handzo GF, Galek K, Silton NR, Carlson M. A national study of chaplaincy services and end-of-life outcomes. BMC Palliat Care. 2012;11:10.
17. Edwards A, Pang N, Shiu V, Chan C. The understanding of spirituality and the potential role of spiritual care in end-of-life and palliative care: a meta-study of qualitative research. Palliat Medicine. 2010;24(8):753–70.
18. Puchalski C. ibid p.894.
19. Massey K and Barnes M. The Advocate Health Care Chaplain Taxonomy. Advocate Health Care, March 2014, www.advocatehealth.com/chaplaincyresearch.

ARTICLE 4

Communicating Chaplains' Care: Narrative Documentation in a Neuroscience–Spine Intensive Care Unit

Rebecca Johnson, Buehler Center on Aging, Health & Society, Northwestern University, Chicago, Illinois, USA

M. Jeanne Wirpsa, Northwestern Memorial Hospital, Chicago, Illinois, USA

Lara Boyken, Buehler Center on Aging, Health & Society, Northwestern University, Chicago, Illinois, USA

Matthew Sakumoto, Northwestern University Feinberg School of Medicine, Chicago, Illinois, USA

George Handzo, HealthCare Chaplaincy Network, New York, New York, USA

Abel Kho, Northwestern University Feinberg School of Medicine, Chicago, Illinois, USA

Linda Emanuel, Buehler Center on Aging, Health & Society, Northwestern University, Chicago, Illinois, USA

Address correspondence to Rebecca Johnson, Buehler Center on Aging, Health & Society, Northwestern University, 750 N Lake Shore Drive Suite 601, Chicago, IL 60611, USA. E-mail: Rebecca.Johnson@northwestern.edu

Copyright © 2016 Taylor & Francis Group, LLC

ISSN: 0885-4726 print/1528-6916 online

DOI: 10.1080/08854726.2016.1154717

Abstract

Chaplaincy care is different for every patient; a growing challenge is to ensure that electronic health records function to support personalized care. While ICU healthcare teams have advanced clinical practice guidelines to identify and integrate relevant aspects of the patient's story into whole person care, recommendations for documentation are rare. This qualitative study of over 400 free-text EHR notes offers unique insight into current use of free-text documentation in ICUs by six chaplains integrated into the healthcare team. Our research provides insight

---

Johnson, R.M., Wirpsa, M.J., Boyken, L., Sakumoto, M., Handzo, G., Kho, A., and Emanuel, L. (2016) "Communicating chaplains' care: narrative documentation in a neuroscience-spine intensive care unit." *Journal of Health Care Chaplaincy*, 22, 4, 133–150.

into the phenomena chaplains record in the electronic record. Content analysis shows recurrent report of patient and family practices, beliefs, coping mechanisms, concerns, emotional resources and needs, family and faith support, medical decision making and medical communications. These findings are important for healthcare team discussions of factors deemed essential to whole person care in ICUs, and, by extension have the potential to support the development of EHR designs that aim to advance personalized care.

Key words: chaplaincy care, documentation, electronic health record, spiritual care, team communication

Introduction

A patient's medical record is usually a compilation of entries from multiple care providers. In hospitals where healthcare chaplaincy is an established service, the chaplain aspires to document information relevant to a patient's overall care. While general standards of practice exist, specific clinical practice guidelines on the function of spiritual care documentation are evolving. The Intensive Care Unit (ICU) is an exception to this rule, with clinical practice guidelines for patient-centered care recommending that the "*spiritual needs of the patient are assessed by the health-care team, and findings that affect health and healing incorporated into the plan of care*" (Davidson et al., 2007). Such an assessment would be expected to include data about explicit religious beliefs and practices, the role played by spirituality and religion in coping with illness, and spiritual and existential suffering caused by illness, accident, or the anticipated death of a loved one (Puchalski, 2010; World Health Organization, 2015). Further, the inclusion of spiritual needs of both patient and family is considered essential to whole person care (Davidson et al., 2007) and, moreover, is increasingly recognized as a key factor impacting ICU length of stay, aggressive/life-prolonging care, and patient/family satisfaction (Balboni et al., 2010; Osborn et al., 2012). How chaplains in the ICU setting are documenting these needs and what is being documented is insufficiently studied.

To date, research on chaplain free-text documentation is limited. A survey of professional medical chaplains in major medical centers showed chaplain access and note entry into the electronic health records (EHR) to be standard practice (Goldstein, Marin, & Umpierre, 2011). Another similar survey observes that chaplains are variably integrated into the larger clinical team (Cadge, Calle, & Dillinger, 2011). However, despite growing consensus on items required for statistical reliability (Borneman, Ferrell, & Puchalski, 2010; Derrickson, 1995; Fitchett, 1993; VandeCreek

& Lucas, 2014), little data exists on what is being recorded in free-text. This study adds to existing data by exploring the free-text records of a pastoral consult template collated as part of the electronic health record by chaplains integrated into a healthcare team.

The study uses inductive content analysis (Elo & Kyngas, 2008; Hsieh & Shannon, 2005); this is a methodology effectively implemented in research areas such as healthcare communication, decision-making, and whole person care (Auton et al., 2015; Bishop & Cregan, 2015; Graneheim & Lundman, 2004; Heid, Zarit, & Van Haitsma, 2016; Roscigno et al., 2012). We chose to sample over 400 free-text notes recorded in an 18-month period by six chaplains well integrated in an ICU care team, because teams in these settings are increasingly looking at ways to identify and integrate relevant aspects of the patient's story into whole-person care (Davidson et al., 2007).

Charting for spiritual need and care in an acute care hospital context

Northwestern Memorial Hospital (NMH) is a 900+ bed tertiary care academic medical center in downtown Chicago, Illinois. The Pastoral Services and Education Department (PSE) consists of two Association for Clinical Pastoral Education (ACPE) supervisors, three board certified staff chaplains, five residents, four associate (volunteer, professionally trained) chaplains, a part-time Catholic priest, and chaplain interns, as well as contract chaplains who work on a periodic basis. Chaplains are assigned primarily to areas of high acuity, including the Emergency Department, and the Departments of Palliative Care, Psychiatry, Cardiac Care, Transplant, Oncology, Perinatal Loss, Neonatal Intensive Care, Medical Intensive Care and the Neuroscience-spine Intensive Care. Chaplains are paged to all Level One traumas, cardiac arrests, and deaths. PSE also oversees a team of qualified volunteers (Advance Directive Experts) who have been trained to assist patients in advance care planning. All chaplains document in the EHR, and are also responsible for documenting the work of Advance Directive Experts. The EHR is used to record, in closed-ended fields, source of referral, religious affiliation, level of importance and faith community, spiritual resources, practices, concerns, and the plan of care. Consults for chaplain services may be generated through this record, as well as through direct communication, crisis pages, and as a result of interdisciplinary care team meetings.

The EHR was first implemented at NMH in 2002. In 2003, chaplains designed their own structured template for the EHR; an unstructured component was added to the template in 2004. The free-text pastoral care narrative note supplemented what had been a design solely composed of checkboxes.

The structured template had proved an insufficient tool to document the complexity of patient/family spiritual issues or capture important patient and family values, cultural context, or history that impact medical decision making and care. As narrative methods are central to chaplaincy identity and practice, members of the department argued that narrative is a more appropriate means to communicate their contribution to the care of patients and, indirectly, promote the "personhood" of the patient (Charon, 2006; Frank, 1995; Risk, 2013).

Chaplains at NMH receive an orientation in accessing the EHR, using the pastoral care template, and writing a free-text narrative note. A five-part model for narrative charting is taught in keeping with best practices in professional chaplaincy: Reason for Referral, Comprehensive Spiritual Assessment, Care Provided, Outcome, and Plan of Care, with examples provided for each of these categories (Peery & Roberts, 2012). These guidelines also include recommendations for the use of terms that will be accessible to non-chaplains, how to address issues of clergy confidentiality, and how to document in specific cases of threatened homicide or suicide, conflict within a family, or conflict between patient/family and staff. No standardized format or uniform style is required (Association of Professional Chaplains, 2010).

Within NMH, the 23-bed Neuroscience-spine Intensive Care Unit (NSICU) receives admissions for patients with stroke, head trauma, and peri-operative neurosurgical care. Chaplaincy care is fully integrated into this intensive care setting. Chaplains attend daily interdisciplinary rounds and family meetings when they occur, receive referrals through the EHR and in direct consultation with other members of the healthcare team, provide hands-on education during the course of work to staff about spiritual/religious issues specific to this patient population, and facilitate debriefings with staff for cases that cause moral or emotional stress. Furthermore, procedures for withdrawal of life support specify the presence of a chaplain. On-call resident or intern chaplains provide overnight and weekend crisis coverage. One would expect this degree of integration to be reflected in chaplains' documentation practices in the EHR, if this record serves to support patient-centered care by the interdisciplinary team.

Methods

Data was taken from patient records (n = 426) over an eighteen month period. The free-text components of the Power Chart (Cerner) EHR template were extracted from Northwestern's Enterprise Data Warehouse (EDW). To avoid over-sampling for individual chaplain notes, analysis was further restricted to the last pastoral care note for each unique patient. Analysis excluded narrative notes of interns and Catholic priests as these chaplains are not fully integrated into the NISCU team and/or are contacted for specific denominationally-based ritual care. Following initial coding and word frequency searches to identify popular nouns and verbs, two detailed analyses were conducted on the sets of free-text notes. The first was thematic coding for spiritual care evident in the free-text notes. The second was axial coding for evidence of professional practice. Guided by healthcare chaplaincy research and the experience of the chaplain on the coding team, the research team coded for professional practice evidence as assessment, intervention or outcome (Roberts, 2012). Both coding processes were completed by a small research group of one chaplain with a background in anthropology and qualitative research methodology, a fifth-year medical student trained in informatics, and a PhD-level qualitative researcher with NVivo training. Initial, thematic, and axial coding was shared by telephone conference call or in person with a multidisciplinary research team to validate item assignment and domain definitions (Davidson et al., 2007; Puchalski, Vitillo, Hull, & Reller, 2014; World Health Organization, 2015). This team included two healthcare chaplains and one MD with track records in research.

To achieve inter-rater reliability, members of the small research group read the collated sets of free-text notes several times, marking up possible spiritual care categories, subcategories, codes and subcodes. One researcher used NVivo 10 (Bazeley & Jackson, 2013) to code subsets of documented notes while two other members of the team coded the same subsets by hand. All stages of the coding process were shared with the full research team by weekly conference call and discrepancies were discussed and resolved by consultation with the wider team. Once themes and categories had been agreed, the experienced qualitative health researcher completed coding in NVivo 10 using an agreed upon coding book that can be obtained from the first author at Rebecca.Johnson@northwestern.edu. An additional column "Pastoral Consult Template categories" was added to the code book in an effort to map the quantitative components of the pastoral consult to the free-text core themes. However, the group decided not to pursue this associative line of enquiry given recent evidence that placement of topics on the pastoral care template impacted chaplain use of the quantitative categories. Chaplains were more likely to complete items grouped at the top of the template (Sakumoto et al., 2015).

Table 1 provides a summary of the eight themes most frequently coded in the ICU free-text data grouped by domain categories determined by the research team. Final domain and thematic terms owe provenance to those used to guide practice in ICU guidelines (Bosslet et al., 2015; Curtis & White, 2008; Osborn et al., 2012) and emergent practice norms for healthcare chaplaincy. Our decision to distinguish non-spiritually sourced emotional resources and needs from spiritually prompted ones was in part due to cross referencing whole patient care guidelines and frameworks which factor out these domains. Free-text notes included recurrent reports of patients' spiritual and religious practices and beliefs; coping mechanisms, concerns, family and faith community support systems; patient and family narratives; reports of medical decision making and medical communication. Additional axial coding was undertaken by the chaplain member of the coding team who does not routinely see patients in the ICU but teaches narrative record. Coding for three core professional practices—chaplaincy assessment, intervention and outcome record—showed assessment to be the most prevalent identifiable practice. In what follows, we describe the main findings of our initial and thematic coding before considering the three professional practice categories.

Table 1: Domain definitions with examples grouped by chaplaincy process categories

Domain	Theme	Chaplaincy process categories		
		Assessment	Intervention	Outcome
Spiritual/ religious	Practices & beliefs	Ritual, prayer, scripture, meditation	Facilitate ritual, prayer	Faith sustained
		Faith tradition and identity, specific beliefs about illness and healing, cultural taboos, dietary restrictions	Provide information regarding pastoral resources	Express trust that beliefs known and respected
	Coping mechanisms	Hope, acceptance of illness, trust in God, peace, healing, meaning, purpose, practices that sustain stability in face of uncertainty	Validate faith as resource for coping Encourage hope, trust, sense of value/dignity	Expresses gratitude, hope Identified spiritual coping strategies

cont.

Domain	Theme	Chaplaincy process categories		
		Assessment	Intervention	Outcome
Spiritual/ religious cont.	Concerns	Fear, loss of control, despair, suffering, spiritual distress, forgiveness, doubt, abandonment by God or faith community	Normalize spiritual doubt, fear Encourage lamentation, expression of anger	Still questioning role of divine in illness Finds hope, strength
Emotional	Emotional resources and needs	General coping, anxiety, grief, happiness, depression, weariness, distrust	Assist in venting, expressing feelings Offer bereavement and grief counseling	Observed to be less anxious Adopting self-care activities
Support systems	Family/Faith community	Clergy, family, friends, financial	Contact faith community, family	Identifies value of support
	Patient/Family story	Biographical information, history of illness and family loss	Identify factors that impact culturally appropriate care	Narrates important elements of identity and story
Decision making	Medical decision making	Capacity, decision makers, treatment preferences, conflict in family about goals of care	Facilitate conversation about decision maker Clarify values that impact decision making	Advance directives completed Values/beliefs integrated into goals of care
	Medical communication	Communication issues (system and interpersonal)	Inform patient/ family about palliative care	Possess needed knowledge, relationships

Results

We describe what we found of the frequently coded items in Table 1. Idiosyncratic features unique to individual chaplains and therefore not generalizable included self-reporting time spent with a patient and specific records of context, for example what the patient was watching on TV at the time of the visit, were excluded.

Spiritual practices and beliefs

All six chaplains used their notes to directly connect spiritual practices and services to medical goals of care for all patients. Examples of spiritual care records that directly relate to goals of care include the need for Catholic last rites before a family will proceed with the withdrawal of life support, assessment for end-of-life rituals and beliefs that impact the disposition of body for a dying Muslim patient, and documentation of a belief in miraculous healing and divine intervention. Chaplains' notes are most authoritative and clear when offering this specialized and immediately relevant knowledge to the healthcare team.

Coping mechanisms

Narrative notes in this data set were also rich in descriptions of patient and family spiritual coping mechanisms. Examples include records of personal struggle and reflection on divine presence: *"Father acknowledges a distant relationship to God, struggling to find meaning in the patient's illness, and suffering of her young children. He is disturbed by lack of divine intervention in this world and the man's inhumanity to man."* All six chaplains offer substantive documentation on how patients and families deploy spiritual and religious resources to cope with illness, injury, and treatment, for example, *"Her connection to her church and Catholic faith has been helping her cope."* They also recorded multiple examples of the impact illness, injury, and treatment can have on the faith of the patient or family, for example: *"Patient expresses feeling of 'terror,' fearful of not being able to walk. Feelings of guilt: being punished b/c did not listen to his parents who were Holocaust survivors."*

Spiritual concerns

In their documentation of more general spiritual or existential concerns, such as feelings of uncertainty, powerlessness, and hope or hopelessness, chaplaincy report was more variable and less specific. A word frequency query across all notes showed that hopefulness is an adjective frequently deployed by chaplains to key into a factor that matters to a patient. The following three patient notes are illustrative of clinically-sourced hope, colloquially-sourced hope, and spiritually-sourced hope: *"Couple thanked chaplain for attempt, expressed feeling more hopeful today after receiving encouraging news from attending physician;" "Patient's father said family is still doing well, hopeful that mother will be visiting tomorrow;"* and *"Patient and family coping well, using faith as a source of strength and hope."* Chaplains' ability to identify what matters to patients and to record this may be particularly valuable in settings such as NISCU, where heightened emotional states are likely to be prevalent and identifying what matters most crucial to patient-centered care.

Emotional resources and needs

The main emotional states recorded by chaplains are anxiety, feeling emotional, coping, struggling [with emotion], grieving/grief/tearfulness/sadness, denial, upset, feeling overwhelmed, distress, and anger. Analysis suggests that these emotions are prompted by a range of factors, including family, faith, a medical event, medical communication, or patient responsiveness, and that it can be difficult to pinpoint one particular source. In this example, the chaplain uses the narrative note to document a patient's anxiety about recovery and goals of care beyond the hospital:

> *Patient placed on consult list by nurse; chaplain followed up with patient and spouse. Patient, accompanied by spouse, expressed a mixture of gratitude and anxiety. Patient grateful for successful surgery, but remains anxious about recovery and managing when she gets home. Patient also especially grateful for the ways spouse has been supporting her and walking with her. Patient was able to identify the ways she is coping and taking things one step at a time.*

In an effort to source the factors causing the anxiety rather than to diagnose the condition, anxiety is being reported in a colloquial way here, rather than as a clinical term such as that informing the Hospital Anxiety Scale or other such measurements (Bjelland, Dahl, Haug, & Neckelmann, 2002).

Medical decision making and communication

Chaplaincy free-text report of decision making included chaplain assessment of patient/family wishes, treatment preferences, impact of religious beliefs on end-of-life decisions, family conflict around goals of care, communication with the medical team, and most prevalently, whether the patient possessed the relevant advance directives documentation.

There were two distinct uses of the narrative note by chaplains for communicating decision making. The first was the use of the note to indicate to other members of the healthcare team whether or not the patient/family has received requested information about advance directives, to record the completion of this documentation, and to thank other members of the team for updating and keeping this note live. It is the one example we found where chaplains may direct their note to a member of the team, suggesting a shared understanding and clarity about their role and what needs to be communicated in these circumstances. A typical note of this type is: "*Chaplain consulted 2/2 DNR order. Appreciate Dr. X's chart note indicating that patient's POA, confirmed DNR as being in accord with patient's wishes.*"

However, there was a second use of the narrative note in evidence within the domain of decision making. This was a verbatim report of the patient's wishes or a summary of patient values drawn from conversations with families. For example:

> X states: "we have done enough, we should stop this." Y states that patient would not want to be "like this," describes patient as very active and that X would want to be able to go out with friends and be independent even if she could not resume working. Y concerned that patient is not waking up.

In some instances, the beliefs or values named were explicitly religious; in many instances, as in those mentioned previously, the chaplain attended to the patient's story to "*lift up*" experiences, values, and character traits that might be considered relevant in deciding the direction of medical care.

Also, the narrative notes the chaplain reported patient responsiveness. Common phrases in the notes include "*patient alert*," "*aphasic*," or "*patient non-responsive*." Occasionally the note implies an association between the observation of patient responsiveness and capacity for decision making; for instance, "*patient alert and oriented, able to say yes and no, otherwise aphasic. Patient does not appear to be able to name a POA at the present time.*" These examples suggest that a function of chaplains in the domain of decision making may be assessing for capacity to make decisions, but the purpose of the communication and for whom it is intended was unclear.

Family/Faith support systems

The fourth domain covered by the unstructured narrative note is chaplain documentation of family and faith-based support systems. This domain includes chaplains' assessment of the presence or absence of family, friends and community support, the continuation of spiritual/religious practices, and the use of prayer or referral to priests or other clergy for religious reasons (for example, "*family requested to have priest say a blessing and prayer for patient*"). Narrative notation of family and faith support also frequently highlighted emotional, psychological, and interpersonal characteristics of the patient/family, providing insight into how well the family and patient are dealing with the medical crisis, as illustrated here:

> *Chaplain followed up with patient's spouse. She is feeling positive about how patient's procedure went today, though still disappointed at the slow pace of progress. Patient and spouse feel support from faith community and family; Spouse still hopes for dx soon to hospital closer to their home. Patient spouse struggling with needing so much help from family members, but ready to receive what help they can offer. Chaplain affirmed spouses coping and promised further prayer in the hopes of patient's progression toward dx. Spouse thanked chaplain for support and encouragement, noted that chaplain had helped her focus on present and near future "without getting too far ahead of myself."*

More particularly, narrative notes such as this one cast light on the patient/family and faith community's active engagement. Chaplains record factors that impact the patient and family personally.

Patient/Family story

Chaplains in our study often elected to record biographical detail to provide context, what coders called *"the patient story."* These included references to the patient's character, the meaning of illness and suffering to the patient/family, as well as the documentation of anecdotes and significant life events. In ways idiosyncratic to each chaplain, details about the patient and family members' ages, occupations, roles in the family, history of health and illness, as well as culturally-specific behaviors or beliefs, were woven into the narrative documentation.

Core professional practices

Three core professional areas related to practice were evident from our axial coding of content: descriptive assessments, records of active behaviors (interventions), and records of outcomes resulting from care provided. Findings are summarized in the following section.

Assessment

For the chaplain, the purpose of a spiritual assessment, in contrast to a screening, is to provide an overview of the whole patient within a care setting. As stated in the Standards of Practice for Professional Chaplains in Acute Care settings, assessment is a core part of chaplaincy practice: *"Assessment is a fundamental process of chaplaincy practice. Provision of effective care requires that chaplains assess and reassess patient needs and modify plans of care accordingly"* (Association of Professional Chaplains, 2010). Although our notes were unstructured and stylistically variable, entries coded as assessments were characteristically descriptive; for example: *"Daughter struggling with timing of dying process, as she does not want to see her mother suffer any more and it is difficult to sit by and not be able to do anything;"* and *"Patient states he does not have enough 'spirituality' to cope with surgery and possibility of not walking since he is a 'physical' person. Tearful during visit."* Chaplains also included in their assessments details of the patient's physical state and prognosis, spiritual resources and needs, cultural framework and practices, family reaction to illness, strategies for coping, and patient/family hopes and fears.

Intervention

Analysis of interventions recorded in the narrative notes showed congruence between verbs used by chaplains to record care provided (for example, affirmed, acknowledged, validated, normalized, identified, explored, clarified, encouraged, reassured, and provided) and those found in the examples cited in current literature on chaplain activities and interventions (Donovan, 2012; Massey et al., 2015). Notably, chaplains provided substantial detail and specificity about the care provided, generally avoiding phrases such as *"pastoral presence"* or *"spiritual care provided"* whose meaning is less transparent.

Records of interventions focusing on patient and family spiritual/religious needs and resources far exceeded those to address emotional needs, decision making issues or support systems. The type of interventions recorded also showed congruence between this study and others in terms of the concrete interventions made, with the provision of prayer, scripture, blessings, and spiritual/religious resources being the items most frequently recorded (Goldstein, 2012; Idler, Binney, Grant, Perkins, & Quest, 2015; Massey et al., 2015; Roberts, 2012).

Coders also found some, albeit limited, evidence of chaplains intentionally linking the intervention or care provided directly to a hoped for or achieved outcome: *"Mrs. L seemed more peaceful and quiet after prayer."*

Outcomes

Records of outcomes were the most sparsely found in the free notes. Coders observed three types of outcome records. First, they noted those that used the normative medical usage of the term patient-centered outcomes. Within this literature, a patient-reported outcome is *"any report of the status of a patient's health condition that comes directly from the patient, without interpretation of the patient's response by a clinician or anyone else"*

(Snowden, Telfer, Kelly, Burniss, & Mowat, 2013). The outcome can be measured in absolute terms (e.g., severity of a symptom, sign, or state of a disease) or as a change from a previous measure (Food and Drug Administration, 2009). The following are illustrative of the kinds of patient-reported outcomes that appeared in our data set: "*Patient reported feeling a great sense of relief and increased peace as a result of this intervention today;*" "*Ms. B noted that prayer and chaplain visit helps her feel relaxed and hopeful;*" and "*Mrs. H noted that chaplain had helped her focus on present and near future 'without getting too far ahead of myself.'*"

Second, the narrative notes contained references to what chaplains observed or believed was the impact of their care on the patient's emotional and spiritual condition. This alternative approach to outcomes is grounded in the seminal work of VandeCreek and Lucas (2014). Here, chaplaincy care aligns itself with evidence-based medicine while also acknowledging the therapeutic and interpretive role of the chaplain. As VandeCreek and Lucas note:

> *Outcomes are simply the observable results of our care... [outcome-oriented care] is concerned with the objective. Receiving the patient's narrative thread—seeing, hearing, listening are examples of the empathetic turn—the belief in chaplaincy terms that it is important to try to imagine what it's like to be in the patient's shoes... to gain an experiential understanding of what is behind the emotional response.*

The following examples demonstrate this interpretive role of the chaplain: "*Having the Sabbath candles on hand is very comforting and hopeful for patient;*" and "*Chaplain acknowledged conflict and affirmed Ms. X's sense of authority about her role in relation to husband. Ms. X seemed self-assured after conversation.*"

A third type of outcome found in these notes was the chaplain's observation of the emotional or spiritual processing that the patient or family were able to accomplish as a result of the chaplain's visit. Examples of this type of outcome in chaplain documentation included statements such as: "*Patient able to identify hoped for outcomes;*" "*Daughter is able to express her anger at 'being robbed' but also gratitude for the past 20 years;*" and "*Family verbally processed grief.*"

Finally, coders also observed that free-text notes of impact were often accompanied by patient and family expressions of gratitude to the chaplain; for example: "*Chaplain offered listening presence, encouragement and reassurance and prayer. Wife grateful and comforted.*" Expressions of thanks for the chaplain and/or visit were sometimes divorced from any record of a change in the patient's emotional or spiritual state, such as in this reference: "*Patient, father and stepmother thanked chaplain 'for listening to my story.*'" The outcome was not entirely clear: How was the family's well-being or coping impacted by the chaplain's act of listening?

Discussion

One of the limitations of our study—its necessary single site restriction—is also a strength. Focusing on a single site enabled us to cross-reference coding domain categories and items with evolving standards of ICU whole patient care as well as the evidence of professional practice of chaplains integrated into an ICU healthcare team. One reason for focusing on one unit of care is that the feasibility of comparing chaplaincy use of free-text notation recorded within EHRs across systems and care units remains a distant goal for the field of chaplaincy healthcare. Currently, there are no standardized forms or procedures. Some chaplaincy health teams use checkboxes only; others are strictly free-text users. Many are still in the process of determining best local practice. The feasibility of comparing experienced with less experienced chaplaincy documentation also remains to be determined. Our study contributes descriptive data to these long-term goals.

Our analysis of chaplain narrative notes supports the conclusion that a potentially important function of chaplains' free-text notes in an EHR is to document evidence of factors which matter to the person being cared for by the medical team and which fall beyond the scope of a generic quantitative spiritual assessment. This is a function for notation supported by proponents of narrative medicine (Charon, 2006; Frank, 1995), who argue that attention to the patient's story makes for better medical outcomes, lessens conflict between patients, families, and the medical team, and upholds or sustains patient dignity. Although short, our narrative notes were used to record more than visitation by the chaplain. This contrasts with Cadge's (2009) observation on the history of shared documentation and may represent an evolving practice in the field over the past few years or simply a site variation. Future research might usefully focus on the optimum length of a narrative note and whether free-text boxes deliver the right "contextual" evidence useful to healthcare team decision making. How free-text contributes meaningfully to communicating basic components of a spiritual assessment or plan in conjunction with quantitative assessment merits further investigation as well.

Our study's findings have a number of implications for the documentation and delivery of personalized care designed to deliver medical outcomes. The record of religious and spiritual factors impacting medical decision making, goals of care, and advance care planning in our study, for example, suggests that free-text notes may be the main avenue available to chaplains to elaborate on the significance of spiritual issues for care in the NISCU setting. This raises the question of what happens to those notes and how much weight they should be given in the final integrated plan. (In a study by Balboni et al. (2010), investigators examining goals of care conversations in the ICU found that religious and spiritual values were rarely integrated into the medical plan by physicians even when the patient or family indicated their high level of significance.) A secondary question is who is processing the information in the notes. When a chaplain records a family comment such as *"we should stop this"* how is that written notation acted upon, and by whom? Is it important to record the reasoning behind a patient's wishes as chaplains often do—and if so, for whom? Is a verbatim record or a record of documentation more or less effective in contributing to goals of personalized care? Which approach do other members of the team find most informative (Curtis & White, 2008)? If, as it appears to be the case in our analysis, chaplains are documenting patient responsiveness in part to assess patient ability to be involved in medical decision making, it would be important to clarify the role the chaplain plays in that process. Finally, would a shared goals-of-care or advanced care planning document better facilitate integration of patients' religious beliefs, values, and preferences into the overall care plan rather than the current discipline-specific model of most EHR templates?

Additional clinical implications of this study concern how chaplains can best communicate with medical colleagues. Within healthcare chaplaincy, there is currently no normative, standardized language for talking about or documenting outcomes, as the recent research in the field testifies (Cadge, 2009; Cadge et al., 2011; Handzo, Cobb, Holmes, Kelly, & Sinclair, 2014; Massey et al., 2015; Peery & Roberts, 2012) or for achieving inter-professional consensus on terms such as "hope," "anxiety," or "distress." Our study found that the term anxiety, for example, was used colloquially rather than in a strict clinical understanding of the term, such as that informing the Hospital Anxiety Scale or other such measurements accepted by the disciplines of psychology, psychiatry, and medicine (Bjelland et al., 2002; Herth, 1992). In a similar manner, the terms hope, hopeful, and hopefulness found in these narrative notes are examples of terms shared by chaplains, clinical health professionals, and the patient, all of which have their own discipline-specific meaning and research literature (Bay, Beckman, Trippi, Gunderman, & Terry, 2008; Gaeeni, Farahani, Mohammadi, & Seyedfatemi, 2014; Herth, 1992; Nolan, 2011; Olver, 2012; Piccinelli, Clerici, Veneroni, Ferrari, & Proserpio, 2015;

Rawdin, Evans, & Rabow, 2013). Chaplaincy usage of terms of hope and anxiety raise the question of whether a shared lexicography and shared conceptual application could improve inter-professional communication. Is there a role for an inter-professional consensus on such terms not only to facilitate communication between different members of the care team, but potentially to measure the impact of our care itself?

In conclusion, free-text notes capture evidence of factors that matter to patients and are recorded outside the scope of quantitative assessment. Although there is evidence of emergent professional practice across them, the notes are not standardized and are personal to each individual chaplain. While on the one hand this freelance practice delivers personalized records of critical factors impacting care, it also raises questions about the function of notes within a healthcare setting. As both chaplaincy documentation practice and the use of the EHR evolve, it will be important to establish best practices for healthcare chaplains at the same time as crafting emerging technology to support whole person, patient-centered care.

Acknowledgments

The authors wish to note that Abel Kho, MD and Linda Emanuel, MD, PhD share the designation of senior author.

Funding

The authors wish to thank the Smart Family Foundation for its support.

References

Association of Professional Chaplains. (2010). *Standards of practice for chaplains in acute care.* Retrieved from www.professionalchaplains.org/files/professional_standards/standards_of_practice/standards_practice_professional_ chaplains_acute_care.pdf

Auton, M. F., Patel, K., Carter, B., Hackett, M., Thornton, I., Lightbody, C. E.,...Watkins, C. L. (2015). Motivational interviewing post-stroke: An analysis of stroke survivors' concerns and adjustment. *Qualitative Health Research, 26*(2), 264–272. Advance online publication. doi: 10.1177/1049732315582197

Balboni, T. A., Paulk, M. E., Balboni, M. J., Phelps, A. C., Loggers, E. T., Wright, A. A.,... Prigerson, H. G. (2010). Provision of spiritual care to patients with advanced cancer: Associations with medical care and quality of life near death. *Journal of Clinical Oncology, 28*(3), 445–452. doi:10.1200/jco.2009.24.8005

Bay, P. S., Beckman, D., Trippi, J., Gunderman, R., & Terry, C. (2008). The effect of pastoral care services on anxiety, depression, hope, religious coping, and religious problem solving styles: A randomized controlled study. *Journal of Religion and Health, 47*(1), 57–69. doi:10.1007/s10943-007-9131-4

Bazeley, P., & Jackson, K. (2013). *Qualitative data analysis with NVivo*. Los Angeles: Sage Publications Limited.

Bishop, A. C., & Cregan, B. R. (2015). Patient safety culture: Finding meaning in patient experiences. *International Journal of Health Care Quality Assurance, 28*(6), 595–610. doi:10.1108/ijhcqa-03-2014-0029

Bjelland, I., Dahl, A. A., Haug, T. T., & Neckelmann, D. (2002). The validity of the hospital anxiety and depression scale. An updated literature review. *Journal of Psychosomatic Research, 52*(2), 69–77. doi:10.1016/s0022-3999(01) 00296-3

Borneman, T., Ferrell, B., & Puchalski, C. M. (2010). Evaluation of the FICA tool for spiritual assessment. *Journal of Pain and Symptom Management, 40*(2), 163–173. doi:10.1016/j.jpainsymman.2009.12.019

Bosslet, G. T., Pope, T. M., Rubenfeld, G. D., Lo, B., Truog, R. D., Rushton, C. H., ... White, D. B. (2015). An official ATS/AACN/ACCP/ESICM/SCCM policy statement: Responding to requests for potentially inappropriate treatments in intensive care units. *American Journal of Respiratory Critical Care Medicine, 191*(11), 1318–1330. doi:10.1164/rccm.201505-0924ST

Cadge, W. (2009). A profession in process. *Chaplaincy Today, 25*(2), 26–27.

Cadge, W., Calle, K., & Dillinger, J. (2011). What do chaplains contribute to large academic hospitals? The perspectives of pediatric physicians and chaplains. *Journal of Religion and Health, 50*(2), 300–312. doi:10.1007/ s10943-011-9474-8

Charon, R. (2006). *Narrative medicine: Honoring the stories of illness*. New York, NY: Oxford University Press.

Curtis, J. R., & White, D. B. (2008). Practical guidance for evidence-based ICU family conferences. *Chest Journal, 134*(4), 835–843. doi:10.1378/chest.08-0235

Davidson, J. E., Powers, K., Hedayat, K. M., Tieszen, M., Kon, A. A., Shepard, E., ... Armstrong, D. (2007). Clinical practice guidelines for support of the family in the patient-centered intensive care unit: American college of critical care medicine task force 2004–2005. *Critical Care Medicine, 35*(2), 605–622. doi:10.1097/01.ccm.0000254067.14607.eb

Derrickson, P. E. (1995). Screening patients for pastoral care: A preliminary report. *The Caregiver Journal, 11*(2), 14–18. doi:10.1080/1077842x.1995.10781716

Donovan, D. (2012). Assessments. In S. Roberts (ed.), *Professional spiritual and pastoral care: A practical clergy and chaplain's handbook* (pp.42–60). Woodstock, VT: Skylight Paths.

Elo, S., & Kyngas, H. (2008). The qualitative content analysis process. *Journal of Advanced Nursing, 62*(1), 107–115. doi:10.1111/j.1365-2648.2007.04569.x

Fitchett, G. (1993). *Assessing spiritual needs: A guide for caregivers*. Minneapolis, MN: Augsburg Fortress.

Food, & Drug Administration. (2009). Guidance for industry patient-reported outcome measures: Use in medical product development to support labeling claims. *Federal Register, 74*(235), 65132–65133.

Frank, A. (1995). *The Wounded Storyteller: Body, Illness, and Ethics*. Chicago, IL: University of Chicago Press.

Gaeeni, M., Farahani, M. A., Mohammadi, N., & Seyedfatemi, N. (2014). Sources of hope: Perception of Iranian family members of patients in the intensive care unit. *Iranian Journal of Nursing and Midwifery Research, 19*(6), 635.

Goldstein, H. R. (2012). Chaplains and charting. In D. Donovan & S. Roberts (Eds.), *Professional spiritual and pastoral care: A practical clergy and chaplain's handbook* (pp.81–91). Woodstock, VT: Skylight Paths.

Goldstein, H. R., Marin, D., & Umpierre, M. (2011). Chaplains and access to medical records. *Journal of Health Care Chaplaincy, 17*(3–4), 162–168. doi:10.1080/08854726.2011.616172

Graneheim, U. H., & Lundman, B. (2004). Qualitative content analysis in nursing research: Concepts, procedures and measures to achieve trustworthiness. *Nurse Education Today, 24*(2), 105–112. doi:10.1016/j.nedt.2003.10.001

Handzo, G. F., Cobb, M., Holmes, C., Kelly, E., & Sinclair, S. (2014). Outcomes for professional health care chaplaincy: an international call to action. *Journal of Health Care Chaplaincy, 20*(2), 43–53. doi:10.1080/08854726.2014.902713

Heid, A. R., Zarit, S. H., & Van Haitsma, K. (2016). Older adults' influence in family care: How do daughters and aging parents navigate differences in care goals? *Aging & Mental Health, 20*(1), 46–55. doi:10.1080/13607863.2015.1049117

Herth, K. (1992). Abbreviated instrument to measure hope: Development and psychometric evaluation. *Journal of Advanced Nursing, 17*(10), 1251–1259. doi:10.1111/j.1365-2648.1992.tb01843.x

Hsieh, H. F., & Shannon, S. E. (2005). Three approaches to qualitative content analysis. *Qualitative Health Research, 15*(9), 1277–1288. doi:10.1177/1049732305276687

Idler, E., Binney, Z., Grant, G., Perkins, M., & Quest, T. (2015). Practical matters and ultimate concerns, "doing" and "being": A diary study of the chaplain's role in the care of the seriously ill in an urban acute care hospital (S710). *Journal of Pain and Symptom Management, 2*(49), 412. doi:10.1016/j.jpainsymman.2014.11.191

Massey, K., Barnes, M. J., Villines, D., Goldstein, J. D., Pierson, A. L., Scherer, C., ... Summerfelt, W. T. (2015). What do I do? Developing a taxonomy of chaplaincy activities and interventions for spiritual care in intensive care unit palliative care. *BMC Palliative Care, 14*, 10. doi:10.1186/s12904-015-0008-0

Nolan, S. (2011). *Spiritual care at the end of life: The chaplain as a "hopeful presence."* London, UK: Jessica Kingsley.

Olver, I. N. (2012). Evolving definitions of hope in oncology. *Current Opinion in Supportive and Palliative Care, 6,* 236–241. doi:10.1097/spc.0b013e3283528d0c

Osborn, T. R., Curtis, J. R., Nielsen, E. L., Back, A. L., Shannon, S. E., & Engelberg, R. A. (2012). Identifying elements of ICU care that families report as important but unsatisfactory: decision-making, control, and ICU atmosphere. *Chest Journal, 142*(5), 1185–1192. doi:10.1378/chest.11-3277

Peery, B., & Roberts, S. (2012). Outcome oriented chaplaincy: Intentional caring. In D. Donovan & S. Roberts (eds.), *Professional spiritual and pastoral care: A practical clergy and chaplain's handbook* (pp.342–361). Woodstock, VT: Skylight Paths.

Piccinelli, C., Clerici, C., Veneroni, L., Ferrari, A., & Proserpio, T. (2015). Hope in severe disease: A review of the literature on the construct and the tools for assessing hope in the psycho-oncologic setting. *Tumori Journal, 101*(5), 491–500. doi:10.5301/tj.5000349

Puchalski, C. M. (2010). Formal and informal spiritual assessment. *Asian Pacific Journal of Cancer Prevention, 11*(Suppl 1), 51–57.

Puchalski, C. M., Vitillo, R., Hull, S. K., & Reller, N. (2014). Improving the spiritual dimension of whole person care: Reaching national and international consensus. *Journal of Palliative Medicine, 17*(6), 642–656. doi:10.1089/jpm.2014.9427

Rawdin, B., Evans, C., & Rabow, M. W. (2013). The relationships among hope, pain, psychological distress, and spiritual well-being in oncology outpatients. *Journal of Palliative Medicine, 16*(2), 167–172. doi:10.1089/jpm.2012.0223

Risk, J. L. (2013). Building a new life: A chaplain's theory based case study of chronic illness. *Journal of Health Care Chaplaincy, 19*(3), 81–98. doi:10.1080/08854726.2013.806117

Roberts, S. (2012). *Professional spiritual and pastoral Care: A practical clergy and chaplain's Handbook.* Woodstock, VT: Skylight Paths.

Roscigno, C. I., Savage, T. A., Kavanaugh, K., Moro, T. T., Kilpatrick, S. J., Strassner, H. T., ... Kimura, R. E. (2012). Divergent views of hope influencing communications between parents and hospital providers. *Qualitative Health Research, 22*(9), 1232–1246. doi:10.1177/1049732312449210

Sakumoto, M., Johnson, R., Wirpsa, J., Handzo, G., Emanuel, L., & Kho, A. (2015). *An empirical analysis of chaplain charting practices to inform electronic health record template redesign.* Paper presented at the American Medical Informatics Association 2015 Annual Symposium. San Francisco, CA.

Snowden, A., Telfer, I., Kelly, E., Burniss, S., & Mowat, H. (2013). The construction of the Lothian PROM. *Scottish Journal of Healthcare Chaplaincy, 16*(1), 3–16.

VandeCreek, L., & Lucas, A. M. (2014). *The discipline for pastoral care giving: Foundations for outcome oriented chaplaincy.* London, UK: Routledge.

World Health Organization. (2015). *People-centred and integrated health services: An overview of the evidence: Interim report.* Retrieved from www.who.int/servicedeliverysafety/areas/people-centred-care/en

ARTICLE 5

Determining Best Methods to Screen for Religious/Spiritual Distress

Stephen D.W. King[1] • George Fitchett[2] • Patricia E. Murphy[2] • Kenneth I. Pargament[3] • David A. Harrison[4] • Elizabeth Trice Loggers[5]

Correspondence: Stephen D. W. King. sking@seattlecca.org

1 Chaplaincy, Child Life, & Clinical Patient Navigators, Seattle Cancer Care Alliance, PO Box 19023, K1-104, Seattle, WA 98109, USA

2 Department of Religion, Health & Human Values, Rush University Medical Center, Chicago, IL 60612, USA

3 Department of Psychology, Bowling Green State University, Bowling Green, OH 43403, USA

4 Department of Psychiatry and Behavioral Sciences, University of Washington School of Medicine, Seattle, WA 98195, USA

5 Clinical Research Division, Fred Hutchinson Cancer Research Center, Seattle, WA 98109, USA

Received: 3 May 2016 / Accepted: 19 September 2016 / Published online: 6 October 2016

Copyright © 2016 Springer-Verlag Berlin Heidelberg

Abstract

Purpose: This study sought to validate for the first time a brief screening measure for religious/spiritual (R/S) distress given the Commission on Cancer's mandated screening for psycho-social distress including spiritual distress.

Methods: Data were collected in conjunction with an annual survey of adult hematopoietic cell transplantation (HCT) survivors. Six R/S distress screeners were compared to the Brief RCOPE, Negative Religious Coping subscale as the reference standard. We pre-specified validity as a sensitivity score of at least 85%. As no individual measure attained this, two post hoc analyses were conducted: analysis of participants within 2 years of transplantation and of a simultaneous pairing of items. Data were analyzed from 1449 respondents whose time since HCT was 6 months to 40 years.

King, S.D., Fitchett, G., Murphy, P., Pargament, K.I., Harrison, D.A., and Loggers, E.T. (2017) "Determining best methods to screen for religious/spiritual distress." Supportive Care in Cancer, 25, 471–479.

Results: For the various single-item screening protocols, sensitivity ranged from 27 (spiritual/religious concerns) to 60% (meaning/joy) in the full sample and 25 (spiritual/religious concerns) to 65% (meaning/joy) in a subsample of those within 2 years of HCT. The paired items of low meaning/joy and self-described R/S struggle attained a net sensitivity of 82% in the full sample and of 87% in those within 2 years of HCT but with low net specificities.

Conclusions: While no single-item screener was acceptable using our pre-specified sensitivity value of 85%, the simultaneous use of meaning/joy and self-described struggle items among cancer survivors is currently the best choice to briefly screen for R/S distress. Future research should validate this and other approaches in active treatment cancer patients and survivors and determine the best times to screen.

Key words: screening, oncology, cancer, religious/spiritual, distress, hematopoietic cell transplant

Introduction

Religious and/or spiritual distress is a common and difficult problem, occurring in up to 50% of cancer patients[1, 2, 3] and 27% of long-term survivors.[4] Defined as religious or spiritual (R/S) tensions and struggles within oneself, with others, and with what one holds to be sacred,[5] R/S distress may include feeling abandoned by God, being in conflict with others about R/S beliefs or practices, or struggling with ultimate meaning.[4, 6, 7, 8, 9] R/S distress is also identified as R/S struggle,[10] R/S pain,[11] and negative religious coping.[5] This type of distress has been associated with physical and emotional pain and poorer quality of life in longitudinal as well as cross-sectional studies among cancer patients and those with other conditions.[1, 6, 12, 13, 14, 15] The negative effects of R/S struggle on emotional distress and quality of life appear consistent across cancer types and phases of cancer treatment, including survivors of hematopoietic cell transplantation (HCT).[1, 2, 3, 4, 15, 16]

Acknowledging the importance of psychosocial distress, including R/S distress, the American College of Surgeons' Commission on Cancer (CoC) mandated screening for all cancer patients effective January 1, 2015.[17, 18] Leaders in psycho-oncology agreed with the CoC's new focus in a joint position statement of the American Psychosocial Oncology Society, the Association of Oncology Social Work, and the Oncology Nursing Society. Furthermore, they reinforced the importance of screening and appropriate referrals for treatment for cancer patients and survivors suffering from R/S distress.[19] Recognizing the importance of this issue, many cancer care organizations are using a variety of brief screens for R/S distress.[11, 20, 21, 22, 23, 24, 25]

Despite the known importance of R/S distress, there is little or no information regarding the validity or reliability of the R/S distress screeners commonly in use. Therefore, this study was designed to rigorously test for the first time a variety of methods of R/S distress screening to identify the best very brief screening items. We used the Brief RCOPE, Negative Religious Coping (NRC) subscale[5] as the reference standard. The NRC is the most commonly used measure of R/S distress, has good validity and reliability, and has been used in diverse patient populations (e.g., age, diagnoses).[5, 15, 26] While most of what is known about R/S distress comes from studies that employed the Brief RCOPE or the NRC subscale, the subscale contains seven items that may be burdensome for vulnerable cancer patients who are being subjected to greater volumes of surveys and screening tools. Therefore, we compared results from the NRC to the commonly used screening tools for R/S distress to validate a single-item screening tool. Some of these screening tools use explicitly spiritual-religious language, e.g., a self-identified spiritual/religious struggle item. Others, such as items for meaning/joy or peace, use psycho-spiritual language, that is, they use psychologically meaningful constructs inviting spiritual reflection. This more implicit spiritual exploration may be especially useful for those with no explicit religious identity.[27]

Methods

Data were collected as part of an annual Patient Recovery Questionnaire (PRQ) of adult survivors of hematopoietic cell transplantation (HCT) at a major cancer center in the northwest United States. Survivors who were 18 to 89 years old inclusive, could read and write English, and were treated at this center were included. HCT survivors represent a reasonable sample for distress screening across the broader care continuum of cancer patients in treatment and cancer survivors because most HCT survivors do not return to their original baseline, continuing to face medical, physical, emotional, and existential threats[28, 29, 30] increasing the likelihood of encountering R/S distress. Further, as previously stated, studies suggest that HCT survivors experience similar effects of R/S distress on emotional distress and quality of life as do other cancer patients.[4, 15, 16]

The 2011–2012 PRQ included an additional R/S coping module that incorporated the NRC subscale of the Brief RCOPE and a number of R/S screening items. The PRQ and the module were paper surveys that were mailed at the same time to the long-term follow-up (LTFU) program's survivors during the month of their transplant anniversary with a request that they be completed and returned by mail. The study compared various screening questions to the NRC subscale. Items for comparison were selected on the basis of both a literature review and clinical experience.

The data collection for this study was approved by the local Institutional Review Board.

Measures

R/S struggle

The 7-item NRC subscale assesses struggle with the sacred (e.g., feeling unloved or abandoned by God/Higher Power) and interpersonal R/S struggle (e.g., feeling abandoned by one's R/S community) using response options of "not at all," (scored 0) to "a great deal" (scored 3). A dichotomous variable of no R/S distress versus R/S distress was used in these analyses. The typical approach to scoring is to sum the item scores with any non-zero sum indicating some degree of R/S distress.[13, 31] However, to ensure that participants with very low R/S distress were not misclassified, we used a more stringent measure: to be identified as having R/S distress, participants had to score 1 (i.e., "somewhat") on at least three items or have a score of at least 2 (i.e., "quite a bit") on any one item.

Six screening measures were studied based upon their prevalence in the literature and/or clinical experience. (1) "Do you struggle with the loss of meaning and joy in your life?" (meaning/joy) and (2) "Do you currently have what you would describe as religious or spiritual struggles?" (self-described struggle) were created with response options "not at all," "somewhat," "quite a bit," and "a great deal." (3) Steinhauser and colleagues developed a single item, "Are you at peace" (peace), with responses in a 5-point Likert scale format of "not at all" "a little bit," and "a moderate amount," "quite a bit," and "completely."[25] (4) The Revised Rush Religious Struggle Protocol (Rush Protocol) screens for R/S distress by asking about the importance of R/S in the person's life and, depending upon the response, asks one of two follow-up questions. Pathway 1 asks those for whom R/S is important, how much support it is providing them as they cope. If not all they need, possible R/S distress is indicated. Pathway 2 asks those for whom R/S is not important if that has always been the case with the assumption that perhaps R/S distress triggered the change.[24] (5) A single item similar to Pathway 1 of the Rush Protocol, "Does your religion/spirituality provide you all the comfort and strength you need from it right now?" (comfort/strength) was created with response options of "not applicable" (n/a), "not at all," "somewhat," "quite a bit," and "a great deal." (6) Finally, one of the most well-known screeners is the checklist item, "spiritual/religious concerns" (R/S concerns) in The National Comprehensive Cancer Network's (NCCN) distress thermometer and problem checklist.[20] It was used here with a yes or no option. Given the low prevalence of individual items of the NRC, they were not considered further as individual screeners.

Disease information and socio-demographics

To help insure accuracy, the study used data from the long-term follow-up database for medical information such as diagnosis, year of diagnosis, and year of transplant and demographics such as age, gender, and race. For ethnicity and when the database had missing information, this study used self-reported information that the study had collected in the survey. Religious identity (e.g., faith tradition) and spiritual identity (e.g., spiritual and religious, spiritual only, religious only, or neither) were also collected in the survey.

Statistical methods

Descriptive statistics were used to characterize the sample and the prevalence of responses to each screening item. Screening item responses were grouped based on degree of distress they appeared to indicate. Dichotomous variables were then created for each item. Sensitivity and specificity percentages are reported for each item. Because we wanted to identify as many of those with potential R/S distress as possible even at the expense of having false positives, the study team determined that sensitivity was the most important factor in screening for R/S distress. Therefore, we set sensitivity of 85% as the threshold for "screening positive," with the expectation that this would lead to a referral to a chaplain, or other team member with appropriate expertise, for further assessment for R/S distress.

Still, because of the expense in staff time and the potential additional burden to patients of further face-to-face assessment, specificity or correctly identifying persons without distress is important as well. Consequently, a specificity as close to 85% as possible was desired. These thresholds are common[33] and are similar to those for the widely used Patient Health Questionnaire-9 (PHQ-9) (e.g., sensitivity and specificity both of 88%).[33] The finding of relatively low sensitivity and specificity for all the screeners in the initial analyses led us to conduct two post hoc analyses. Because R/S distress, and factors associated with it, may vary for very long-term survivors, our first post hoc analysis restricted the sample to participants who were 2 years or less since their transplant. We chose 2 years because of its proximity to active treatment, increasing the likelihood that any observed R/S distress would be cancer associated (rather than associated with other stressors). It is widely recognized that the simultaneous use of two screening questions (distress indicated by at least one of two items) can increase net sensitivity.[33] Thus, the second post hoc analysis tested the net sensitivity and specificity of various combinations of two of the screening questions.

Of 2113 survivors who returned the PRQ (52% response rate), 83% returned the R/S module survey ($n=1745$). Eighty-one survivors completed the surveys twice due to the nature of their transplant; our analysis omitted their second survey leaving 1664 first surveys returned. Of the 1664 R/S surveys that were returned, 215 (13%) were omitted from the analysis: 73 either did not receive HCT or did not receive HCT at our center, and 142 cases had missing data on one of the study variables, including 54 cases with more than three missing NRC items. In 38 returns, data were missing for either one or two NRC items. For these cases, regression equations were used to predict parameter estimates for each of the missing items based on the responses to the remaining NRC items. The final sample for these analyses was 1449. All analyses were done using SPSS 19.

Results

Fifty percent of the subjects were between ages 50 and 64 inclusive, 51% male, 93% White people, 68% Christian (with 19% atheist/agnostic/none/no preference) (Table 1). The responses of the study participants to negative religious coping items indicated that 14% had some R/S distress. Across the various screening protocols, the proportion with potential R/S distress ranged from 38% (meaning/joy) to 13% (R/S concerns) (Table 2). For the various screening protocols, the sensitivity ranged from 60% (meaning/joy) to 27% (R/S concerns), and specificity ranged from 89% (R/S concerns) to 65% (meaning/joy). As can be seen in Table 3, though two of the screeners had a specificity of at least 85%, none of the very brief screeners approached our pre-specified minimum of 85% for sensitivity.

Since there were no acceptable single item measures for R/S distress, our first post hoc analysis focused on the subsample of participants who had received their transplant within the last 2 years. In this subsample, the sensitivity of the various screeners was somewhat higher than for the whole sample. Sensitivity ranged from 65% (meaning/joy) to 25% (R/S concerns). Specificity ranged from 90% (Rush Protocol) to 58% (meaning/joy). Again, though some of the screeners had a specificity of at least 85%, none of the screening protocols provided sensitivity that approached our criteria of 85% (Table 3).

In our second post hoc analysis, the simultaneous use of two screening items was assessed (the Rush Protocol was omitted from these analyses because it is not a single-item screener, single items being necessary for this type of analysis). Combining the meaning/joy item with the self-described struggle produced the highest sensitivity (82% sensitivity) followed by the pair of meaning/joy and the peace item (78% sensitivity) in the whole sample (Table 4).

In the sample of participants within 2 years of transplant, those same pairs were the best at identifying people with R/S distress with the meaning/joy and self-described struggle paired items at 87% net sensitivity (net specificity 44%) and the meaning/joy and peace paired items at 84% (net specificity 47%). The combination of the peace and self-described struggle items produced relatively high net specificity, especially in the subsample (sensitivity 83%; specificity 60%) (Table 4).

Table 1: Sample characteristics (n=1449)

Age category	
• 18–39	172 (12%)
• 40–49	228 (16%)
• 50–64	724 (50%)
• ≥ 65	325 (22%)
Gender	
• Male	744 (51%)
• Female	705 (49%)
Race (n=1413)	
• White people	1316 (93%)
• [a]Other	97 (7%)
Religion (n=1435)	
• Christian	980 (68%)
• [b]Other	188 (13%)
• No preference/none	179 (13%)
• Agnostic/Atheist	88 (6%)

Spirituality	
• Both spiritual and religious	729 (50%)
• Religious/not spiritual	85 (6%)
• Spiritual/not religious	472 (33%)
• Neither spiritual nor religious	163 (11%)
Diagnosis	
• Leukemia	678 (47%)
• Lymphoma/Hodgkin's disease	263 (18%)
• Multiple myeloma	218 (15%)
• Aplastic anemia	63 (4%)
• MDS	157 (11%)
• Other	44 (3%)
• Solid tumors	26 (2%)
Year of diagnosis (n=1446)	
• 1966–1994	421 (29%)
• 1995–2004	531 (37%)
• 2005–2011	494 (34%)
Years since transplant	
• 2 years or less	341 (24%)
• 3–10 years	498 (34%)
• 11–20 years	387 (27%)
• 21 or more years	223 (15%)

[a]Other includes Black or African American, 21 (1.5%), Asian, 50 (3.5%), Mixed, 15 (1.1%), American Indian or Alaskan Native, 8 (.6%), Native Hawaiian, 3 (.2%).
[b]Other includes Jewish, 60 (4.2%), LDS 27 (1.9%), Buddhist 19 (1.3%), Muslim 8 (.6%), Native American/Aboriginal 4 (.3%), Hindu 2 (.1%), other affiliation, 68 (4.7%).

Table 2: Distribution of scores for religious/spiritual (R/S) screeners

	Number (percent)
Do you struggle with the loss of meaning and joy in your life? (n=1447)	
• Not at all	895 (62%)
• Somewhat	467 (32%)
• Quite a bit	64 (4%)
• A great deal	21 (2%)

	Number (percent)
Do you currently have what you would describe as religious or spiritual struggles? (n=1444)	
• Not at all	1052 (73%)
• Somewhat	334 (23%)
• Quite a bit	41 (3%)
• A great deal	17 (1%)
Are you at peace? (n=1445)	
• Not at all	16 (1%)
• A little bit	67 (5%)
• A moderate amount	224 (16%)
• Quite a bit	651 (45%)
• Completely	487 (34%)
Rush Screening Protocol	
Path 1 (R/S is currently important but issues with strength/comfort) (n=1037)	
• Yes	151 (15%)
• No	886 (85%)
Path 2 (R/S not currently important was important in the past) (n=360)	
• Yes	155 (43%)
• No	205 (57%)
Possible struggle either Path 1 or Path 2 (n=1397)	
• Yes	306 (22%)
• No	1091 (78%)
Does your religion/spirituality provide you all the strength and comfort you need from it right now? (n=1441)	
• Not applicable	219 (15%)
• Not at all	36 (3%)
• Somewhat	234 (16%)
• Quite a bit	359 (25%)
• A great deal	593 (41%)
Do you have any spiritual/religious concerns? (n=1437)	
• No	1248 (87%)
• Yes	189 (13%)

Shaded rows were coded as indicators of possible R/S struggle, unshaded rows as no R/S struggle.

Table 3: Properties of religious/spiritual (R/S) screeners whole sample and subsample 2 years or less since transplant

Screening items	Whole sample					Subsample: 2 years or less since transplant				
	Total Sample n (percent)	Struggle (14%)	No struggle (86%)	Sensi-tivity	Speci-ficity	Total Sample n (percent)	Struggle (14%)	No struggle (86%)	Sensi-tivity	Speci-ficity
Do you struggle with the loss of meaning and joy in your life?										
• Somewhat/Quite a bit/A great deal	552 (38%)	119 (22%)	433 (78%)	60%	65%	153 (45%)	32 (21%)	121 (79%)	65%	58%
• Not at all	895 (62%)	78 (9%)	817 (91%)			187 (55%)	17 (9%)	170 (91%)		
Do you currently have what you would describe as religious or spiritual struggles?										
• Somewhat/Quite a bit/A great deal	392 (27%)	106 (27%)	286 (73%)	54%	77%	103 (30%)	30 (29%)	73 (71%)	61%	75%
• Not at all	1052 (73%)	90 (9%)	962 (91%)			237 (70%)	19 (8%)	218 (92%)		
Are you at peace?										
• Not at all/A little bit/A moderate amount	307 (21%)	88 (29%)	219 (71%)	45%	83%	85 (25%)	27 (32%)	58 (68%)	55%	80%
• Quite a bit/Completely	1138 (79%)	109 (10%)	1029 (90%)			256 (75%)	22 (9%)	234 (91%)		
Rush protocol										
• Potential struggle	306 (22%)	80 (27%)	226 (74%)	42%	81%	42 (13%)	15 (36%)	27 (64%)	31%	90%
• No struggle	1093 (78%)	110 (10%)	983 (90%)			287 (87%)	33 (11%)	254 (89%)		
Does your religion/spirituality provide you all the strength and comfort you need from it right now?										
• Not at all/Somewhat	270 (19%)	81 (30%)	189 (70%)	42%	85%	64 (19%)	21 (33%)	43 (67%)	43%	85%
• "Not applicable/Quite a bit/A great deal	1171 (81%)	113 (10%)	1058 (90%)			277 (81%)	28 (10%)	249 (90%)		
Do you have any spiritual/religious concerns?										
• Yes	189 (13%)	52 (28%)	137 (73%)	27%	89%	50 (15%)	12 (24%)	38 (76%)	25%	87%
• No	1248 (87%)	141 (11%)	1107 (89%)			287 (85%)	36 (13%)	251 (88%)		

Table 4: Two screening items used simultaneously

Items	Full sample		Less than or equal to 2 years	
	Net sensitivity	Net specificity	Net sensitivity	Net specificity
Meaning/joy and self-described struggle	82%	50%	87%	44%
Peace and meaning/joy	78%	54%	84%	47%
Comfort/strength and meaning/joy	77%	56%	80%	50%
Peace and self-described struggle	75%	64%	83%	60%
Comfort/strength and self-described struggle	73%	65%	78%	64%
R/S concerns and meaning/joy	71%	58%	74%	51%
Comfort/strength and peace	68%	70%	74%	68%
R/S concerns and self-described struggle	66%	69%	71%	65%
Peace and R/S concerns	60%	73%	66%	70%
Comfort/strength and R/S concerns	58%	76%	57%	74%

Full sample and less than or equal to 2 years after transplant.

Discussion

This study is the first to evaluate the validity of various screening items to identify R/S distress in cancer survivors. While no single item was acceptable using our predetermined sensitivity value of 85%, the two-item combination of meaning/joy and self-described R/S distress is promising based on a net sensitivity of 82% in the full sample and of 87% in those within 2 years of hematopoietic cell transplantation. Furthermore, the meaning/joy item may discover some spiritual/existential distress not revealed by the NRC. Unfortunately, the net specificity was low for this pairing which may have important implications for resource use in cancer care organizations attempting to efficiently screen for R/S distress.

Given this, the higher net specificity of the peace/self-described struggle dyad might suggest use of this pairing for a screener. While there may be some merit to this choice as one attempts to balance the value of sensitivity relative to that of specificity, one concern might be the timing. In our clinical experience, cancer patients who were newly diagnosed were much more likely to screen positive for R/S distress using the peace question than those who are months along in active treatment [King S. One Department's Collection and Use of Data to Advance Chaplaincy Care. Presented at the Association of Professional Chaplains Annual Conference, Orlando, Florida, June 28, 2013]. This suggests that using the peace question early in the treatment trajectory may lead to more false positives due to confounding of anxiety with R/S distress.

While this study is the first to examine the validity of diverse approaches to R/S distress screening, it also has several limitations. Although the percentage of Christians in our sample is similar to the USA,[36] our sample is more White than the national census.[37] Our sample is limited by the racial distribution within the LTFU program that we studied and this may limit generalizability. In addition, although the Brief RCOPE, NRC subscale has been the gold standard for identifying and studying R/S distress, it has some limitations. Six of its seven items focus on struggles with the sacred (including one item that mentions the demonic) and one item focuses on conflict with an R/S community. R/S struggles in other domains such as ultimate meaning, doubts, and morals are not included in this measure.[38] Because of this, R/S struggle may be underestimated, especially among those who are more spiritual rather than religious or have more existential concerns as opposed to theistic concerns. This study's best single screening item, meaning/joy, is limited in that it measures two themes simultaneously. This study also does not include those in active treatment, and we have not studied how well these screeners will generalize to that population. Further, there is limited literature on the trajectory of R/S distress in either survivors or those in active treatment.[15, 39] Consequently, we do not know the best times to screen, how often to screen, or how having different types of cancer may impact this trajectory. Further research is needed that addresses these lacunae.

Unlike many other studies, we identified clear cut-off values for each screening item and pre-specified our target sensitivity and specificity. Other strengths of the study include the large and geographically diverse sample used in the analyses and consistency of the findings in the full sample and the subsample.

Despite this, there is much more to study and learn. First, our results should be replicated (with or without other potential screeners), including using clinical interviews by a chaplain or other professional with expertise in R/S distress as a reference standard. Furthermore, a new Religious and Spiritual Struggles Questionnaire[38] has been developed which assesses six domains of R/S distress rather than the Brief RCOPE's three domains, thus expanding the comprehensiveness of R/S distress measurement.

Assessing the performance of this questionnaire in comparison to the NRC subscale, clinical interviews and brief screening tools will be important.

While this study did not identify a valid single item screener for R/S distress, the simultaneous use of the meaning/joy and self-described distress items is currently the best choice for screening for R/S distress in cancer patients and survivors. Until further study identifies another method, we recommend this pair be considered for all clinical screening for R/S distress, even among cancer patients in active treatment, when only a minimal number of items are permitted.

Acknowledgments

We express great appreciation to Dr. Paul Martin for his support for the conduct of the survey that produced the data for this study and for his helpful comments regarding this paper. We also express appreciation to those within the Long-Term Follow Up program at Fred Hutchinson Cancer Research Center, including Peggy Adams Myers, Kathleen Meeth, Kevin Bray, and Carey Fudurich. The collection of the survey data for this project was supported by the ALC grant CA018029.

Compliance with ethical standards

Ethical approach: All procedures in this study were in accordance with the ethical standards of the institutional review committee and with the 1964 Helsinki declaration and its later amendments or comparable ethical standards.

Conflict of interest: The authors declare no conflict of interest. We do not have full control of all the primary data.

Disclaimers: The views expressed in the submitted article are the authors' and not an official position of their respective institutions.

References

1. Fitchett G, Murphy PE, Kim J et al. (2004) Religious struggle: Prevalence, correlates, and mental health risks in diabetic, congestive heart failure, and oncology patients. Int J Psychiatry Med 34: 179–196.
2. Tarakeshwar N, Vanderwerker LC, Paulk E et al. (2006) Religious coping is associated with quality of life of patients with advanced cancer. J Palliat Med 9:646–657.
3. Thune-Boyle ICV, Stygall J, Keshtgar MRS et al. (2013) Religious/ spiritual coping resources and their relationship with adjustment in patients newly diagnosed with breast cancer in the UK. Psycho-Oncology 22:646–658.

4. King SDW, Fitchett G, Murphy P et al. (2015) Spiritual or religious struggle in hematopoietic cell transplant survivors. Psycho-Oncology. doi:10.1002/pon.4029.
5. Pargament KI, Feuille M, Burdzy D (2011) The Brief RCOPE: Current psychometric status of a short measure of religious coping. Religions 2:551–576.
6. Exline JJ (2013) Religious and spiritual struggles. In: Pargament KI, Exline JJ, Jones J (eds) APA handbook of psychology, religion, and spirituality (vol 1). American Psychological Association Press, Washington DC, pp.459–475.
7. Pargament KI (1997) The psychology of religion and coping: Theory, research, practice. Guilford Press, New York.
8. Pargament KI, Murray-Swank N, Magyar G et al. (2005) Spiritual struggle: A phenomenon of interest to psychology and religion. In: Miller WR, Delaney H (eds) Judeo-Christian perspectives on psychology: Human nature, motivation, and change. APA Press, Washington, DC, pp.245–268.
9. Exline JJ, Park CL, Smyth JM et al. (2011) Anger toward God: Social-cognitive predictors, prevalence, and links with adjustment to bereavement and cancer. J Pers Soc Psychol 100:129–148.
10. Pargament KI, Koenig HG, Tarakeshwar N et al. (2001) Religious struggle as a predictor of mortality among medically ill elderly patients. Arch Intern Med 161:1881–1885.
11. Mako C, Galek K, Poppito SR (2009) Spiritual pain among patients with advanced cancer in palliative care. J Palliat Med 9:1106–1113.
12. Hebert R, Zdaniuk B, Schulz R et al. (2009) Positive and negative religious coping and well-being in women with breast cancer. J Palliat Med 12:537–545.
13. Pargament KI, Koenig HG, Tarakeshwar N et al. (2004) Religious coping methods as predictors of psychological, physical and spiritual outcomes among medically ill elderly patients: A two-year longitudinal study. J Health Psychol 9:713–730
14. Park CL, Wortmann JH, Edmondson D (2011) Religious struggle as a predictor of subsequent mental and physical well-being in advanced heart failure patients. J Behav Med 34:426–436.
15. Sherman AC, Plante TG, Simonton S et al. (2009) Prospective study of religious coping among patients undergoing autologous stem cell transplantation. J Behav Med 32:118–128.
16. Sherman AC, Simonton S, Latif U et al. (2005) Religious struggle and religious comfort in response to illness: Health outcomes among stem cell transplant patients. J Behav Med 28:359–367.
17. American College of Surgeons. About CoC accreditation. www.facs.org/quality%20 programs/cancer/accredited/about. Accessed 21 Sept. 2015.
18. American College of Surgeons (2012) Commission on Cancer. Cancer Program Standards. Ensuring Patient Centered Care, Standards 3.2 and E10. www.facs.org/~/media/files/quality%20 programs/cancer/coc/programstandards2012.ashx. Accessed 11 April 2016.
19. Pirl WF, Braun IM, Deshields TL et al. (2013) Implementing screening for distress: The joint position statement from the American Psychosocial Oncology Society, Association of Oncology Social Work and Oncology Nursing Society. www.apos-society.org/docs/APOS.AOSW.ONS.StmtDistressScreening.16July13.pdf. Accessed 11 April 2016.
20. National Comprehensive Cancer Network (NCCN): NCCN distress thermometer for patients. www.nccn.org/patients/resources/life_with_cancer/pdf/nccn_distress_thermometer.pdf.Accessed 11 April 2016.
21. Bultz BD, Groff SL, Fitch M et al. (2011) Implementing screening for distress, the 6th vital sign: A Canadian strategy for changing practice. Psycho-Oncology 20:463–469.
22. Loscalzo M, Clark KL, Holland J (2011) Successful strategies for implementing biopsychosocial screening. Psycho-Oncology 20: 455–462.
23. Wells-Di GS, Prensky EK, Minotti M et al. (2013) The James Supportive Care Screening: Integrating science and practice to meet the NCCN guidelines for distress management at a comprehensive cancer center. Psycho-Oncology 22:2001–2008.

24. King SDW, Fitchett G, Berry D (2013) Screening for religious/spiritual struggle in blood and marrow transplant patients. Support Care Cancer 21:993–1001.
25. Steinhauser KE, Voils CI, Clipp EC et al. (2008) Are you at peace? One item to probe spiritual concerns at the end of life. Arch Intern Med 166:101–105.
26. Pargament KI, Smith BW, Koenig HG et al. (1998) Patterns of positive and negative religious coping with major life stressors. JSSR 37:710–724.
27. Pargament KI (2007) Spiritually integrated psychotherapy: Understanding and addressing the sacred. Guilford Press, New York.
28. Andrykowski MA, Bishop MM, Hahn EA et al. (2005) Long-term health-related quality of life, growth, and spiritual well-being after hematopoietic stem-cell transplantation. J Clin Oncol 23:599–608.
29. Syrjala KL, Langer SL, Abrams JR et al. (2005) Late effects of hematopoietic cell transplantation among 10-year adult survivors compared with case-matched controls. J Clin Oncol 23:6596–6606.
30. Syrjala KL, Martin PJ, Lee SJ (2012) Delivering care to long-term adult survivors of hematopoietic cell transplantation. J Clin Oncol 30:3746–3751.
31. Fitchett G, Winter-Pfändler U, Pargament KI (2014) Religious struggle in Swiss patients visited by chaplains: Prevalence and correlates. J Health Psychol 19:966–976.
32. Smets IHGJ, Kempen GIJM, Janssen-Heijnen MLG et al. (2014) Four screening instruments for frailty in older patients with and without cancer: A diagnostic study. BMC Geriatr 14:26.
33. Kroenke K, Spitzer RL, Williams JB (2001) The PHQ-9: The validity of a brief depression severity measure. JGIM 16:606–616
34. Gordis L (2014) Epidemiology, 5th edn. Elsevier Saunders, Philadelphia.
35. Roth PL, Switzer FS, Switzer DM (1999) Missing data in multiple item scales: A Monte Carlo analysis of missing data techniques. Organ Res Methods 2:211–232.
36. Pew Research Center: America's Changing Religious Landscape. www.pewforum.org/2015/05/12/americas-changing-religious-landscape. Accessed 5 Sept. 2016.
37. United States Census Bureau: QuickFacts. United States. www.census.gov/quickfacts. Accessed 5 Sept. 2016.
38. Exline JJ, Pargament KI, Grubbs JB et al. (2014) The religious and spiritual struggles scale: Development and initial validation. Psycholog Relig Spiritual 6:208–222.
39. Gall TL, Guirguis-Younger M, Charbonneau C et al. (2009) The trajectory of religious coping across time in response to the diagnosis of breast cancer. Psycho-Oncology 18:1165–1178.

ARTICLE 6

The Spiritual Distress Assessment Tool: An Instrument to Assess Spiritual Distress in Hospitalised Elderly Persons

Stefanie M Monod[1*], Etienne Rochat[1,2], Christophe J Büla[1], Guy Jobin[3], Estelle Martin[1], Brenda Spencer[4]

* Correspondence: stefanie.monod-zorzi@chuv.ch

1 Service of Geriatric Medicine & Geriatric Rehabilitation, University of Lausanne Medical Center (CHUV), 1011 Lausanne, Switzerland

2 Chaplaincy Service, University of Lausanne Medical Center (CHUV), 1011 Lausanne, Switzerland

3 Faculty of Theology and Religious Sciences, University of Laval, QC G1V 0A6 Quebec, Canada

4 Institute of Social and Preventive Medicine (IUMSP), University Hospital Center and University of Lausanne, Bugnon 17, 1005 Lausanne, Switzerland

Copyright © 2010 Monod et al; licensee BioMed Central Ltd. This is an Open Access article distributed under the terms of the Creative Commons Attribution License (http://creativecommons.org/licenses/by/2.0), which permits unrestricted use, distribution, and reproduction in any medium, provided the original work is properly cited.

Abstract

Background: Although spirituality is usually considered a positive resource for coping with illness, spiritual distress may have a negative influence on health outcomes. Tools are needed to identify spiritual distress in clinical practice and subsequently address identified needs. This study describes the first steps in the development of a clinically acceptable instrument to assess spiritual distress in hospitalized elderly patients.

Methods: A three-step process was used to develop the Spiritual Distress Assessment Tool (SDAT): 1) Conceptualisation by a multidisciplinary group of a model (Spiritual Needs Model) to define the different dimensions characterizing a patient's spirituality and their corresponding needs; 2) Operationalisation of the Spiritual Needs Model within geriatric hospital care leading to a set of questions (SDAT) investigating needs related to each of the defined dimensions; 3) Qualitative assessment of the instrument's acceptability and face validity in hospital chaplains.

Monod, S.M., Rochat, E., Büla, C.J., Jobin, G., Martin, E., and Spencer, B. (2010) "The spiritual distress assessment tool: an instrument to assess spiritual distress in hospitalized elderly persons." *BMC Geriatrics*, 10, 88–96.

Results: Four dimensions of spirituality (Meaning, Transcendence, Values, and Psychosocial Identity) and their corresponding needs were defined. A formalised assessment procedure to both identify and subsequently score unmet spiritual needs and spiritual distress was developed. Face validity and acceptability in clinical practice were confirmed by chaplains involved in the focus groups.

Conclusions: The SDAT appears to be a clinically acceptable instrument to assess spiritual distress in elderly hospitalised persons. Studies are ongoing to investigate the psychometric properties of the instrument and to assess its potential to serve as a basis for integrating the spiritual dimension in the patient's plan of care.

Background

The relationship between spirituality and medicine is a field of growing interest.[1, 2, 3] In palliative care, the spiritual dimension is considered as an important component of care along with physical, psychological, and social or existential support.[4] Spirituality is also considered an essential component of the multidimensional approach used in geriatric care of elderly patients who face illness, disability, and potentially life-threatening events.[5]

Spirituality has been shown to influence, usually in a positive way, coping with illness, disability, or life-threatening events.[6, 7, 8, 9, 10] Many studies have documented significant associations between spirituality and better mental, physical, and functional health, especially in cancer, HIV, and hospice patients.[11, 12] Some studies have, however, shown that negative manifestations of spirituality may be associated with poorer health outcomes. Religious struggle, defined as negative feelings towards God, feeling punished by God, or believing that « the devil is at work in the illness », has been associated with increased mortality in elderly patients.[13] Spiritual distress, that can be defined as "a state in which the individual is at risk of experiencing a disturbance in his/her system of belief or value that provides strength, hope, and meaning to life"[14], seems also associated with more severe depression and desire for hastened death in end-of-life patients.[15, 16] Spiritual distress might have a potentially harmful effect on patients' prognosis and quality of life.[17, 18, 19, 20]

Despite evidence suggesting an association between spiritual distress and worse health outcome, very few intervention studies have been conducted to improve patients' spiritual health.[21, 22] This may be explained by the lack of consensus on the definition of spirituality, and, as a consequence, of spiritual distress, within health care research.[23, 24, 25]

Numerous instruments have been developed to assess spirituality. Most currently available describe behaviours, beliefs or attitudes towards spirituality.[26, 27, 28] Although some instruments measuring spiritual well-being or spiritual needs might equally reflect spiritual distress,[29, 30, 31] none of these instruments has been designed for this specific purpose. Moreover, conceptual models on which to base spiritual assessment, spiritual distress recognition and spiritual intervention in hospital settings are essentially lacking, and are called for in order to improve patient care.[25] These conceptual models should also be congruent with other bio-psycho-social processes of care in order to promote integrative models of care in hospital settings. These shortcomings need to be addressed as a prerequisite to conducting intervention studies.

The present paper describes work to address this issue and presents: a) an operational definition of spiritual distress; b) the successive steps in the development of an instrument to assess spiritual distress in hospitalized elderly patients; c) the subsequent assessment of this instrument's face validity and acceptability in clinical practice.

Methods

Basic concepts

There are different ways to assess spirituality; this research focuses on assessment of the patient's *spiritual state*. Spiritual state is here defined as the patient's feelings regarding his or her spirituality. Spiritual state is dynamic: it fluctuates according to a hypothesised spectrum of spiritual wellness, ranging from spiritual well-being to spiritual distress. A spiritual state might be worse because of external stressors such as illness or bereavement; it may also be improved by spiritual intervention. This concept of spiritual state appeared as the most appropriate way to assess spirituality within the hospital setting. The intention is that assessment of a patient's spiritual state should serve to determine the need for specific interventions.

Based on this definition of a spiritual state, an operational definition of *spiritual distress* was hypothesised. The hypothesis was made that spiritual distress arises from unmet spiritual needs and that the greater the degree to which a spiritual need remains unmet, the greater the disturbance in spiritual state and the greater the level of spiritual distress experienced by the patient.

Development of the Spiritual Distress Assessment Tool (Figure 1)

The development of the Spiritual Distress Assessment Tool (SDAT) was based on a conceptual model of spiritual needs assessment previously published under the name of the Spiritual Needs Model.[32]

Development of the Spiritual Distress Assessment Tool was yet carried out in three stages.

a) Conceptualisation of spirituality and spiritual needs in hospitalised persons: definition of the Spiritual Needs Model[32]

An interdisciplinary group of health professionals (one physician, four nurses, and three chaplains), working in five different geriatric hospitals in Switzerland, met on fourteen occasions over a two-year period to define and conceptualise spirituality in the hospitalised person. The group was directed by one of the co-authors (ER).

A literature search and review in PubMed and Google, using "spirituality" and "religiosity" as search terms, was performed to select and define candidate dimensions that could characterize spirituality in hospitalised persons. Candidate dimensions were discussed and consensus was achieved through the sharing of spiritual care experiences, role play and case analysis. Finally, using the same process, the working party further defined the spiritual needs corresponding to each selected dimension of spirituality.

The work of the interdisciplinary group resulted in a definition of *spirituality in hospitalised persons*, of the *dimensions that characterize a patient's spirituality* and of the *needs corresponding to each of these dimensions*.

The overall concept was defined as **The Spiritual Needs Model.**[32]

b) Definition of the Spiritual Distress Assessment Tool (SDAT) and guidelines for administration

Two of the authors (SM and ER) decided to integrate the Spiritual Needs Model into hospital geriatric care over a six-month period in order to assess its practicability in clinical care.

This phase of the research was conducted in the post-acute care unit of the Department of Geriatric Medicine, University of Lausanne Medical Center. This 66-bed unit admits patients aged 65 years and older and provides interdisciplinary care to restore the highest possible level of functional independence and quality of life. Eighty percent of patients report a Judaeo-Christian religious background.

During this phase, the leader of the working party (ER) was integrated into the interdisciplinary team. He performed systematic bedside assessments of patients' spirituality using the framework of the Spiritual Needs Model and participated in weekly interdisciplinary team meetings to share the results of this assessment with health professionals.

Over the six-month period, 69 patients were assessed by the chaplain using the framework of the Spiritual Needs Model. Of those patients proposed a meeting with the chaplain, only one refused. Characteristics of the participants are described in Table 1.

Based on this experience, spiritual needs assessment with use of the Spiritual Needs Model was progressively structured and systematised. In the course of this process, a set of questions was gradually devised for use in the interview to investigate the patient's spiritual needs and guidelines to conduct spiritual needs assessment (e.g. patient's consent, confidentiality) were defined. In parallel, a structured analytical framework was developed to assess the severity of unmet spiritual needs, as manifested in the interview.

This process resulted in the definition of the SDAT, that is, a formalised assessment procedure to identify unmet spiritual needs, to score the degree to which spiritual needs remained unmet and to determine the presence of spiritual distress.

This part of the SDAT development was approved by the institutional Ethical Review Board of the University of Lausanne.

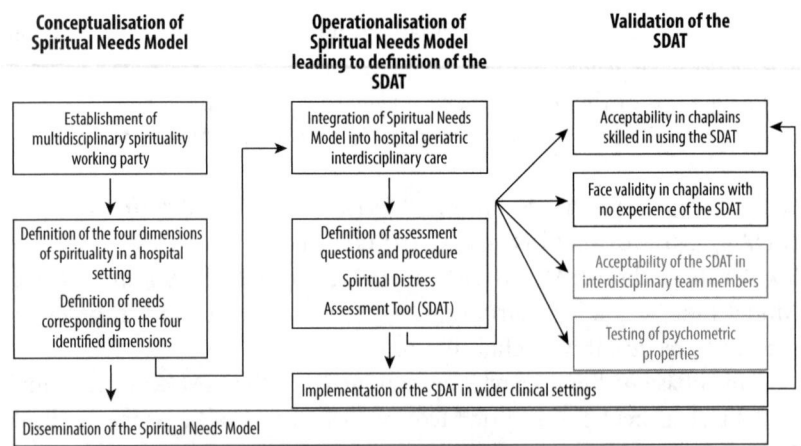

Figure 1: Process of SDAT development and assessment of face validity and acceptability of the SDAT

Table 1: Patients' characteristics

Characteristics	Population (N = 69)
Age (years)	82.5 ± 8.3
Women (%)	78.3
Living alone (%)	62.5
Cognitive impairment* (%)	30.4
Depressive symptoms †	12.1
Basic ADL at admission ¥	2.5 ± 1.6

* defined as a score < 24 at the Mini Mental State Examination (score ranging from 0 to 30, with higher scores indicating better cognition).

† defined as a score ≥ 6 at the 15-item Geriatric Depression Scale (score ranging from 0 to 15, with higher scores indicating more depressive symptoms).

¥ Katz's basic Activities of Daily Living (score ranging from 0 to 6, with higher score indicating better function).

c) Assessment of the face validity and acceptability of the SDAT

It was considered important to assess the validity of the SDAT. However, as no consensus exists regarding the definition of spirituality and the dimensions that characterize spirituality, no real "definitional standard" could be said to exist.[33] Thus, true assessment of the content validity of the SDAT against a gold standard would not have been possible. However, face validity, considered as being a particular type of content validity, was assessed. Face validity refers to whether persons not involved in the development of an instrument perceive it as measuring what it is deemed to measure. In this case, we established whether hospital chaplains experienced in hospital pastoral care, who had not been in any way involved in the development or use of the SDAT, perceived the instrument as able to measure a patient's spirituality.

Face validity of the SDAT in chaplains with no experience of the SDAT, but experienced in providing hospital pastoral care

In order to assess these characteristics, a moderated structured discussion group was conducted with chaplains practising at the chaplaincy of the University of Lausanne Medical Center (see Appendix) who were unfamiliar both with the Spiritual Needs Model and with the SDAT. Of the six chaplains invited, four protestant chaplains accepted the invitation, one declined and one catholic chaplain was not available. Participants were invited to watch a video of a pastoral interview using the SDAT and subsequently participated in a moderated discussion lasting two hours. Chaplains were asked to compare the interview with their own way of conducting a first pastoral encounter with a patient, to determine whether all dimensions of a patient's spirituality were addressed in the SDAT interview and to express their view on the structured approach used to assess a patient's spirituality in the hospital setting.

ACCEPTABILITY OF THE SDAT IN CHAPLAINS ALREADY SKILLED IN USING THE SDAT

Assessment of *acceptability* is commonly made in health services research with a view to determining the potential impact of proposed services, since services can only be effective if delivered and taken-up as intended. It is therefore important during implementation to assess acceptability in both service providers and service users.

As the SDAT was specially designed to be used by chaplains, the acceptability of the SDAT was assessed in members of the chaplaincy of the University of Lausanne Medical Center who were already trained in use of the instrument. In this case, the aim was to ascertain to what extent these chaplains perceived the instrument as relevant to their work and to what extent they considered its use feasible within the hospital setting.

Assessment of acceptability of the SDAT's use in other interdisciplinary team members (medical and paramedical) has also been performed and is to be published separately.

All four chaplains skilled in application of the SDAT, and working in different hospital departments, participated in two structured, moderated group discussions, each lasting two hours. Topics covered included: methods and level of appropriation of the SDAT by the chaplains; acceptability of the sets of questions proposed for the patient's interview; definition of skills necessary to identify and score unmet spiritual needs.

Results

a) Conceptualisation of spirituality and spiritual needs in hospitalised persons: definition of the Spiritual Needs Model (Table 2)

Overall, spirituality in the hospitalised elderly person was defined as the particular coherence expressed when describing one's meaning of life, referring to one's transcendence and explaining one's values.

Spirituality, in the particular context of hospital setting, was defined as a multidimensional concept that includes four dimensions considered to be interrelated: *Meaning, Transcendence, Values* and *Psycho-social Identity*.

The *Meaning* dimension was defined as that which provides orientation to an individual's life and promotes his or her overall life balance.

The *Transcendence* dimension was defined as an anchor point exterior to the person; the relationship with an external foundation that provides a sense of grounding.

The *Values* dimension was defined as the system of values that determines goodness and trueness for the person, as made apparent in his or her actions and life choices.

The *Psycho-social Identity* dimension was defined as the patient's environment; those elements, such as society, caregivers, family, and close relationships that together make up a person's singular identity.

In hospital care, the patient's medical, psychological and social needs are systematically defined, assessed and addressed. The same approach has therefore been applied regarding the patient's spiritual needs. Needs corresponding to each dimension of spirituality were thus defined.

The four defined dimensions of spirituality and their corresponding needs are summarized in Table 2.

b) Definition of the SDAT (Additional file 1: Table S1)

Using the Spiritual Needs Model, a set of questions was developed to facilitate investigation of the patient's needs (Additional file 1: Table S1). These questions serve as prompts to be used only if the patient does not spontaneously mention anything related to the investigated need.

Guidelines for administering the SDAT

The SDAT is administered according to the following procedure:

First, in order to identify unmet spiritual needs, a 20–30-minute semi-structured interview is conducted by the chaplain with the patient after having obtained his/her *consent*.

Second, immediately following the interview, the chaplain conducts an assessment of how the patient spoke about his or her five spiritual needs, using the analytical framework to determine the eventual presence of spiritual distress.

Third, needs are scored on a four-point Likert scale ranging from 0 (no unmet spiritual need) to 3 (severe unmet spiritual need). A global score of spiritual distress may therefore range from 0 (no spiritual distress) to 15 (severe spiritual distress). Examples of statements made by patients experiencing unmet needs are provided in Table 3.

At the end of the interview, the chaplain tells the patient precisely what information he or she intends to relay to the interdisciplinary team members, and requests the patient's consent to proceed. When presenting results of spiritual assessments to the team, special attention is taken to avoid unnecessarily sharing intimate information and to ensure *confidentiality*.

Table 2: Spiritual Needs Model: dimensions of spirituality and corresponding needs in hospitalized patients

Dimension of spirituality	Definition of dimension	Needs associated with dimension
Meaning	The dimension that provides orientation to an individual's life and promotes his or her overall life balance.	**The Need for life balance:** The need to rebuild a new life balance and the need to learn how to better cope with illness or disability.
Transcendence	An anchor point exterior to the person; the relationship with an external foundation that provides a sense of grounding. The group considered that everyone has an external foundation, even if different from God. For example, for some people, this transcendence might be found in nature, beauty, or art.	**The Need for connection:** The need for connection with his or her existential foundation and the need for Beauty (aesthetic sense).
Values	The system of values that determines goodness and trueness for the person; it is made apparent in the person's actions and life choices.	***The Need for values acknowledgement:** The need that health professionals know and respect one's values. ***The Need to maintain control:** The need to understand and to feel included in decision-making processes and to be associated with health professionals' decisions and actions.
Psycho-social Identity	The patient's environment; those elements, such as society, caregivers, family, and close relationships that together make up the person's singular identity.	**The Need to maintain identity:** The need to be loved, to be heard, to be recognized, to be in touch, to have a positive image of oneself and to feel forgiven.

*According to the hospital setting, two different needs were clearly distinguished to translate the values dimension.

c) Assessment of the face validity and acceptability of the SDAT

FACE VALIDITY OF THE SDAT IN CHAPLAINS WITH NO EXPERIENCE OF THE SDAT, BUT EXPERIENCED IN HOSPITAL PASTORAL CARE
Chaplains reported overall positive appraisal of the SDAT.

The *Meaning*, *Transcendence* and *Psycho-social Identity* dimensions were clearly acknowledged by this group. The *Values* dimension and, in particular, its related needs (need to maintain control; need for values acknowledgement) were more debated. The group mostly acknowledged that chaplains do not systematically address this dimension unless they perceive some discomfort around these issues for the patient. Nevertheless, they generally agreed that this dimension was part of the patient's spirituality, as it reflects the patient's need to make meaningful life choices. Some chaplains also commented that certain aspects of religiosity, such as connection with the faith community and the need for ritual, should have been more clearly assessed in the video interview. They considered that these aspects should not simply be subsumed under the *Transcendence* dimension, but viewed as an additional dimension.

Their appraisal of the structured format for spiritual assessment differed from that of the group of chaplains skilled in using the SDAT (see below). They raised the question of the overall goal of a pastoral interview; for most, it is to engage with the patient and not to assess or to evaluate disturbance in their spiritual health. They argued that a spiritual interview should be tailor-made for each patient, and should, therefore, be less directive or restrictive than the SDAT. Some reluctance was expressed about using a structured format, as this seemed to imply that spirituality could be reduced to an assessment instrument. They perceived a risk of "medicalising"[34, 35] spirituality and limiting its assessment to a health perspective. Nevertheless, it was agreed that the structured format of the SDAT would be of use when integrating pastoral care into health care and could help chaplains synthesise their evaluation and transmit meaningful information to health professionals. The group also agreed that a structured format could stimulate the assessment of dimensions that are not systematically addressed by chaplains, such as the *Values* dimension.

ACCEPTABILITY OF THE SDAT IN CHAPLAINS ALREADY SKILLED IN USING THE SDAT

Overall, the SDAT was perceived by the chaplains as a useful adjunct to their pastoral interviews. They reported that the instrument allowed for more precise assessment of patients' spiritual needs. They also reported that the SDAT facilitated the communication of their observations to health professionals, and helped them clarify their potential role as well as their own implication in patient care. The structured format of the SDAT emerged as both an advantage (more efficient use of time, better organisation of the interview, systematic investigation of the four dimensions) and a disadvantage (restricts the flexibility of the interview, conveys the impression that spirituality can be "put in a box"). The group related that they tended to use the SDAT when asked by health professionals to visit a patient, the instrument allowing for a better synopsis and transfer of relevant information.

The set of standardised SDAT questions for the patient's interview was considered as acceptable and appropriate by the group. Chaplains felt comfortable enough with the instrument to consider potential useful applications in other settings or with younger patients (assuming that additional questions such as how they saw their future in terms of work, family life, or children were used).

Chaplains considered that it was not difficult to identify unmet spiritual needs during the patient interview. In contrast, assessing the *severity* of unmet spiritual needs proved more problematic. In particular, they pointed to the issue of adequately distinguishing between the severity of unmet spiritual needs and the availability of resources to cope with these needs. A patient with a severe unmet need for life balance may either be with or without resources to face this unmet need (e.g., he may or not have a good social network). The chaplains noted that when coping resources were absent, they tended to score more highly on the level of spiritual distress than when these resources were present.

Numerous skills necessary to use the SDAT were outlined by the group, the most important being good communication skills, such as the ability to build a meaningful relationship with the patient before going ahead with the semi-structured interview, and having empathetic listening skills. A second group of required skills was more related to knowledge, such as familiarity with the four spiritual dimensions and their related spiritual needs, and theological and pastoral skills. A third group of skills included the capacity to analyse and synthesise the interview, and, a fourth group, the capacity to transmit relevant information to other team members.

Table 3: Examples of statements made by patients experiencing unmet needs

Need for life balance	"I know I've got to find a way to cope, but I just can't manage. I just don't have the strength any longer."
Need for connection	"I think that God has abandoned me." "I am no longer able to paint and it was the painting that kept me in touch with the force that kept me going."
Need for values acknowledgement	"I'm just a number here. The staff don't know who I am."
Need to maintain control	"I don't know what I'm doing here in the hospital. Why hasn't anyone given me any medicine?"
Need to maintain identity	"My friends don't come and visit me; my family has no idea of what I'm going through here; I just don't know myself any longer."

Discussion

This paper presents in detail the different steps in the development of an instrument aimed to assess spiritual distress in hospitalised older persons.

Overall, results show that the proposed conceptualisation of spirituality in hospitalised elderly patients as defined in the Spiritual Needs Model and the corresponding assessment instrument (SDAT) have face validity in chaplains providing hospital pastoral care and prove acceptable to those experienced in their application. Furthermore, chaplains did not report a feeling of confusion with psychological assessment, a criticism sometimes made of other spirituality constructs.[39] Certain reservations were, however, expressed.

Some chaplains felt that the definition of the different dimensions was somewhat unusual. The *Meaning* dimension is widely recognised as central components of spirituality.[37, 38] In the literature, *Meaning* generally refers to the finding of a global meaning to life and death, and is generally associated with purpose in life.[3] Elderly patients often mention that because of their "old age," they have no purpose in life, but still see meaning in life. Thus, the definition of *Meaning* given in the Spiritual Needs Model refers to what provides orientation to an individual's life and promotes his or her overall life balance, rather than to definitions of the individual's new projects. Special attention was also given to the *Values* dimension. This dimension is less frequently identified as a specific dimension of spirituality. However, this dimension was warranted by the importance of recognising each patient's personal values so as to ensure respect for the patient's autonomy, dignity and integrity.[39, 40] This was considered especially important in the hospital setting, given the vulnerability of elderly patients in this respect.

Second, some chaplains would have attributed a stronger, more explicit, place to religious practice, considering, for example, that rituals should be viewed as an additional spirituality dimension. Third, an additional important reservation concerned the *raison d'être* of pastoral hospital work: several chaplains expressed their concern that pastoral care could become medicalised and then be seen as a simple adjunct to health care. These reservations will need to be adequately addressed when attempting to further integrate spirituality assessment and management into routine care.

Interestingly, chaplains did not challenge our initial assumption that spiritual distress results from unmet spiritual needs. In fact, chaplains commonly recognized that the most promising way to integrate spirituality into health care is to be consistent with the other care processes established by the interdisciplinary team and the established institutional policy. This approach implies that the same approach be applied to spiritual needs as to bio-psycho-social needs. It seemed therefore rational to define spiritual distress as unmet needs.

Although not formally assessed, information obtained from patient contact during the development process indicates the feasibility and acceptability to patients of a systematic and structured bedside assessment of their spirituality. Also, the chaplain's participation in weekly interdisciplinary team meetings to share the results of his assessment has demonstrated the feasibility of integrating spirituality assessment into routine interdisciplinary geriatric care. A survey enquiring about interdisciplinary team members' appraisal of systematic spirituality assessment was conducted and showed that the contribution of the chaplain to improving patient care through weekly team meetings was considered essential.

It is, however, acknowledged that the feasibility and acceptability demonstrated is context-specific. Whether similar acceptance will be observed in other settings requires further study. This work was performed in a clinical setting already familiar with a comprehensive approach to patients' needs; these conditions may prove to be a prerequisite for successful integration of spirituality assessment and for the participation of chaplains in routine care. The Christian origin and advanced age of patients enrolled in this phase of the development probably facilitated the acceptability of the encounter with the chaplain. Further assessment of acceptability will therefore be needed in larger, more diverse, elderly populations.

Besides these acknowledged limitations, the present work also has several strengths. The SDAT was developed according to a rigorous structured process: spirituality in hospitalized older patients was conceptualized through a consensus process, and its dimensions and their corresponding needs were then specified. The model was subsequently implemented within a clinical setting in order to operationalize further the assessment process. This process, going from the definition of spirituality to the definition of an instrument to assess spirituality, has previously been adopted in the development of other spirituality assessment instruments (e.g. The spirituality Index of Well-Being[41]) and strengthens the relevance of the instrument. Finally, face validity and acceptability in experienced chaplains were assessed. Though relatively long and complex, this approach had the advantage of ensuring contextual relevance for the instrument since issues regarding implementation could be dealt with progressively and *in situ*.

Although the SDAT was developed specifically in a population of hospitalized elderly patients, chaplains working with different populations saw considerable potential for use in other settings and in other age groups. Our procedure of assessment (a semi-structured interview) enables the patient to speak about spirituality with his or her own words and from very different perspectives. This should ensure relevancy of the SDAT for every patient, whatever their age or religious or spiritual background. Ultimately, the quality and limitations of the SDAT will be judged by the sustainability and dissemination of its use: by other chaplains, in other Departments and institutions, in research and evaluation, and, ultimately, in different cultural and religious contexts. Furthermore, as previously mentioned, the instrument's use is conditional on the availability of staff experienced in interdisciplinary care and with access to appropriate training facilities.

As yet, very few instruments have been developed on the basis of a spiritual needs construct. Two instruments, coming from nursing research, have been identified.[31, 42] These two instruments were based on qualitative studies of patients who were asked to describe their specific spiritual needs. The approach presented here is unique because spiritual needs were assessed on the basis of a previously defined concept of spirituality. This structured approach ensures coherence between theoretical work and the investigative process.

Conclusions

These preliminary results suggest that the SDAT is an acceptable instrument to assess spiritual distress in hospitalised persons. The instrument provides a tool for communication between disciplines, based on a shared vocabulary, and provides a new basis for integrating spirituality into the patient's plan of care. Further research is underway to assess the SDAT's acceptability in a larger sample of elderly patients and to investigate its psychometric properties. These are necessary steps before its application in intervention studies; that is, before using the SDAT to assess the impact of spiritual distress on health outcomes and patient prognosis.

Appendix

The chaplaincy of the University of Lausanne Medical Center

This chaplaincy was created by the hospital management together with both the Catholic and Protestant churches and has responsibility for pastoral care within the hospital and for hospital pastoral training.

Chaplains work in all departments of the hospital, regardless of the patient's religious affiliation.

The chaplaincy is composed of 7 ordained chaplains (2 Catholic; 5 Protestant) and 5 lay chaplains (4 Catholic; 1 Protestant).

External chaplains from other religious affiliations (rabbis, imams, Greek orthodox priests) are solicited on patient request.

Additional material

Additional file 1: Table S1: Structure of the Spiritual Needs Model and the Spiritual Distress Assessment Tool.

Acknowledgements

Source of research support: Service of Geriatric Medicine and Geriatric Rehabilitation, University of Lausanne Medical Center (CHUV), CH-1010 Lausanne, Switzerland.

Authors' contributions

SM planned the study, supervised the development of the tool, supervised the validation procedure, and wrote the paper. ER conceptualized the tool, and helped write the paper. CB helped planned the study and contributed to revising the paper. GJ contributed to conceptualization of the tool and revising the paper. EM contributed to revising the paper. BS conceptualized the overall qualitative methodology, performed the validation and revised the manuscript.

All authors read and approved the final manuscript.

Competing interests

The authors declare that they have no competing interests.

References

1. Thoresen CE, Harris AHS: Spirituality and health: What's the evidence and what's needed? *Ann Behav Med* 2002, 24:3–13.
2. Miller WR, Thoresen CE: Spirituality, religion, and health: An emerging research field. *Am Psychol* 2003, 58:24–35.
3. Vachon M, Fillion L, Achille M: A conceptual analysis of spirituality at the end of life. *J Palliat Med* 2009, 12:53–59.
4. Sulmasy DP: A biopsychosocial–spiritual model for the care of patients at the end of life. *Gerontologist* 2002, 42 (Special Issue 3):24–33.

5. Monod S, Rochat E, Bula C: Is there a place for spirituality in the care of elderly patients? In *Religion and Psychology*. Edited by: Michael T Evans Walker, Emma D Walker. New York: Nova Publishers; 2009.
6. Koenig HG, Pargament KI, Nielsen J: Religious coping and health status in medically ill hospitalized older adults. *J Nerv Ment Dis* 1998, 186:513–521.
7. Kirby SE, Coleman PG, Daley D: Spirituality and Well-Being in Frail and Nonfrail Older Adults. *J Gerontol B Psychol Sci Soc Sci* 2004, 3:P123–P129.
8. Crowther MR, Parker MW, Achenbaum WA, Larimore WL, Koenig HG: Rowe and Kahn's model of successful aging revisited: positive spirituality – the forgotten factor. *Gerontologist* 2002, 42:613–620.
9. Krause N: Religious meaning and subjective well-being in late life. *J Gerontol B Psychol Sci Soc Sci* 2003, 3:S160–S170.
10. Idler EL, Kasl SV: Religion among disabled and nondisabled persons II: attendance at religious services as a predictor of the course of disability. *J Gerontol Soc Sci* 1997, 52(6):S306–S316.
11. Koenig HG, McCullough ME, Larson DB: *Handbook of Religion and Health*. New York: Oxford University Press; 2001.
12. Koenig HG, Larson DB, Larson SS: Religion and coping with serious medical illness. *Ann Pharmacother* 2001, 35:352–359.
13. Pargament KI, Koenig HG, Tarakeshwar N, Hahn J: Religious struggle as a predictor of mortality among medically ill elderly patients: a 2-year longitudinal study. *Arch Intern Med* 2001, 161(15):1881–1885.
14. Carpenito-Moyet: *Nursing Diagnosis: Application to Clinical Practice*. 10th edition. Philadelphia: Lippincott Williams & Wilkins; 2004.
15. McClain CS, Rosenfeld B, Breitbart W: Effect of spiritual well-being on end-of-life despair in terminally-ill cancer patients. *Lancet* 2003, 361:1603–1607.
16. Rodin G, Lo C, Mikulincer M, Donner A, Gagliese L, Zimmermann C: Pathways to distress: the multiple determinants of depression, hopelessness, and the desire for hastened death in metastatic cancer patients. *Soc Sci Med* 2009, 68:562–569.
17. Grant E, Murray SA, Kendall M, Boyd K, Tilley S, Ryan D: Spiritual issues and needs: perspectives from patients with advanced cancer and nonmalignant disease. A qualitative study. *Palliat Support Care* 2004, 2:371–378.
18. Monod S, Rochat E, Martin E, Bula C: Spiritual assessment in older patients undergoing post-acute rehabilitation: A pilot study. *Gerontologist* 2007, 47:S774.
19. Astrow AB, Wexler A, Texeira K, He MK, Sulmasy DP: Is failure to meet spiritual needs associated with cancer patients' perceptions of quality of care and their satisfaction with care? *J Clin Oncol* 2007, 25:5753–5757.
20. Hills J, Paice JA, Cameron JR, Shott S: Spirituality and distress in palliative care consultation. *J Palliat Med* 2005, 8:782–788.
21. Miller DK, Chibnall JT, Videen SD, Duckro PN: Supportive-Affective Group Experience for persons with life-threatening illness: reducing spiritual, psychological, and death-related distress in dying patients. *J Palliat Med* 2005, 8:333–343.
22. Tarakeshwar N, Pearce MJ, Sikkema KJ: Development and implementation of a spiritual coping group intervention for adults living with HIV/AIDS: A pilot study. *Mental Health, Religion & Culture* 2005, 8:179–190.
23. Moberg DO: Assessing and measuring spirituality: Confronting dilemmas of universal and particular evaluative criteria. *J Adult Dev* 2002, 9:47–60.
24. Sloan RP, Bagiella E, VandeCreek L, Hover M, Casalone C, Jinpu HT, et al.: Should physicians prescribe religious activities? *N Engl J Med* 2000, 342(25):1913–1916.
25. Vivat B: Measures of spiritual issues for palliative care patients: a literature review. *Palliat Med* 2008, 22:859–868.
26. Sinclair S, Pereira J, Raffin S: A thematic review of the spirituality literature within palliative care. *J Palliat Med* 2006, 9:464–479.

27. Mularski RA, Dy SM, Shugarman LR, Wilkinson AM, Lynn J, Shekelle PG, et al.: A systematic review of measures of end-of-life care and its outcomes. *Health Serv Res* 2007, 42:1848–1870.
28. Stefanek M, McDonald PG, Hess SA: Religion, spirituality and cancer: current status and methodological challenges. *Psycho-Oncology* 2005, 14:450–463.
29. Brady MJ, Peterman AH, Fitchett G, Mo M, Cella D: A case for including spirituality in quality of life measurement in oncology. *Psycho-Oncology* 1999, 8:417–428.
30. Ellison CW: Spiritual well-being: Conceptualization and measurement. *J Psychol Theol* 1983, 11:330–340.
31. Taylor EJ: Prevalence and associated factors of spiritual needs among patients with cancer and family caregivers. *Oncol Nurs Forum* 2006, 33:729–735.
32. Brennan M, Heiser D: Introduction: Spiritual Assessment and Intervention: Current Directions and Applications. *J Religion Spirituality Aging* 2004, 17:1–20.
33. Monod S, Rochat E, Bula C, Spencer B: The Spiritual Needs Model: Spirituality Assessment in the Geriatric Hospital Setting. *J Religion Spirituality Aging* 2010, 22:271–282.
34. Stewart AL: Psychometric Considerations in Functional Status Instruments. In *Functional Status Measurement in Primary Care.* Edited by: Wonca Classification Committee. New York: Springer-Verlag; 1990:3–26.
35. Anastasi A: *Psychological Testing.* Toronto, Canada: The Macmillan Company; 1968.
36. Monod S, Rochat E, Martin E, Bula C: Spirituality in post-acute rehabilitation: Appraisal by interdisciplinary team members. *J Am Gerioatr Soc* 2008, 56(S4):S110.
37. Illich I: The medicalization of life. *J Med Ethics* 1975, 1:73–77.
38. Conrad P: *The Medicalization of Society: On the Transformation of Human Conditions into Treatable Disorders.* Baltimore, MD, US: Johns Hopkins University Press; 2007.
39. Moreira-Almeida A, Koenig HG: Retaining the meaning of the words religiousness and spirituality: a commentary on the WHOQOL SRPB group's "a cross-cultural study of spirituality, religion, and personal beliefs as components of quality of life". *Soc Sci Med* 2006, 63:843–845.
40. Koenig HG, Larson DB, Matthews DA: Religion and psychotherapy with older adults. *J Geriatr Psychiatr* 1996, 29:155–184.
41. Blazer D: Spirituality and aging well. *Generations: J Am Soc Aging* 1991, 15:61–65.
42. Kemp P, Rendtorff JD, Mattsson N: *Bioethics and Biolaw* Vols 1 and 2. Copenhague: Rhodos 2000.
43. Muldoon M, King N: Spirituality, health care, and bioethics. *Journal of Religion & Health* 1995, 34:329–349.
44. Daaleman TP, Kuckelman CA, Frey BB: Spirituality and well-being: an exploratory study of the patient perspective. *Soc Sci Med* 2001, 53:1503–1511.
45. Daaleman TP, Frey BB, Wallace D, Studenski S: The Spirituality Index of Well-Being: Development and testing of a new measure. *J Fam Pract* 2002, 51(11):952.
46. Hermann C: Development and testing of the spiritual needs inventory for patients near the end of life. *Oncol Nurs Forum* 2006, 33:737–744.

Pre-publication history

The pre-publication history for this paper can be accessed here:
http://www.biomedcentral.com/1471-2318/10/88/prepub
doi:10.1186/1471-2318-10-88
Cite this article as: Monod et al.: The spiritual distress assessment tool: an instrument to assess spiritual distress in hospitalised elderly persons. BMC Geriatrics 2010 10:88.

Additional file 1: Table S1: Structure of the Spiritual Needs Model and the Spiritual Distress Assessment Tool

SPIRITUAL NEEDS MODEL		SPIRITUAL DISTRESS ASSESSMENT TOOL (SDAT)		
		PATIENT INTERVIEW	INTERVIEW ANALYSIS	
Spiritual dimension	Need associated with the spiritual dimension	Set of questions for patient interview	Questions for analysing the interview and identifying unmet spiritual need	Scoring of unmet spiritual need (range from 0 to 3*)
MEANING Overall life balance	**NEED FOR LIFE BALANCE** • need to maintain and/or rebuild an overall life balance • need to learn to "live with" an illness or disability	Does your hospitalisation have any repercussions on the way you live usually? Is your overall life balance disturbed by what is happening to you now (hospitalisation, illness)? Are you having difficulties coping with what is happening to you now (hospitalisation, illness)?	How does the patient speak about his or her need for life balance? Is the overall life balance of this patient disturbed?	To what degree does the *Need for Life Balance* remain unmet? ☐ 0 ☐ 1 ☐ 2 ☐ 3
TRANSCENDENCE Anchor point exterior to the person	**NEED FOR CONNECTION** • need for Beauty • need to be connected with the personal existential anchor	Do you have a religion, a particular faith or spirituality? Does what is happening to you now change your relationship to God /or to your spirituality? (closer to God, more distant, no change) Is your religion / spirituality / faith challenged by what is happening to you now? Does what is happening to you now change or disturb the way you live or express your faith / spirituality / religion?	How does the patient speak about his or her need for connection? Is his or her need for connection disturbed?	To what degree does the Need for Connection remain unmet? ☐ 0 ☐ 1 ☐ 2 ☐ 3

cont.

SPIRITUAL NEEDS MODEL		SPIRITUAL DISTRESS ASSESSMENT TOOL (SDAT)		
		PATIENT INTERVIEW	INTERVIEW ANALYSIS	
Spiritual dimension	Need associated with the spiritual dimension	Set of questions for patient interview	Questions for analysing the interview and identifying unmet spiritual need	Scoring of unmet spiritual need (range from 0 to 3*)
VALUES System of values that determine goodness and trueness for the person; the system is made apparent in the person's actions and life choices	**NEED FOR VALUES ACKNOWLEDGEMENT** • need that caregivers understand what has value and significance in his or her life **NEED TO MAINTAIN CONTROL** • need to understand and be involved in caregivers' decisions and actions	Do you think that the health professionals caring for you know you well enough? Do you have enough information about your health problem, and on the goals of your hospitalisation and treatment? Do you feel that you are participating in the decisions made about your care? How would you describe your relationship with the doctors and other health professionals?	How does the patient speak of his or her need that caregivers understand what has value and significance in his or her life? How does the patient speak of his or her need to understand and be involved in caregivers' decisions and actions?	To what degree does the *Need for Values Acknowledgement* remain unmet? ☐ 0 ☐ 1 ☐ 2 ☐ 3 To what degree does the *Need to Maintain Control* remain unmet? ☐ 0 ☐ 1 ☐ 2 ☐ 3
PSYCHO-SOCIAL IDENTITY The environment (society, caregivers, family, close relations) that maintain the person's particular identity.	**NEED TO MAINTAIN IDENTITY** • need to be loved, to be recognised • need to be listened to • need to be in contact (in particular with the person's faith community and other people) • need to have a positive self-image • need to feel forgiven, to be reconciled	Do you have any worries or difficulties regarding your family or other persons close to you? How do people close to behave with you now? Does it correspond with what you expected from them? Do you feel lonely? Could you tell me about the image you have of yourself in your current situation (illness, hospitalisation)? Do you have any links with your faith community?	How does the patient speak of his or her need to maintain identity?	To what degree does the Need to Maintain Identity remain unmet? ☐ 0 ☐ 1 ☐ 2 ☐ 3

* **0** = no evidence of unmet spiritual need; **1** = some evidence of unmet spiritual need; **2** = substantial evidence of unmet spiritual need; **3** = evidence of severe unmet spiritual need

SECTION 2

PATIENT/FAMILY SPIRITUAL NEEDS AND SPIRITUAL CARE INTERESTS

Introduction

An important area of chaplaincy research focuses on the religious/spiritual needs of patients and families and their interest in and perceptions about spiritual care services. The studies included in Section 2, like the articles in Section 1, fall into the research categories of chaplaincy process and chaplaincy outcomes. The first article in this section, by Nuzum, Meaney, and O'Donoghue (2017), describes the spiritual pain of bereaved parents who experienced stillbirth. The theme of religious and spiritual coping is also central to the study by Ragsdale et al. (2014) of adolescents and young adults (AYAs) undergoing hematopoietic stem cell transplant. The third study in Section 2 (Grossoehme et al. 2016) also focuses on adolescents. The authors of this study described the relationship between spiritual coping and a specific outcome – that of increased airway clearance treatment adherence of youth with cystic fibrosis.

The next three articles in Section 2 examine the perceptions about chaplains of different groups of patients and families. Donohue et al. (2017) were interested in how parents of hospitalized children perceived chaplaincy services. Raffay, Wood, and Todd (2016) explored the preferences for spiritual care within the seldom researched population of people receiving psychiatric care. These two articles are from US and UK contexts respectively, while the sixth article in this section of the *Reader*, by Schultz, Lulav-Grinwald, and Bar-Sela (2014) comes from Israel, where the team asked oncology patients about their interest in spiritual care. The final article in Section 2, by Hui et al. (2011), also focuses on cancer patients but in an acute palliative care unit in the US, describing the prevalence and correlates of chaplains' assessments of spiritual distress.

The articles in Section 2 illustrate some overlapping themes that inform an evidence-based approach to chaplaincy care. For instance, chaplain research can clarify the role of religion and spirituality for people living with specific health issues. Raffay et al. (2016) studied this theme for mental health service users, while Ragsdale et al. (2014) considered the role of religion and spirituality for AYAs coping with hematopoietic stem cell transplants.

Chaplains also use research to learn how recipients of care evaluate their services and their suggestions for improving them. This theme was taken up by the Donohue team (2017) who investigated whether parents saw chaplains as members of the healthcare team and whether it was better if chaplains were at least somewhat autonomous from that team. The participants in the Raffay et al. study (2016) also described the pros and cons of the chaplain being part of the team.

Another important theme in Section 2 is describing the unique experiences of specific populations across the life course. The articles by Hui et al. (2011) and Schultz, Lulav-Grinwald and Bar-Sela (2014) focused on the experiences of oncology patients. The studies by Grossoehme et al. (2016) and Ragsdale et al. (2014) examined religious/spiritual coping with illnesses faced by adolescents, cystic fibrosis and blood and marrow transplant respectively. The issue of treatment adherence was central in Grossoehme et al.'s article (2016). Those with cystic fibrosis (CF) experienced the challenges of coping with a chronic disease and with carrying through on daily treatment. This study looked at the role of spirituality among 11–19-year-olds diagnosed with CF, while the participants in Ragsdale et al.'s study (2014) ranged in age from 15 to 28.

The issue of spiritual distress is a shared theme in both Nuzum et al. (2017) and Schultz et al. (2014). Their work points to the importance of building chaplain capacity to identify the presence and intensity of spiritual distress.

We were struck by the similarity of spiritual themes expressed by the parents in Nuzum et al.'s study (2017) and by those articulated by the AYAs in Ragsdale et al.'s article (2014). While there seem to be spiritual experiences and theological reflections unique to populations and diagnoses, participants in both these studies sought meaning, asking why, and using faith practices to find comfort and hope. Exploration of such similarities is part of the future research agenda as chaplains seek to identify best practices for the profession.

Diverse research designs help to improve chaplaincy care. For instance, Ragsdale et al.'s (2014) use of grounded theory is both similar to and different from Nuzum et al.'s (2017) use of the phenomenological method. Both are qualitative approaches, but each has a different goal for the data. Grounded theory is often used as a first step when very little is known on a given topic or population. It is a helpful model for developing theory. A phenomenological approach is used to better understand the subjective meaning-making processes of people facing significant life challenges. Both approaches are useful ways to collect rich data about topics such as the religious/spiritual issues associated with illness or loss.

Each of the articles in Section 2 make important contributions to chaplaincy by helping us consider the unique experiences and perceptions of patients and families with specific illnesses. Their findings have implications for how chaplains assess diverse spiritual and religious needs and develop care plans that address specific outcomes for their patients. We hope you find information from these articles directly applicable to your work with your patient populations.

Article 7: Nuzum, D., Meaney, S., and O'Donoghue, K. (2017) The Spiritual and Theological Challenges of Stillbirth for Bereaved Parents

The article by Nuzum, Meaney, and O'Donoghue (2017) provides compelling evidence that perinatal bereavement is associated with intense spiritual pain and unmet spiritual needs. This qualitative study focused on the spiritual and theological struggles of bereaved parents who experienced stillbirth. While several quantitative studies have noted the potential for spiritual distress caused by perinatal death, the few earlier qualitative studies on pregnancy loss documented the importance of pastoral and ritual care in the midst of that experience (Kelly 2007 and Newitt 2014).

Nuzum and team studied the spiritual struggle of bereaved parents through interpretive phenomenological analysis (IPA). IPA is a useful approach for researchers interested in examining highly sensitive topics, such as spiritual distress in the midst of stillbirth. IPA seeks to gain in-depth empathic understanding of how a person in a particular context makes sense of life events or relationships. The semi-structured interviews provided the flexibility to invite parents to talk at length about their spiritual needs and the care they received. The authors made a strong recommendation for well-trained chaplains to be part of the perinatal bereavement care team.

A clinical pastoral education (CPE) supervisor in Ireland, Nuzum also completed research on the impact of stillbirth on chaplains (Nuzum, Meaney, and O'Donoghue 2015 and 2016a) and obstetricians and their faith (Nuzum, Meaney, and O'Donoghue 2016b). He contributed to new national standards for bereavement care following pregnancy loss and perinatal death in Ireland (National Standards for Bereavement Care 2015).

A few limitations of this article (Article 7) are worth noting. The authors tell us very little about their sample and methods. Details of who agreed to be interviewed (e.g., parents' age, other children, time since loss) would provide helpful background information for interpreting their findings. Additionally, the report could have included their interview questions and a description of how the interview transcripts were coded.

Given their findings—that care provided to bereaved parents can shape their grieving process—further research is indicated. A longitudinal study that interviewed the parents annually for five years would help us understand their ongoing spiritual and theological needs and any changes to such needs. Alternatively, researchers could retrospectively interview parents and enquire about their spiritual pain and any changes they had experienced over time (see Bradshaw and Fitchett 2003 for an example of a retrospective approach). This approach has possible limitations, such as selection and recall biases. However, a retrospective design is less expensive than a longitudinal study and is, therefore, more feasible; it is a helpful place to begin to engage the question of change over time.

We also wondered about using research to understand spiritual needs throughout the course of pregnancy. Given how life-altering pregnancy can be for parents—whether it involves complications or not—there may be important roles for chaplains throughout the pregnancy, birth, and early infancy experiences. Research is needed to assess the types of spiritual needs parents face along this continuum and possible variations across different populations.

What is the role of culture in shaping the faith and spiritual pain described by this sample of parents in Ireland? If replicated in the US, Canada, or a more secular European nation such as the Netherlands, what would research reveal? And what about different family configurations—for example, single or same-gender parents—or those for whom pregnancy was unplanned or traumatic, as in the case of rape, or protracted illness of the fetus or birth mother? How might spiritual needs differ among these populations, and what are the implications of any possible differences for chaplaincy care?

Article 8: Ragsdale, J.R., Hegner, M.A., Mueller, M., and Davies, S. (2014) Identifying Religious and/or Spiritual Perspectives of Adolescents and Young Adults Receiving Blood and Marrow Transplants: A Prospective Qualitative Study

One of the unique aspects of this paper by Ragsdale and her team (2014) is that their findings led them to rethink their approach to routine spiritual care with adolescents and young adults (AYAs) who were undergoing hematopoietic stem cell transplants (HSCT). Reflecting on their interviews with the study participants, the team realized they were unaware of the importance of religion and spirituality for the AYAs coping with HSCT. They concluded that chaplains not only needed to provide emotional support to AYAs with this diagnosis but also needed to initiate conversations with them about the role their faith played in supporting them through their diagnosis and treatment. The study findings also led the investigators to recommend that the medical team routinely assess the religious and spiritual resources and concerns of these patients.

It is helpful to put this paper in the context of research about religion/spirituality and coping with illness and other crises. Thirty years ago, little research about this topic existed, but since then there has been dramatic growth in this research. Nonetheless, there still is a need for additional research about how people with specific types of illness or loss use religion/spirituality to cope with their experiences and especially for research about any variations in that coping for important subgroups of people (e.g., age, gender, race/ethnicity, religion). Along with the papers by Nuzum et al. (2017) and Raffay et al. (2016), this article by Ragsdale and colleagues (2014) demonstrates how qualitative research can be used to expand our understanding of how patients or families—in this case, AYAs facing HSCT—make meaning and cope with their illnesses.

This paper comes from investigators at Cincinnati Children's Hospital and Medical Center, where Daniel Grossoehme also works. The department is a leader in spiritual care research, especially in pediatrics. Judy Ragsdale, the first author of this article, is a Certified Educator (ACPE) and an experienced qualitative researcher whose work has focused on the education and certification of CPE educators (Ragsdale et al. 2012 and Ragsdale et al. 2016).

Does this article reflect the paradigm shift we have been describing in this *Reader*, that is, from chaplains relying mainly on a ministry of presence to a more intentional assessment of religious/spiritual needs? To be sure about this, it would have been helpful if the authors had outlined what they meant by "routine spiritual care" and described what specific strategies they recommend to facilitate discussion about religious/spiritual concerns with these AYAs. Does "routine spiritual care" mean ministry of presence?

We recommend this study as a useful model to explore the religious and spiritual needs or issues experienced by patients or families who are coping with any illness or loss. The authors used grounded theory, which is a strong qualitative approach for deriving in-depth preliminary data on a previously unexplored subject. They also relied on information from two points in time that allowed observations about changes over time in the role of religion/spirituality in coping with illness. Some chaplains worry that asking patients to participate in research imposes a burden. In contrast, several of the patients in this study reported appreciating the interview because it gave them time to think and talk about their faith. The question of whether participation in research can be a chaplaincy intervention is examined further in an article by Grossoehme (2011). Areas for future research include whether some AYAs experience ongoing struggles with religion and spirituality and what factors predict that trajectory.

Article 9: Grossoehme, D.H., Szczesniak, R.D., Mrug, S., Dimitriou, S.M., Marshall, A., and McPhail, G.L. (2016) Adolescents' Spirituality and Cystic Fibrosis Airway Clearance Treatment Adherence: Examining Mediators

Daniel Grossoehme, the lead author for this study, is a nationally recognized chaplaincy researcher from Cincinnati Children's Hospital and Medical Center. His research about the role of religion/spirituality in parents coping with a child diagnosed with cystic fibrosis (CF) and in adolescents coping with CF has been funded by the US National Institutes of Health.

This article explored whether and how adolescent religious/spiritual beliefs and coping may be associated with adherence to recommended airway clearance (AC) among adolescents with CF. Adherence to recommended treatment for adolescents and adults with chronic illnesses plays an important role in the progression of many illnesses as well as quality of life, yet adherence is often less than optimal. This study is important because it tests whether religious/spiritual beliefs and coping may be associated with this important health outcome. One of the strengths of the paper is integrating specific religious/spiritual beliefs and coping in a well-established model of health behavior, the Theory of Reasoned Action (TRA).

The team found significant pathways from religious/spiritual beliefs and coping to adherence to prescribed AC activities. Specifically, adolescents with "engaged spirituality" were more likely to perceive the value of AC activities and to perceive that their AC efforts were supported by their close friends. Both of these were linked to greater treatment adherence. However, spiritual struggle was associated with lower perceived value of AC and with lower treatment adherence. The findings point to the possibility that chaplaincy interventions with adolescents with CF, especially interventions that address spiritual struggle, may affect their adherence to this important health behavior.

Replication of a study, often with some modifications, is important in building a body of informative research. What do you think we would find if we explored whether an adolescent's developmental stage influenced the association between religious/spiritual beliefs and perceived treatment utility and peer norms? Do you think these associations vary with disease intensity? Would we see similar findings in adolescents with other chronic conditions such as childhood diabetes, a growing diagnosis in the US, or leukemia or lymphoma?

Article 10: Donohue, P.K., Norvell, M., Boss, R.D, Shepard, J., Frank, K., Patron, C., and Crowe, T.Y (2017) Hospital Chaplains: Through the Eyes of Parents of Hospitalized Children

What do patients and families know about chaplains—who we are and what we do? Some existing research suggests that potential recipients of chaplaincy care do not have a very clear or positive image of chaplains (Kelly 2007). Donohue et al. (2017), a multidisciplinary team of researchers from Johns Hopkins Hospital in Baltimore, Maryland, United States, conducted a survey to get feedback from parents who had received care from a chaplain.

The authors surveyed families of hospitalized children to see whether they considered chaplains to be part of the medical team, what their perceptions were of the roles chaplains play in providing care, how they view unsolicited visits by chaplains, and whether satisfaction with chaplains influenced satisfaction with their hospital experience. The majority of parents saw positive benefits of chaplain visits as part of the overall care they received, regardless of their religiosity. You may wish to compare their findings about chaplaincy care and parents' satisfaction with their child's hospitalization with the findings in Article 14 (Marin et al. 2015).

One of the reasons we selected this article is because these researchers were seeking information to guide their future practice. However, the low response rate (29%) and other characteristics of the sample (mostly religious mothers of children who had been seriously ill) point to selection bias. Selection bias, a component of external validity, occurs when the study sample does not represent the population from which it is drawn (in this case, parents of any child who had been hospitalized in 2013 who had received a chaplain visit). Because we do not have information from those who did not participate, the ability to generalize from those who did participate is limited.

If we want the views of a more representative sample of parents, how can we design future studies that reduce the problem of selection bias?

In a large enough study, we could also examine whether different subgroups of parents had different views about chaplaincy care. What are your hypotheses about any differences in views regarding chaplaincy care among parents who were more or less religiously involved? And among parents whose children had more or less serious illnesses than those described in this study?

Article 11: Raffay, J., Wood, E., and Todd, A. (2016) Service User Views of Spiritual and Pastoral (Chaplaincy) in NHS Mental Health Services: A Co-Produced Constructivist Grounded Theory Investigation

Julian Raffay, a researcher, chaplain, and the first author of this study, led this effort within mental health chaplaincy, an area where there has been limited research. He and his colleagues studied the Spiritual and Pastoral Care Services (SPC) being provided through the Mersey Care NHS Foundation Trust in Liverpool, England. The authors recognize the importance of research to identify specific outcomes in order to help SPC justify their funding, survive, and grow. They used a qualitative approach to conduct interviews about what service users valued in chaplaincy services. Specifically, they conducted this study using a constructivist grounded theory—a research methodology that builds theory from the data.

The authors were committed to co-production, an approach to research not unlike participatory action research and transformative research, which are scientific paradigms that rely on collaboration and collective reflection. This is the only chaplaincy study that we are aware of that has used this method; wider use in chaplaincy research should be considered (see Wood, Raffay, and Todd 2016). For this team, co-production meant involving service users and carers (family members of service users) throughout the study, including designing the interview schedule, pilot testing the interview, and interpreting the findings. Though the sample was small and largely Christian, their findings indicate the value of spiritual and religious care for mental health service users.

They conclude that in order for chaplains to be effective, they need to sensitively explore patients' experiences of their illnesses in relation to the spiritual dimension. In other words, the spiritual dimension helps patients make sense of their experiences of anxiety and frustration. Respecting individual needs is a part of care planning.

The results of this study described mental health service users' perspectives regarding chaplains' care. How do their perspectives compare with those of the parents surveyed by Donohue et al. (2017)? How might insights from Nolan (2016) inform research that builds on Raffay et al.'s (2016) observation that more work needs to be done on how to provide the most effective support to those without faith?

Article 12: Schultz, M., Lulav-Grinwald, D. and Bar-Sela, G. (2014) Cultural Differences in Spiritual Care: Findings of an Israeli Oncologic Questionnaire Examining Patient Interest in Spiritual Care

Spiritual care in healthcare in Israel is relatively new. Nonetheless, spiritual care providers in Israel (incidentally, *spiritual care provider* is the preferred term in Israel) are making a serious effort to develop an evidence-based approach to their care. In addition to this study, see a recent related study describing several approaches to screening for religious/spiritual distress (Schultz et al. 2017).

Do patients and their loved ones want and need spiritual care? Do patients and families understand what spiritual care providers (SCPs) and chaplains do? Do only patients who are very religious want spiritual care? And, if so, do they receive this service from their clergy? Do people have universal spiritual care needs? These are the big questions asked by this team from Israel made up of Schultz, Lulav-Grinwald, and Bar-Sela (2014). They were interested in cultural differences in how to approach screening for spiritual care. Specifically, they wanted to see if they could identify patients who were open to receiving spiritual care. They were also interested in whether there are universal spiritual care needs for which screening instruments could be developed.

Despite spiritual care being relatively new in Israel, the authors found a substantial proportion of oncology patients (41%) who reported they were open to a visit from an SCP. This proportion falls within the 35–54 percent who have been found to be interested in spiritual care in studies in the US. An important part of this study is their examination of factors that predicted this interest in spiritual care, especially prior experience with an SCP. These factors say a lot about how possible misunderstandings and stereotypes about SCPs limit people's openness to spiritual care.

As you read this study, note the care the authors took in their design, from the careful translation processes to make the questionnaire available in several languages to the adaptation of existing data collection instruments to fit their setting and to permit examining thematic categories important to them, such as finding meaning, coping, and decision-making.

Their study confirmed the need for a screening protocol that focuses less on demographic variables and more on self-defined religiosity/

spirituality and social factors such as loneliness. As you read through the results, what surprised you (if anything) about the predictors (e.g., illness severity) of wanting spiritual care?

Article 13: Hui, D., de la Cruz, M., Thorney, S., Parsons, H., Delgado-Guay, M., and Bruera, E. (2011) The Frequency and Correlates of Spiritual Distress among Patients with Advanced Cancer Admitted to an Acute Palliative Care Unit

The final paper in Section 2 of the *Reader* by Hui et al. (2011) adds to the literature that reports the prevalence of spiritual distress in a specific clinical population; 44 percent of the patients had what this team defined as spiritual distress. This means that spiritual distress is not rare; clinicians need to be on the lookout for it, and responsible clinical programs need to have the spiritual care resources to address it. A growing body of research describes the association of spiritual distress with factors such as greater emotional distress and poorer quality of life (Hebert et al. 2009 and Pargament et al. 2004).

This paper comes from a team of leading palliative care researchers at one of the US's top cancer treatment centers. Members of this team have published other important papers on the prevalence and correlates of spiritual pain in palliative care patients and their family carers (Delgado-Guay et al. 2011). Their most recent work reports the addition of an item about spiritual pain to a well-known palliative care screening tool, the Edmonton Symptom Assessment Scale (ESAS) (Delgado-Guay et al. 2016). Given the popularity of the ESAS and the respect people have for this team, this addition may mean a significant increase in people being screened for spiritual pain and, hopefully, referred for further assessment and care when indicated.

In this study, the team conducted a retrospective review of patient medical records. Two of the advantages of this approach are time and money; researchers do not have to wait for patients to volunteer for a new study, and it costs less to collect existing data than to conduct interviews to gather new data. The disadvantage is that the quality of the data in charts may be inconsistent; sometimes, data is missing or recorded in diverse ways. For a study like this, the quality of the chaplain assessment notes is critical. Fortunately, the chaplain on this team, Steve Thorney, was an experienced palliative care chaplain who followed a clear assessment protocol and thoroughly documented his assessments, so there was high-quality data for this study.

The authors point to the need to better define spiritual pain and, we would add, spiritual well-being (see Schultz et al. 2017 for one attempt). How do you define—and assess—spiritual pain and well-being with your clinical population? How often should your population be screened for spiritual distress? How do your definitions and assessments compare to those used by the authors in this study? Do you think the patient's proximity to death influences their level of spiritual distress? If so, how? Do you see evidence within the clinical population with whom you work of the interconnectedness of spiritual distress and physical and psychosocial distress?

Since the publication of this article, a conference was held to summarize the state of research about spirituality and spiritual care in palliative care. Readers interested in research about this clinical context, including spiritual assessment in palliative care, should consult the three articles from that conference that summarize their findings (Steinhauser and Balboni 2017, Steinhauser et al. 2017, and Balboni et al. 2017).

The articles in this section provide a good overview of the kinds of research being conducted regarding patient/family spiritual needs and interest in spiritual care. They come from diverse clinical and national contexts. Reading them will help you develop your research literacy—both your understanding of diverse research methods and your familiarity with important contributions to chaplaincy-related research.

References

Balboni, T.A., Fitchett, G., Handzo, G.F., Johnson, K.S., et al (2017) "State of the science of spirituality and palliative care research part II: screening, assessment, and interventions." *Journal of Pain Management*, 54, 3, 441–453.

Bradshaw, A. and Fitchett, G. (2003) "God, why did this happen to me?: Three perspectives on theodicy." *Journal of Pastoral Care & Counseling*, 57, 2, 179–189.

Delgado-Guay, M.O., Chisholm, G., Williams, J., Frisbee-Hume, S., Ferguson, A.O., and Bruera, E. (2016) "Frequency, intensity, and correlates of spiritual pain in advanced cancer patients assessed in a supportive/palliative care clinic." *Palliative Supportive Care*, 14, 4, 341–348.

Delgado-Guay, M.O., Hui, D., Parsons, H.A., Govan, K., et al. (2011) "Spirituality, religiosity, and spiritual pain in advanced cancer patients." *Journal of Pain Symptom Management*, 41, 6, 986–994.

Donohue, P.K., Norvell, M., Boss, R.D., Shepard, J., et al. (2017) "Hospital chaplains: through the eyes of parents of hospitalized children." *Journal of Palliative Medicine*, 20, 2, 1352–1358.

Grossoehme, D. (2011) "Research as a chaplaincy intervention." *Journal of Health Care Chaplaincy*, 17, 3–4, 97–99.

Grossoehme, D.H., Szczesniak, R.D., Mrug, S., Dimitriou, S.M., Marshall, A., and McPhail, G.L. (2016) "Adolescents' spirituality and cystic fibrosis airway clearance treatment adherence: examining mediators." *Journal of Pediatric Psychology*, 41, 19, 1022–1032.

Hebert, R., Zdaniuk, B., Schulz, R., and Scheier, M. (2009) "Positive and negative religious coping and well-being in women with breast cancer." *Journal of Palliative Medicine*, 12, 6, 537–545.

Hui, D., de la Cruz, M., Thorney, S., Parsons, H.A., Delgado-Guay, M., and Bruera, E. (2011) "The frequency and correlates of spiritual distress among patients with advanced cancer admitted to an acute palliative care unit." *American Journal of Hospice and Palliative Medicine*, 28, 4, 264–270.

Kelly, E.R. (2007) *Marking Short Lives: Constructing and Sharing Rituals Following Pregnancy Loss.* Bern: Peter Lang Publishing.

Marin, D.B., Sharma, V., Sosunov, E., Egorova, N., Goldstein, R., and Handzo, G. (2015) "Relationship between chaplain visits and patient satisfaction." *Journal of Health Care Chaplaincy*, 21, 1, 14–24.

National Standards for Bereavement Care Following Pregnancy Loss and Perinatal Death (2015) Health Service Executive. Accessed on 1/13/18 at www.hse.ie/eng/about/Who/acute/bereavementcare/standardsBereavementCarePregnancyLoss.pdf.

Newitt, M. (2014) "Chaplaincy support to bereaved parents—Part 1: liturgy, ritual and pastoral presence." *Health and Social Care Chaplaincy*, 2, 2, 179–194.

Nolan, S. (2016) "'He needs to talk!': a chaplain's case study of nonreligious spiritual care." *Journal of Health Care Chaplaincy*, 22, 1, 1–16.

Nuzum, D., Meaney, S., and O'Donoghue, K. (2016b) "The place of faith for consultant obstetricians following stillbirth: a qualitative exploratory study." *Journal of Religion & Health*, 55, 1519–1528.

Nuzum, D., Meaney, S., and O'Donoghue, K. (2016a) "The provision of spiritual and pastoral care following stillbirth in Ireland: a mixed methods study." *BMJ Supportive & Palliative Care*, 6, 2, 194–199.

Nuzum, D., Meaney, S., and O'Donoghue, K. (2017) "The spiritual and theological challenges of stillbirth for bereaved parents." *The Journal of Religion & Health*, 56, 1081–1095.

Nuzum, D., Meaney, S., and O'Donoghue, K. (2015) "The spiritual and theological issues raised by stillbirth for healthcare chaplains." *Journal of Pastoral Care & Counseling*, 69, 3, 163–170.

Pargament, K.I., Koenig, H.G., Tarakeshwar, N., and Hahn, J. (2004) "Religious coping methods as predictors of psychological, physical and spiritual outcomes among medically ill elderly patients: a two-year longitudinal study." *Journal of Health Psychology*, 9, 6, 713–730.

Rattay, J., Wood, E., and Todd, A. (2016) "Service user views of spiritual and pastoral (chaplaincy) in NHS mental health services: a co-produced constructivist grounded theory investigation." *BMC Psychiatry*, 16, 200.

Ragsdale, J.R., Hegner, M.A., Mueller, M., and Davies, S. (2014) "Identifying religious and/or spiritual perspectives of adolescents and young adults receiving blood and marrow transplants: a prospective qualitative study." *Biological Blood Marrow Transplantation*, 20, 8, 1242–1257.

Ragsdale, J.R., Orme-Rogers, C., Bush, J.C., Stowman, S.L., Seeger, R.W. (2016) "Behavioral outcomes of supervisory education in the Association for Clinical Pastoral Education: a qualitative research study." *Journal of Pastoral Care & Counseling*, 70, 1, 5–15.

Ragsdale, J.R., Steele-Pierce, M.E., Bergeron, C., and Scrivener, W.E. (2012) "Mutually engaged supervisory processes: a proposed theory for ACPE supervisory education." *Journal of Pastoral Care & Counseling*, 66, (3–4), 3.

Schultz, M., Lulav-Grinwald, D., and Bar-Sela, G. (2014) "Cultural differences in spiritual care: findings of an Israeli oncologic questionnaire examining patient interest in spiritual care." *BMC Palliative Care*, 13, 1, 19–29.

Schultz, M., Meged-Book, T., Mashiach, T., and Bar-Sela, G. (2017) "Distinguishing between spiritual distress, general distress, spiritual well-being, and spiritual pain among cancer patients during oncology treatment." *Journal of Pain Symptom Management*, 54, 1, 66–73.

Steinhauser, K.E. and Balboni, T.A. (2017) "State of the science of spirituality and palliative care research: research landscape and future directions." *Journal of Pain Management*, 54, 3, 426–427.

Steinhauser, K.E., Fitchett, G., Handzo, G.F., Johnson, K.S., et al. (2017) "State of the science of spirituality and palliative care research part I: definitions, measurement, and outcomes." *Journal of Pain Management*, 54, 3, 428–440.

Wood, E., Raffay, J., and Todd, A. (2016) "How could co-production principles improve mental health, spiritual and pastoral care (chaplaincy) services?" *Journal of Health and Social Care Chaplaincy*, 4, 1, 51–56.

ARTICLE 7

The Spiritual and Theological Challenges of Stillbirth for Bereaved Parents

Daniel Nuzum[1] • Sarah Meaney[2] • Keelin O'Donoghue[1,3]

Correspondence: Daniel Nuzum

Daniel.nuzum@ucc.ie

1 Department of Obstetrics and Gynaecology, University College Cork, Cork University Maternity Hospital, Wilton, Cork, Ireland

2 National Perinatal Epidemiology Centre, University College Cork, Cork, Ireland

3 Irish Centre for Fetal and Neonatal Translational Research (INFANT), Department of Obstetrics and Gynaecology, University College Cork, Cork University Maternity Hospital, Cork, Ireland

Published online: 2 February 2017

© Springer Science+Business Media New York 2017

Abstract

Stillbirth is recognized as one of the most challenging experiences of bereavement raising significant spiritual and theological questions. Semi-structured qualitative interviews were conducted with bereaved parents cared for in a tertiary maternity hospital to explore the spiritual impact of stillbirth. Data were analysed using interpretative phenomenological analysis. Stillbirth was identified as an immensely challenging spiritual and personal experience with enduring impact for parents. The superordinate themes to emerge were searching for meaning, maintaining hope and questioning core beliefs. Most parents reported that their spiritual needs were not adequately addressed while in hospital. The faith of all parents was challenged with only one parent experiencing a stronger faith following stillbirth. This study reveals the depth of spiritual struggle for parents bereaved following stillbirth, with a recommendation that spiritual care is provided as part of comprehensive perinatal bereavement care in the obstetric setting.

Key words: spirituality, stillbirth, bereavement, spiritual care, chaplaincy

---

Nuzum, D., Meaney, S., and O'Donoghue, K. (2017) "The spiritual and theological challenges of stillbirth by bereaved parents." *The Journal of Religion & Health*, 56, 1081–1095.

Introduction/Background

The death of a baby through stillbirth is recognized as one of life's most challenging bereavements with long-lasting consequences (Burden et al. 2016; Froen et al. 2011; Leon 1990; Leoni et al. 1998; Worden 2009). In pregnancy, parents begin a journey of expectancy and hope, with immense personal investment in a new future with their baby. New life is expected and experienced as pregnancy progresses, and for most couples, it is a time of great joy as bonds of attachment are formed with a new baby (Condon and Corkindale 1997; Lumley 1982; Tsartsara and Johnson 2006). At an early stage, this new baby takes his or her place within the story of their family. It is a sad reality, however, that not all babies will survive. The diagnosis that a baby has a life-limiting condition or has already died ruptures the experience of expectancy and hope for parents with the unwanted presence of death and grief. Stillbirth is defined as the death of a baby during pregnancy and varies internationally from the period from 20 to 24 weeks of gestation up to birth. In Ireland, where this study was conducted, stillbirth is defined in the Stillbirths Registration Act 1994 as 'a child born weighing 500 grammes or more or having a gestational age of 24 weeks or more who shows no sign of life' (Eireann 1994).

Birth and death are the two most significant life events in their own right: in stillbirth they fuse inseparably, with devastating impact not just for the baby who has died but also for parents, families, healthcare professionals, communities and wider society (Burden et al. 2016; Heazell et al. 2016; Newitt 2015; Nuzum et al. 2015a, 2015b, 2016). The care that bereaved parents receive during this time can shape their whole grieving process and recovery (Kingdon et al. 2015; Leon 1990; Leoni et al. 1998). The psychosocial burden of stillbirth is well documented in the published literature and has had heightened awareness following a renewed global focus on stillbirth as a global public health challenge to be addressed (Cacciatore 2013; Flenady et al. 2014; Heazell et al. 2016). What is less studied is the spiritual impact of stillbirth whether anticipated following a diagnosis of a life-limiting condition or anomaly during pregnancy or the sudden unanticipated death of a baby during an otherwise healthy pregnancy. In stillbirth, the 'natural order' of birth, life and death is disrupted raising existential questions (Jones 2001).

Most published studies in the wider field of pregnancy loss have been quantitative and have identified that perinatal death is a source of spiritual distress and challenge for parents but are inconclusive concerning the place of religious support and practice in bereavement recovery (Cowchock et al. 2010, 2011). Qualitative studies by Kelly and Newitt have identified the relationship with pastoral care and ritual following perinatal death (Kelly 2007; Newitt 2015). For those of faith, stillbirth can rock belief structure to its core especially where there is negative religious coping and expressed religious distress (Cowchock et al. 2010, 2011). Conversely for others, the death of a baby can invite a deeper reliance on faith as a supportive anchor in the turbulence of grief (Cacciatore and Ong 2011).

This study explores qualitatively the spiritual and theological struggle of stillbirth for bereaved parents.

Methods

Qualitative methods are used to understand complex social processes, and capture essential dimensions of a phenomenon from the perspective of study participants, and were therefore seen as appropriate for this study (Biggerstaff and Thompson 2008; Smith et al. 2009). Phenomenology is concerned with the study of experience and how experiences are understood. Interpretative phenomenological analysis (IPA) focuses on the specific and particular nature of a phenomenon or experience at depth and what it means for each individual participant (Smith *et al.* 2009). The researcher is tasked with entering as far as possible in an empathic way into the world of the participant (Biggerstaff and Thompson 2008). IPA as a methodology complements the approach of theological reflection as a hermeneutical tool to reveal new insight into spiritual care and practice in a healthcare environment (Ballard and Pritchard 2006; Green 2009; Nuzum et al. 2005b).

A semi-structured interview schedule was developed by the authors informed by the literature in the field and the professional experience of the research team who work in a specialist perinatal bereavement team as a healthcare chaplain (DN), consultant obstetrician (KOD) and a social researcher (SM).

Following Ethical Approval from the Clinical Research Ethics Committee of the Cork Teaching Hospitals (Ref. No: ECM 4 (pp) 06/03/12), a purposive sample of bereaved parents of twelve babies who had died following stillbirth were invited to participate in the study. Inclusion criteria were that the participants had been cared for at the study hospital, were not currently pregnant, were over 18 years old and had not previously indicated that they did not wish to be contacted by the hospital for study purposes.

Initial contact to participate in the study was made to bereaved mothers by a bereavement and loss midwife specialist known to them. Following agreement, each bereaved mother then received a personal invitation from the researcher to participate in a semi-structured in-depth interview with the stated aim to explore the spiritual and pastoral needs of bereaved parents following stillbirth and what their experiences of care were. Each participating mother was invited to extend the invitation to her partner to participate in the study.

Sample

IPA as a research methodology focuses on the depth of data, and by their nature, IPA studies have small sample sizes to allow experience to be studied at depth (Smith et al. 2009).

Twelve mothers and five fathers participated in the study. Half of the babies ($n = 6$) in the sample had received a diagnosis *in utero* of a life-limiting condition (for example, anencephaly or skeletal dysplasia) and were unlikely to survive up to birth. The remaining babies died through an unanticipated stillbirth.

Data collection

Each interview took place in a private environment without interruption at a location and time of the participants' choosing. Most participants ($n = 14$) were interviewed in their home environment, and the remaining ($n = 3$) chose to return to the study hospital for their interview. Interviews lasted between 31 and 104 mins, were digitally recorded and subsequently transcribed verbatim. Transcripts were anonymized to protect the identity of the participants. Following transcription and before analysis, each transcript was checked for accuracy against the original recordings by the researcher. The researcher kept a reflective journal to capture the experiences of the interviews and to record additional data such as body language and non-verbal communication to aid in personal theological reflection.

Analysis

The data were analysed using IPA. Data analysis is thorough and undertaken using the established five steps of IPA: (1) familiarization of the transcripts, (2) preliminary themes identified, (3) themes are grouped together as clusters, (4) the creation of a master table of superordinate and subordinate themes and (5) the integration of cases – this involves moving from one analysed transcript to the wider sample to compare and contrast themes and identify emerging overall patterns (Nuzum et al. 2014a, 2014b; Smith et al. 2009).

The data were analysed by the research team, and consensus was formed on the emergence of superordinate and subordinate themes. Data were managed using NVIVO version 10 (QSR International).

Results

All participants were emotional as they recalled the experiences surrounding the diagnosis of a life-limiting condition or stillbirth and the care they received in hospital.

The superordinate themes arising from the data relating to faith were: searching for meaning, maintaining hope and questioning core beliefs (Fig. 1).

Theme 1: Searching for meaning

Every parent expressed a deep sense of devastation and shock when they discovered that there was something wrong with their baby. This led to considerable personal reflection and questioning concerning the circumstances of the diagnosis and possible events leading up to diagnosis. The subordinate themes that made up the superordinate theme of searching for meaning were: being chosen, value of their baby's life and spiritual significance (see Fig. 1).

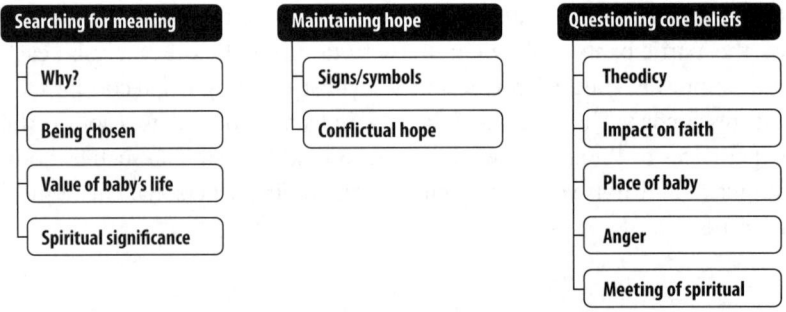

Fig. 1: Superordinate and subordinate themes

Parents demonstrated a strong desire to seek to understand why their baby had an anomaly or died unexpectedly, especially during an otherwise healthy pregnancy. This questioning was expressed most often by 'Why did this happen to our baby, or to us?' In seeking to answer what are in many ways unanswerable and existential questions, parents revisited experiences and events that occurred during their pregnancy. Searching for meaning was an active pursuit. A core part of searching for meaning was honouring the life of a baby, that his or her life was not in vain.

> Like I definitely feel that everything is meant for a reason. I think that's what made us happy, that this was her life cycle. This is all she knew. This was all she was meant for.[2013P1]

> Very important to me was to know that it [baby's death] wasn't in vain.[2010U1]

BEING CHOSEN

The sense of being chosen for this role only arose for mothers. The sense of being chosen was expressed in the data by mothers as an honour and a privilege and yet at the same time carried with it a certain conflict of wishing that they had not been chosen to be the mother of a baby who had died. Those who had time to prepare for the impending death of their baby were more expressive about being chosen for this 'special role' in the life of their baby. For some parents, being chosen was attributed to an intentional act on the part of their baby whom they believed had chosen them. This ascription to an independent identity of a baby also features in a further superordinate theme of personhood.

> She was a little angel and she needed to be born and she picked us to bring her into the world and that was our gift to her, was to bring her into the world. She knew from the outset that wasn't going to last longer than the pregnancy and she needed someone strong to be able to bring her into the world and she picked me and James.[2013P1]

Being chosen also conveyed an interpretation of inner strength on the part of mothers. They expressed a sense of pride that, as mothers, they were able to be parents of a stillborn baby with the inference that not all mothers would. Mothers who had experienced a sudden unexplained stillbirth expressed being chosen more as a posthumous hope as they reflected on their memories than as an experienced reality at the time.

> So when I was chosen there could be reasons he [baby] came into my life to help me on my journey, that maybe he was helping God. He knew my faith was strong enough to go on his way or maybe God called him, I don't know. I got a good sense without any help from anybody; I was sensing all this in hospital.[2010U1]

> I can remember [when people said] 'Oh God, he's chosen you' and I remember saying 'I wish he'd chosen me for something else.' But it was more, in some ways I kind of treasure the fact that we were chosen.[2008U1]

Value of their baby's life

All parents placed a strong emphasis on the value of finding meaning in both the life and death of their baby. For parents who had received a diagnosis of a life-limiting condition, this subordinate theme was especially significant as they used the time between diagnosis and death/birth to create memories, to make the most of every day and experience.

> Getting the diagnosis early I think was a blessing because I was able to enjoy everything.[2013P1]

Even though this was not the life or outcome that parents would have chosen for their baby, they nonetheless sought to find value in the importance of the life of their baby in their own right as they searched for meaning.

> I don't think it would have mattered to me if he had two heads. He was lovely.[2008U1]

Parents who had an unexpected stillbirth recalled the experiences they had during pregnancy. This retrospective grieving and attribution of significance was an important part of honouring the life of their baby and establishing patterns of meaning that provided ongoing comfort.

> I see his life as being the nine months that he lived. He had his own kind of life. He didn't live any kind of life in my world, he lived his own life in another world, that was very real, very his own. He had his own experiences. He got to have all the adventures that I had. He got to go swimming; he got to go to San Francisco. He got to taste funny food. He got to taste bakery cakes. He got to go to the cinema. He got to have all those experiences in his own way. ... He had his own life. We shared in it in a lot of ways and we didn't in other ways…he must have seemed to be another part of me also.[2013U2]

Spiritual significance

All parents were from a Christian faith background although one mother did not now belong to any faith group. She described this as

> I wouldn't call myself religious; I wouldn't attach myself to any particular religion now. I think nature is one of the defining forces in the world, in the planet, in our lives. I would say there is an awful lot going on that we

have no grasp, that I have no grasp on… I don't associate that with a god or something, but I see it as a huge part of us. It's an area I don't have a huge inclination to define…possibly partly because of a lack of interest in a religion.[2013U2]

Most parents had a ceremony of naming/blessing for their baby after their baby was born. Three couples had a baptism for their baby. Some mothers also engaged in spiritual practices during pregnancy such as a service of blessing for their baby *in utero* following a diagnosis of a life-limiting condition. This involved an intentional 'prayer of blessing and protection' by a priest friend and was conducted in the family home with the couple. All parents had a funeral/prayer service for their baby prior to burial or cremation. All parents expressed how these ceremonies helped them to attribute spiritual significance and value to their baby's life. Participation in a ceremony helped parents to express their grief and to confront the reality of physical separation by saying 'goodbye'. A ceremony was also something that parents were able to invest in for their baby as they planned an individualized ceremony. For many parents, it was important that their baby received the same honour as every other baby in terms of ritual and ceremony.

We had him christened, same as the rest of us (very upset).[2013U1]

It was in some way, it was before the service that was the really difficult part, the service was part of the process, you know the really hard parts were before the service because they had to be done before the service could happen. So it kind of pushed us into some things that we really needed to do. The writing of the service was as important as the having of the service. The finding of the painting and the working out the booklet and working out the words that I'd like to put in and things I wanted to say and what things I wanted to remember him by, what music I wanted.[2013U2]

Theme 2: Maintaining hope

All parents reported that hope was an important value that sustained them during their care. Hope was described as something that provoked a level of inner conflict for parents when their wishes for their baby were at odds with the medical evidence or diagnosis. This was particularly so if a baby was diagnosed with a life-limiting condition.

The subordinate themes to emerge in this area were: signs and symbols, and conflictual hope.

SIGNS AND SYMBOLS

Many parents spoke of how they had received various 'signs' which they interpreted as being from their baby or that pointed towards their baby. In addition, parents also mentioned that various symbols had taken on significance for them following the death of their baby. These signs and symbols were interpreted as being very closely connected with their baby's person and were of immense meaning and enduring comfort to parents. Signs and symbols were experienced as an ongoing connection with a deceased baby and were cherished by parents as embodying hope that their baby was still close to them. These signs of hope were described in liminal terms, as of threshold significance between this world and the next. Two signs in particular stood out for bereaved parents: white feathers and butterflies. Two mothers spoke about how butterflies were important symbols for them following the deaths of their babies.

> I remember the week after he was born…there were all these little white feathers on the path ahead of us. There's a lot of places you go and you find these little white feathers. You know, in your head you're thinking, that's him.[2010P2]

> You would go to bed and the next morning you would pull up the blind and there would be butterflies inside the house, it was just very weird. And right up until Christmas, Christmas Eve, there was a butterfly, so we all associate butterflies with the baby… I just always feel like it's baby saying 'hello'.[2010P1]

Other parents shared how they had other experiences that gave them closeness to their baby.

> Sometimes at night-time it happens here, someone blowing into my ear or my head. It's always my head and I think maybe Samuel is present. I don't know. It's very strange. It has happened three times and it wasn't my husband as he wasn't there, so I take comfort in that.[2010U1]

CONFLICTUAL HOPE

Parents reported that they struggled with a sense of conflictual hope when they found it hard to accept the finality of a diagnosis that their baby was unlikely to survive until birth. This was heightened as mothers in particular continued to feel their baby move *in utero*. An inner conflict arose for mothers as they explored whether there was anything they could do to alter the prognosed outcome for their baby. One mother following a diagnosis that her baby had a cardiac anomaly where she was informed that her baby was unlikely to live longer than 2–4 weeks after the diagnosis, expressed this sense of hoping against hope as:

> I started going to a homeopath… I took every remedy and supplement, everything you could think of, everything under the sun to try and make him stronger, that his heart might get stronger. So I felt like I really had to keep going for him. I kept trying to think of ways to make him better. I was reading and everything trying to find out things that might help him but Dr Y said I couldn't do anything.[2013P2]

For parents who received a diagnosis of sudden unanticipated stillbirth, they expressed how they tried to cling on to hope from the moment they suspected that something might be wrong. This created inner conflict and turmoil.

> I think I knew, my gut feeling was like, that I had either lost the baby or whatever, and I just didn't want it to become real. Because I suppose there was a chance they could save him.[2008U2]

Theme 3: Questioning core beliefs

Parents expressed that they questioned their belief structure and practice following the death of their baby. For all parents, the death of their baby caused them to reflect existentially on their life values and belief systems. For all but one, this was based on their Christian understanding of God, and for one, it was based on a more humanistic approach. One mother who was a committed Catholic before her baby died expressed the impact on her faith as:

> My faith has changed. I used to go to mass all the time but I rarely go to mass now… I was very much the traditional, go to mass, sit down and I suppose I always had that kind of spiritual side. The God I believe in is not the same as [formal church]… I went to mass on [last] Sunday, the first time in a long time and I nearly walked out…the priest is doing the Catholic church thing, he said that people who voted for the abortion thing were evil and they should never go to mass…and I'm there thinking 'will we try for another [baby]?'[2008U2]

Subordinate themes that were part of the superordinate theme of questioning core beliefs were theodicy, impact on faith, place of baby and anger.

Theodicy

Theodicy is one of the most challenging aspects of pain and suffering for people of faith. Cooper-White's definition is perhaps the most appropriate for the context of stillbirth. She defines theodicy as 'the tension between three mutually incompatible axioms: divine goodness, divine omnipotence/sovereignty and the existence of suffering…' (Cooper-White 2012).

The struggle of some parents with theodicy found expression in feelings of unfairness and injustice at why their baby died.

> I wondered why this happened to me. I had no baby, Why me? It's beyond my capability of understanding, so I asked questions about God.[2010U1]

> I was angry and I said why is this happening to me? What did I do to deserve this?[2013P2]

> I can always remember the day I found out, that, I had the scan. I went outside the front door and there was a couple of girls there. I know this is a completely horrible thing to say, but they were out smoking out the front and they were as big as buses now and I don't mean to, I was thinking 'they're fine now and here am I, haven't touched a drink. I don't smoke, didn't drink and this is happening to me and these ones out smoking, like, fit to have their babies'. I felt it very unfair.[2008P1]

Parents who were practising their faith found this area particularly hard as it jarred with their sense of devotion and religious commitment. It created an unsettling relationship with their faith and belief in a caring God. This is discussed further under the subordinate theme 'impact on faith'.

> Sure we always went to Mass and everything like, you're kind of saying 'why?' then like, wouldn't you? You'd be wondering what you did wrong, what you did to anybody that drew this down on your doorstep?[2013U1F]

Impact on faith

All parents experienced the death of their baby as challenging to their faith and belief. This challenge for eight mothers and four fathers led them to question their faith and belief in a caring God with four mothers and three fathers expressing that their faith was weaker as a result. One mother felt that her experience of stillbirth led her to a deeper faith. Four parents expressed that their faith, although challenged, remained unchanged following stillbirth.

> I still believe in God and I still believe as I did before but I just (deep sigh) never expected this thing would be so hard. I never thought I would have to go through something like that (voice breaking and emotional) Life can be hard enough without going through something like that. It has made me worry about what's around the corner. It has made me fearful for my three kids that are here with me. I'd still say my prayers but sometimes I feel 'is there any point?' It didn't work with the baby anyway.[2013P2]

> When he died it was like, what? Why is he [God] doing this and 'why would you do this to anyone?'[2010U2]

> I used to go to mass and that sort of stuff; I haven't gone for five or six months. I found it was something I was doing rather then something I was partaking in, I just find religion confusing now. It's like I'd be questioning at times, is there anything after? I just don't know.[2010P2F]

The diagnosis of a life-limiting condition led some parents to express strong feelings of anger towards God yet at the same time feeling a sense of dependence on God to get them through the experience. This led to a confusing sense of dependent ambivalence.

> Oh I screamed at him [God], I gave him the big finger there. I did suffer a long time. I just couldn't leave it, praying went out the door. I found it very hard to pray, but I spoke. I didn't say prayers, I spoke and I screamed and I roared at him…maybe I was given the grace to help me along because I was struggling so much…'Why am I going through this? God, what are you doing?' And at the same time going 'please help me, I'm leaving it in your hands.'[2008P3]

Place of baby?

Many parents reflected on the question about where their baby is now. This subordinate theme was expressed as parents shared their sense of ongoing connection and relationship with their baby. For some parents, it was closely linked with their sense of the after-life. Is my baby still a person? Where is my baby now? Parents wrestled with these questions as they shared how they still felt a close connection and relationship with their baby.

> I felt great frustration and confusion around where like, where would a spirit, where would that spirit go?[2010P2]

> I kept getting reassurances that he's in heaven, and that was great.[2010U1]

One mother connected with her baby through a medium which was a source of comfort.

> She [medium] just said that the baby is very happy where he is and that he doesn't want us to be miserable, to be grieving over him, that he is just feeling loved. He just came to me to be loved, to feel loved and just wants us to be happy.[2013P2]

The experience of loneliness and grief was also part of this subordinate theme. Parents described this as the reality of the absence of their baby, as if they were missing something, yet at the same time feeling close to their baby.

> The first three or four times we got the ferry out to the island, it was just the oddest thing. I got off the ferry and we had our bags and I was going, 'I'm missing something'. I'm missing, I'm missing a bag, there's a bag missing, there's something missing. I'm supposed to be carrying something else off the boat and I went down to the boat again and the man said, 'no, no, no all your bags are up'. And I'm missing something. And then we get everything into the car and went to the house and he's [partner] also saying 'I'm missing something, I'm missing a bag.' I said, 'no, I thought the same thing' and then an hour later it's like, 'I know what it is, I'm missing a baby.'[2013U2]

Anger

Anger was a subordinate theme running through most interviews as parents expressed the pain associated with the death of their baby. As a subordinate theme, anger challenged the world view of parents where the natural order of birth and death is reversed and most especially where there were no identifiable reasons.

> With God you'd be saying 'why my baby? This is a baby that would have been loved', there's the bitter side to it.[2010P1]

> Sometimes you'd be quite angry how God can let something like this happen.[2010P2]

> When he died, it was like, what, why is he [God] doing this? I just stopped doing it [going to Mass] for a good while… I was very angry, angry, just devastated. Just why? Why us? Why anyone? James was almost full term; you know moving around and kicking. So, yeah, very angry.[2010U2]

Parents recalled expressing their anger to God during their pregnancy. Two parents found the experience of labour very difficult and were angry with God and with the healthcare team. One mother expressed:

> My husband was crying, I just went, I discarded God at that point and I shouted to Our Lady saying 'what's wrong with you, why have you left me?'[2008P1]

One father described his anger and sadness from a faith perspective because he and his partner were denied a funeral for their baby son in their church as he had not been baptized.

> I suppose because he hadn't been christened, we couldn't have a service in the church... I remember the priest saying one day, 'you can't pick and choose what parts of being a Catholic you want to be' and I just thought to myself, then everyone in this room will have to get out.[2010P2F]

Two parents expressed that stillbirth had transformed their relationship with God through the awareness of their anger. This transformative growth led to an integration and acceptance of anger as a justified response to the death of their babies.

> She has taught me that it's ok to be angry with God... He's very understanding and that he understands and if you got angry with him and said 'I'm cross' that he'd be ok with that...you can be cross with him and you can go away from him for a while and the door is always open and he's understanding.[2008U2]

Spiritual needs

Parents expressed that they struggled with existential questions following the diagnosis of a life-limiting condition or stillbirth of their baby. All parents shared emotions such as fear, anxiety, sadness and doubt that indicated spiritual distress. Most parents availed of chaplaincy services during their time in hospital; however, these services were reported as being exclusively for ceremonial functions such as naming/blessing ceremony or a baptism. These ceremonies were described in functional terms. While this was valued by parents, most parents ($n = 13$) felt that their deeper spiritual needs were not adequately met while in hospital. The parents of three babies felt that their spiritual needs were met during their time in hospital.

> I met with [chaplain] she came up and had a chat with me and she was lovely... I suppose in a way nobody did address my faith or where I was there... I guess you need somebody to knock off the question to 'why is God so horrible?'[2008P2]

> He [chaplain] blessed the baby but I suppose we didn't really have any... I suppose we could have asked, but we didn't have anyone that sat down and kind of talked about the spiritual side of it.[2013P2]

No parent had received any follow-up pastoral care from the hospital. Of note, only three of the twelve babies had a ceremony/funeral in a church prior to burial/cremation. Most parents had a private ceremony in their home or at the hospital prior to discharge.

Participants were asked if they would have appreciated if their obstetrician had discussed their spiritual needs as part of their care. Only one parent said that they would have valued this. All other parents said that they felt this was not something they would expect from their obstetrician but would like the doctor to recognize that they needed support.

> I would be okay. I don't know whether [partner] would be though... you'd have to use your judgement.[2008U2]

> I would have been shocked if she [consultant] had asked me [if the baby's death was impacting on faith/belief]... I would assume that her job is to look after the mother and the baby...she'd be in there hours if she started asking questions like that.[2008P1]

> I didn't need to go into depth with faith [with consultant] to be perfectly honest with you. At the time, I was more concentrating on the scans, my faith is always there. I didn't need [doctor] to ask me about my faith as such. It was more 'How are you doing overall?'[2008P2]

> I would rather they asked you than not say anything about it and just ignore it, because it did happen and you do want them [doctors] to acknowledge it.[2010U2]

Three parents said that they felt that their obstetrician and bereavement and loss midwives were very sensitive to their deeper needs and provided deep empathic care.

> Every time we went in [for appointments] it was a case of we sat down and we talked for about five minutes or so [about how I am in myself which this participant described as spiritual] before we went into the medical stuff. Not pregnancy related stuff, not up in your head. They were phenomenal...so caring all the way through.[2013P2]

Discussion

The spiritual reality of stillbirth on bereaved parents is immense and impacts significantly on the faith, practice and belief of parents. The findings from this study demonstrate the presence of spiritual distress and ongoing struggle following stillbirth for parents. Bereaved parents voiced strong emotions and spiritual distress towards God as part of the interview process. Parents expressed the tension between trying to believe in a compassionate and caring God on the one hand and yet on the other hand struggling with the reality of theodicy. The expressions of theodicy and lament, while often difficult for people of faith, are close to the strong expression of spiritual distress and existential pain recorded in many sacred writings – not least in the Hebrew psalms where voice is given to the emotions of pain, angst, anger, fear, loneliness and abandonment. The heart-rending lament finds echoes in the words of Psalm 44:20 and 25 '…you have crushed us…and covered us with the shadow of death. Why do you hide your face and forget our grief and oppression?' (*NRSV Anglicized Bible* 1998). These are strong emotions which deserve sensitive spiritual care and attention.

Considering the depth of spiritual distress expressed by parents, it is a concern that only four parents felt that their spiritual needs were met during their time in hospital as they experienced the acute phase of bereavement following stillbirth. The role of spiritual care and chaplaincy is recognized as being of value in perinatal bereavement (Kelly 2012, 2007; Newitt 2016; O'Connell et al. 2016; Pierce 2003). The experiences from bereaved parents outlined above reveal the raw edge of lament and theodicy following the death of a baby. It is in this painful wilderness that healthcare chaplains are best placed to provide sensitive and meaningful spiritual care. Accompanying parents as they acknowledge and give voice to these deep spiritual and heartfelt feelings has positive therapeutic implications for healing and recovery and demands a high level of spiritual and pastoral competence and maturity coupled with the capacity to wrestle theologically with the depths of lament and theodicy (Nuzum et al. 2015b). When the data from this study are compared with a study of the provision of pastoral care in Ireland which identified that 40% of maternity healthcare chaplains are not board-certified, it raises a concern that spiritual need is not being adequately met following stillbirth in Ireland (Nuzum et al. 2016). The findings from bereaved parents concerning the importance of searching for meaning, maintaining hope and questioning core beliefs highlight areas of sensitivity and importance for parents which should be attended to as part of holistic perinatal bereavement care. These areas are best attended to by appropriately trained healthcare chaplains working as integrated members of multidisciplinary perinatal bereavement teams in the acute setting. These findings are also of importance to community clergy and spiritual advisors who provide ongoing care for bereaved parents.

The role of clinicians in the recognition of spiritual distress as part of clinical care is recognized in the published literature, most notably in the area of palliative care (Balboni et al. 2014; Puchalski and Ferrell 2010; Puchalski 2010). The findings from this study, however, identified that parents did not expect that obstetricians would have this responsibility as part of their care. In a related study at the same study site, most consultant obstetricians recognized that stillbirth does cause spiritual distress, but felt unable to address it or respond to it and saw this as something that the wider bereavement team should attend to (Nuzum et al. 2015b). These results further support the recommendation above for the provision of multidisciplinary perinatal bereavement teams in the overall provision of comprehensive bereavement care following stillbirth.

The strengths of this study are the depth of personal spiritual pain and wrestling that have been shared by bereaved parents to contribute to this field. This study explores and gives voice to often unarticulated spiritual distress as parents seek to understand the death of their baby and to find meaning in their loss.

The limitations of the study are that the participants were all from one study site and that the results pertain to one group of parents of whom nearly all are Christian.

The findings from this study suggest that further research should be conducted to explore how spiritual distress is identified by the wider clinical team and following identification and referral how this distress is then attended to both by the wider specialist perinatal bereavement team in general and healthcare chaplains in particular.

Conclusion

The data from this study reveal the depth of spiritual struggle experienced by bereaved parents leading up to and following stillbirth. That this spiritual distress and struggle were not adequately responded to as part of the care experienced by the participating parents highlights the need for professional spiritual care as an important component of overall perinatal bereavement care in the obstetric setting.

Compliance with ethical standards

Conflict of interest

Daniel Nuzum declares that he has no conflict of interest; Sarah Meaney declares that she has no conflict of interest; and Keelin O'Donoghue declares that she has no conflict of interest.

Ethical approval

Ethical approval for this study was received from the Clinical Research Ethics Committee of the Cork Teaching Hospitals (Ref. No: ECM 4 (pp) 06/03/12).

Human and animal rights

All procedures performed in studies involving human participants were in accordance with the ethical standards of the institutional and/or national research committee and with the 1964 Declaration of Helsinki and its later amendments or comparable ethical standards.

Informed consent

Informed consent was obtained from all individual participants included in the study.

References

Balboni, M., Puchalski, C., & Peteet, J. (2014). The relationship between medicine, spirituality and religion: Three models for integration. *Journal of Religion and Health, 53*(5), 1586–1598. doi:10.1007/s10943-014-9901-8

Ballard, P., & Pritchard, J. (2006). *Practical Theology in Action* (2nd ed.). London: SPCK.

Biggerstaff, D., & Thompson, A. R. (2008). Interpretative phenomenological analysis (IPA): A qualitative methodology of choice in healthcare research. *Qualitative Research in Psychology, 5*(3), 214–224. doi: 10.1080/14780880802314304

Burden, C., Bradley, S., Storey, C., Ellis, A., Heazell, A. E., Downe, S., et al. (2016). From grief, guilt pain and stigma to hope and pride—a systematic review and meta-analysis of mixed-method research of the psychosocial impact of stillbirth. *BMC Pregnancy Childbirth, 16,* 9. doi:10.1186/s12884-016-0800-8

Cacciatore, J. (2013). Psychological effects of stillbirth. *Semin Fetal Neonatal Med, 18*(2), 76–82. doi: 10.1016/j.siny.2012.09.001

Cacciatore, J., & Ong, R. (2011). Through the touch of god: Child death and spiritual sustenance in a Hutterian colony. *Omega (Westport), 64*(3), 185–202.

Condon, J. T., & Corkindale, C. (1997). The correlates of antenatal attachment in pregnant women. *British Journal of Medical Psychology, 70*(4), 359–372.

Cooper-White, P. (2012). Suffering. In B. J. Miller-McLemore (ed.), *The Wiley-Blackwell companion to practical theology* (p. 626). Chichester: Wiley.

Cowchock, F. S., Ellestad, S. E., Meador, K. G., Koenig, H. G., Hooten, E. G., & Swamy, G. K. (2011). Religiosity is an important part of coping with grief in pregnancy after a traumatic second trimester loss. *Journal of Religion and Health, 50*(4), 901–910. doi:10.1007/s10943-011-9528-y

Cowchock, F. S., Lasker, J. N., Toedter, L. J., Skumanich, S. A., & Koenig, H. G. (2010). Religious beliefs affect grieving after pregnancy loss. *Journal of Religion and Health, 49*(4), 485–497. doi:10.1007/s10943-009-9277-3

Eireann, O. (1994). *Stillbirths Registration Act*. Dublin: Government Stationery Office. www.irishstatutebook.ie/eli/1994/act/1/enacted/en/print.

Flenady, V., Boyle, F., Koopmans, L., Wilson, T., Stones, W., & Cacciatore, J. (2014). Meeting the needs of parents after a stillbirth or neonatal death. *BJOG: An International Journal of Obstetrics & Gynaecology, 121*(S 4), 137–140. doi:10.1111/1471-0528.13009

Froen, J. F., Cacciatore, J., McClure, E. M., Kuti, O., Jokhio, A. H., Islam, M. et al. (2011). Stillbirths 1 Stillbirths: Why they matter. *Lancet, 377*(9774), 1353–1366. doi:10.1016/s0140-6736(10)62232-5

Green, L. (2009). *Let's do Theology Resources for Contextual Theology*. London: Mowbray.

Heazell, A. E., Siassakos, D., Blencowe, H., Burden, C., Bhutta, Z. A., Cacciatore, J.,. et al. (2016). Stillbirths: economic and psychosocial consequences. *Lancet, 387*(10018), 604–616. doi:10.1016/S0140-6736(15)00836-3

Jones, L. S. (2001). Hope deferred: Theological reflections on reproductive loss (infertility, miscarriage, stillbirth). *Modern Theology, 17*(2), 227.

Kelly, E. R. (2007). *Marking short lives: Constructing and sharing rituals following pregnancy loss*. Bern: Peter Lang AG.

Kelly, E. (2012). *Personhood and presence. In Self as a resource for spiritual and pastoral care* (p. 209). London: T & T Clark International.

Kingdon, C., O'Donnell, E., Givens, J., & Turner, M. (2015). The role of healthcare professionals in encouraging parents to see and hold their stillborn baby: A meta-synthesis of qualitative studies. *PLoS ONE, 10*(7), e0130059. doi: 10.1371/journal.pone.0130059

Leon, I. G. (1990). *When a baby dies: Psychotherapy for pregnancy and newborn loss*. Newhaven: Yale University Press.

Leoni, L. C., Woods, J. R., & Woods, J. E. (1998). Caring for patients after pregnancy loss. *AWHONN Lifelines, 2*(1), 56–58.

Lumley, J. M. (1982). Attitudes to the fetus among primigravidae. *Australian Paediatric Journal, 18*(2), 106–109.

Newitt, M. (2015). Chaplaincy support to bereaved parents – Part 1: Liturgy, ritual and pastoral presence. *Health and Social Care Chaplaincy, 2*(2), 179–194.

Newitt, M. (2016). Healthcare chaplains among the virtues? *Practical Theology, 9*(1), 16–28. doi:10.1080/1756073X.2016.1149303

NRSV *Anglicized Bible*. (1998). Oxford: Oxford University Press.

Nuzum, D., Meaney, S., O'Donoghue, K., & Morris, H. (2015a). The spiritual and theological issues raised by stillbirth for healthcare chaplains. *Journal of Pastoral Care & Counseling, 69*(3), 163–170. doi:10.1177/1542305015602714

Nuzum, D., Meaney, S., & O'Donoghue, K. (2014a). The impact of stillbirth on consultant obstetrician gynaecologists: A qualitative study. *BJOG: An International Journal of Obstetrics & Gynaecology, 121*(8), 1020–1028. doi:10.1111/1471-0528.12695

Nuzum, D., Meaney, S., & O'Donoghue, K. (2014b). The spiritual impact of death on consultant obstetricians following stillbirth. *Journal of Palliative Care, 30*(3), 244–245.

Nuzum, D., Meaney, S., & O'Donoghue, K. (2015b). The place of faith for consultant obstetricians following stillbirth: A qualitative exploratory study. *Journal of Religion and Health*. doi:10.1007/s10943-015-0077-7

Nuzum, D., Meaney, S., & O'Donoghue, K. (2016). The provision of spiritual and pastoral care following stillbirth in Ireland: A mixed methods study. *BMJ Support Palliat Care, 6*(2), 194–200. doi:10.1136/bmjspcare-2013-000533

O'Connell, O., Meaney, S., & O'Donoghue, K. (2016). Caring for parents at the time of stillbirth: How can we do better? *Women Birth.* doi:10.1016/j.wombi.2016.01.003

Pierce, B. (2003). *Miscarriage and Stillbirth: the Changing Response.* Dublin: Veritas & SPCK.

Puchalski, C. M. (2010). Formal and informal spiritual assessment. *Asian Pacific Journal of Cancer Prevention, 11,* 51–58.

Puchalski, C., & Ferrell, B. (2010). *Making healthcare whole. integrating spirituality into patient care.* West Conshohoken: Templeton Press.

Smith, J. A., Flowers, P., & Larkin, M. (2009). *Interpretative phenomonological analysis: Theory, method, research.* London: Sage.

Tsartsara, E., & Johnson, M. P. (2006). The impact of miscarriage on women's pregnancy-specific anxiety and feelings of prenatal maternal-fetal attachment during the course of a subsequent pregnancy: An exploratory follow-up study. *Journal of Psychosomatic Obstetrics and Gynecology, 27*(3), 173–182.

Worden, J. (2009). *Grief counselling and grief therapy* (4th ed.). New York: Springer.

ARTICLE 8

Identifying Religious and/or Spiritual Perspectives of Adolescents and Young Adults Receiving Blood and Marrow Transplants: A Prospective Qualitative Study

Judith R. Ragsdale*, Mary Ann Hegner, Mark Mueller, Stella Davies

Cincinnati Children's Hospital, Cincinnati, Ohio

* Correspondence and reprint requests: Dr. Judith R. Ragsdale, Cincinnati Children's Hospital Medical Center, 3333 Burnet Avenue, MLC 5022, Cincinnati, OH 45229.

E-mail address: Judy.Ragsdale@cchmc.org (J.R. Ragsdale).

© 2014 American Society for Blood and Marrow Transplantation.

http://dx.doi.org/10.1016/j.bbmt.2014.04.013

Abstract

The potential benefits (or detriments) of religious beliefs in adolescent and young adults (AYA) are poorly understood. Moreover, the literature gives little guidance to health care teams or to chaplains about assessing and addressing the spiritual needs of AYA receiving hematopoietic stem cell transplants (HSCT). We used an institutional review board-approved, prospective, longitudinal study to explore the use of religion and/or spirituality (R/S) in AYA HSCT recipients and to assess changes in belief during the transplantation experience. We used the qualitative methodology, grounded theory, to gather and analyze data. Twelve AYA recipients were interviewed within 100 days of receiving HSCT and 6 participants were interviewed 1 year after HSCT; the other 6 participants died. Results from the first set of interviews identified 5 major themes: using R/S to address questions of "why me?" and "what will happen to me;" believing God has a reason; using faith practices; and benefitting from spiritual support people. The second set of interviews resulted in 4 major themes: believing God chose me; affirming that my life has a purpose; receiving spiritual encouragement; and experiencing strengthened faith. We learned that AYA patients were utilizing R/S far

Ragsdale, J.R., Hegner, M.A., Mueller, M., and Davies, S. (2014) "Identifying religious and/or spiritual perspectives of adolescents and young adults receiving blood and marrow transplants: a prospective qualitative study." *Biological Blood Marrow Transplantation*, 20, 8, 1242–1257.

more than we suspected and that rather than losing faith in the process of HSCT, they reported using R/S to cope with illness and HSCT and to understand their lives as having special purpose. Our data, supported by findings of adult R/S studies, suggest that professionally prepared chaplains should be proactive in asking AYA patients about their understanding and use of faith, and the data can actively help members of the treatment team understand how AYA are using R/S to make meaning, address fear, and inform medical decisions.

Key words: religion, spiritual, adolescent, young adult

Introduction

Adolescents/young adults (AYA) receive hematopoietic stem cell transplantation (HSCT) for a variety of illnesses and conditions, all of them life threatening. HSCT offers hope of health and, in some cases, cure. The process of HSCT brings considerable challenge in the form of physical pain and often psychosocial trauma, in addition to the normal developmental challenges of adolescence and young adulthood.[1,2] For many patients facing life-threatening conditions, religion and/or spirituality (R/S) provide support.[3] Unmet spiritual needs are associated with an increase in depression and decrease in spiritual well-being in adults.[2] One study links R/S use with improved quality of life and with longer survival after HSCT for adult patients.[4] Hospitalized adult patients with un-met spiritual needs report less satisfaction with care.[5] Although there is growing evidence linking R/S of adults to health care outcomes, this link has not been as thoroughly explored with AYA.[6]

Religion and spirituality are resources for many AYA. Over 90% of adolescents in the United States report a belief in God; several studies describe adolescents' use of religion and spirituality for coping with health concerns.[7,8] Young adults' religious and spirituality behaviors, such as prayer and service attendance, have been demonstrated to have a relationship with their health behaviors.[9] The way AYA make meaning of their illnesses has been the subject of study, yielding some surprising results; for instance, Haller et al. found several studies indicating that young people had "a wide array of views on the causes of illness that often differ from the biomedical view."[10] An earlier qualitative study found that adult HSCT patients viewed their suffering as a "wake-up call from God," whereas others saw their suffering as a "test from God."[1] Very few studies have examined how AYA use religion to help them understand and cope with their illness and their HSCT. Our study explored how

R/S beliefs provide a way of understanding and coping with illness for AYA patients receiving HSCT, and whether the experience of HSCT led to change in the AYA patients' understanding of R/S. Our goal was to provide data to inform health care teams about R/S as a resource for AYA HSCT patients and to promote evidence-based pastoral care interventions for the chaplains on the health care team.

Religion and spirituality have been defined as distinct from each another in the literature; neither term has a generally accepted definition.[11] For the purposes of our paper, we define *religion* as the formal organization of sacred beliefs, rituals, and traditions held in a community of like-minded believers.[11, 12] We define *spirituality* as any way of seeking or relating to whatever a person considers sacred.[13] In this paper, we combine these concepts and refer to them as R/S.

Methods

We chose to use qualitative methodology as a way to explore the participants' understanding of their R/S and to determine whether and how it helped them, hindered them, and changed from the time they received their HSCT to 1 year after transplantation. We used grounded theory as a way to collect data via interview and to analyze our data by coding.[14] Grounded theory is a method of qualitative research drawn from the premise that not enough is known about the subject to have an informed hypothesis. Grounded theory seeks to explore a little-known subject by gathering data based on the experience of the participants, analyzing the data using iterative coding processes to identify key themes, and proposing hypotheses for further study. The ultimate goal is to develop a theory of how the process—in this case the process of AYA use of R/S—functions. Semistructured interview questions guide the interviewer and help keep the participants focused on the subject of interest for the research question. Interviews provided a way to explore patients' perspectives and ways of making meaning.[15]

We attempted to recruit all 15 patients eligible for our study; which is to say, receiving HSCT, well enough to communicate verbally, and between the ages of 13 and 29 inclusive, from December 1, 2010 until February 1, 2012. Twelve agreed to participate. Although faith development has been demonstrated to begin earlier than adolescence, we sought participants who had a more evolved cognitive understanding of what they believed. Each participant received a description of this study based on our institutional review board-approved protocol. The chaplain on the HSCT service or 1 of the HSCT nurse coordinators worked with staff to determine which patients met the study criteria and were well enough to be interviewed. The chaplain or nurse coordinator explained to the patient and, if a minor, to her or his parents, that we were conducting a study to explore how AYA used faith in the process of their HSCT. Patients either consented or assented to participate. When the patient was a minor and assented, his or her parent or guardian also provided consent. Our study originally proposed to interview HSCT recipients just before they received HSCT, 100 days after HSCT, and 1 year after HSCT. We had a difficult time with this plan because of lack of availability of participants because of illness or being too busy with preparation for treatment to be interviewed. We amended our study to interview participants as close to the date of HSCT as possible and then 1 year after HSCT. Participants received the incentive of $20.00 for the first interview and $50.00 for the second interview.

The interviews were done by a PhD-prepared qualitative researcher with a background in chaplaincy or by a chaplain with master's level course work in qualitative research. The interviews were semi structured; Table 1 contains the interview questions guiding the interview. The interviews lasted between 10 and 50 minutes, depending on the length of time the participant chose to speak. The interviewer asked follow-up questions until the participant indicated he or she had completed addressing a question. Each interview was audiotaped and transcribed by a professional service. Each interview was reviewed for accuracy by 1 of the chaplain researchers by listening to the tape and editing the transcript, as necessary.

Interview texts were coded by an interdisciplinary team of coders using grounded theory methodology. Interviews were not separated by gender, age, faith, or diagnosis for purposes of coding. The first series of codes were open codes; they used the language of the participants. Codes were gathered into subject categories. We compared codes from the first and second set of interviews and arrived at saturation with 5 key themes for the first set series of interviews and 4 key themes for the second set. In grounded theory, saturation is reached when no new themes emerge from the interviews.

Table 1: Interview questions

First interview: semistructured questions for before one hundred days after transplantation
When did you learn you had this illness?
How did you come to be offered the option of receiving a bone marrow transplant?

cont.

Why do you think this has happened to you?
If you were raised with any type of religious belief or practices, how would you describe them?
How would you describe your faith beliefs (using whatever language the patient has used) today?
Has your faith changed since your diagnosis and, if so, how would you describe what's different now?
How is your faith helping you (or not) with what you're going through?
Is there anything about your faith that you question now, or wonder about?
Is there anything about this topic that you'd like to talk about?
How would you describe to someone who's never been through this what it has been like to have a bone marrow transplant?
How has your way of doing faith (using whatever words they have used) changed since your bone marrow transplant?
How do you see God or the Holy or your Higher Power in this experience?
Have you engaged in religious or spiritual activities since receiving your BMT—such as prayer or talking with a spiritual leader or friend? How have these activities been helpful or unhelpful for you?
Has anyone said anything to you of a religious or spiritual nature that has been helpful or unhelpful?
What would you say to a person thinking of receiving a BMT that you found helpful or wish someone had said to you?
If you could ask God or the Holy or your Higher Power any 2 questions, what would they be?
Is there anything else you'd like to say about this subject that I haven't thought to ask about?
Second interview: semistructured questions for 1 year after transplantation
It's been a year now since you received your BMT—what has changed in your life since your treatment?
Did you ever feel any difficult feelings toward God or the Holy or your Higher Power?
Was your way of doing faith changed at all by this experience and if so, how?
If you're a person of faith, what kinds of questions would you want to ask God or the Holy or your Higher Power?
Sometimes in the middle of really hard times, people report having religious experiences. Did you ever have a religious experience you could describe?
Did any spiritual understandings come to you out of this experience that you think might be useful for others to know about?
Is there anything about this topic that you'd like to talk about?

Participants

The demographics of study participants are shown in Table 2. Seven of the 12 participants were female, and ages ranged from 15 to 28 years. Five of the participants were male, and ages ranged from 15 to 19 years. All patients received allogeneic transplantation and 7 of 12 received a reduced-intensity preparative regimen. Six patients underwent transplantation for leukemia and the remainder underwent transplantation for immune deficiency or marrow failure. Nine patients identified themselves as Christian in the first interview, 1 identified having no personal religious affiliation, and 2 were listed as Christian on the admission page of their medical record. Four participants were interviewed before HSCT, 1 at 3 days, 1 at 4 days, 1 at 6 days, and 1 at 12 days before HSCT. The other 8 participants were interviewed after HSCT: 7, 18 (2 participants), 21, 28, 35, 39, and 87 days after HSCT. The participants interviewed at 35, 39, and 87 days after HSCT were quite ill and died within the year. Of the twelve patients who participated in the first interview, 6 participated in the second interview. The diagnoses of these 6 patients participating in the second interview included acute lymphoblastic leukemia (1), acute myeloid leukemia (2), aplastic anemia (2), and non-Hodgkin lymphoma and X-linked lymphoproliferative disorder (1). The other 6 participants died in the course of the year after transplantation.

The 3 patients who declined to participate were 2 males aged 18 and 1 female aged 15. One male was Asian and the other 2 patients were Caucasian; 1 male was Buddhist and the other 2 patients were Christian; all 3 patients were to receive HSCT for immunodeficiency/bone marrow failure. Two refused with no explanation; the other said he was Buddhist and chose not to participate.

Although the data for our study were drawn from interviews, we did consult the patients' medical records to clarify diagnoses. In 2 cases in which the interviewer failed to ask the participants about faith tradition, that information was also accessed via the medical records. Although data for this grounded theory study were drawn exclusively from interviews, we needed to access the medical records to describe the demographics of our participants.

Table 2: Characteristics of patients

UPN	Age, yr	Faith (family)	Faith (personal)	Diagnosis	Race	Gender	Donor source	Conditioning regimen
1	16	Presbyterian	Presbyterian	ALL	Caucasian	M	BM, related donor	CY/TBI/ATG
2	28	Christian	Christian	AML	Afr-Am	F	BM (first); cord (second)* unrelated donors	CAM/FLU/MEL
3	21	Methodist	No response	Schwachman Diamond Anemia	Caucasian	F	BM, unrelated donor	CAM/FLU/MEL
4	23	Christian (per chart)	Christian (per chart)	XLP-like immune deficiency	Caucasian	M	PBSC, unrelated donor	CAM/FLU/MEL
5	15	Baptist	Baptist	NHL and XLP	Caucasian	M	BM, related donor	CAM/FLU/MEL
6	15	None	None	AML	Hispanic	M	BM, unrelated donor	BU/CY/ATG
7	19	Baptist	Baptist	CGD	Caucasian	F	BM, related donor	BU/CY/ATG
8	20	Catholic	Catholic	AML	Hispanic	F	BM, unrelated donor	BU/CY/ATG
9	15	Christian	Christian	Aplastic anemia	Caucasian	F	BM, related donor	CY/ATG
10	19	Roman Catholic	Roman Catholic	HLH	Caucasian	F	BM, unrelated donor	CAM/FLU/MEL
11	19	Christian	Christian	CML	Caucasian	M	BM, unrelated donor	CY/TBI/ATG
12	21	Baptist	Baptist	Aplastic anemia	Caucasian	F	BM, unrelated donor	CAM/FLU/MEL

Afr-Am indicates African American; ATG, antithymocyte globulin; BM, bone marrow; BU, busulfan; Cam, campath; CGD, chronic granulomatous disease; CY, cyclophosphamide; Flu, fludarabine; HLH, hemophagocytic lymphohistiocytosis; Mel, melphalan; NHL, non-Hodgkin lymphoma; PBSC, peripheral blood stem cells; XLP, X-linked lymphoproliferative disorder; UPN, unique patient number; ALL, acute lymphoblastic leukemia; AML, acute myelogenous leukemia; CML, chronic myelogenous leukemia; TBI, total body irradiation.

* UPN 2 received a second graft for treatment of failed engraftment with the first graft

Results

First set of interviews

Review of the first set of interviews (n = 12) resulted in 5 major themes raised by participants: asking, "why me," asking, "what will happen to me," believing God has a reason, using faith practices, and benefiting from spiritual support people.

Asking, "Why me?"

Most participants (n = 11) used R/S to wrestle with the questions of why they had a life-threatening illness and the related question of what would happen to them. Participants offered the following comments exemplifying this category: "I feel like emotional, like why me? (tearful) Like why this point in my life when I'm just about to go off to college and like I've been working so hard and now I can't go right now," and "'Why' was the main thing, why He made me…why it was me. I know I didn't want to play the, 'Woe is me,' but when I first got sick, I was upset about it."

Asking, "What will happen to me?"

The physical question of whether they would live or die was accompanied for some by the spiritual question of whether, if they died, they would go to heaven or hell. One participant said, "I thought there was a chance that this can…the bone marrow transplant, there's a chance that it will kill me and I knew that I had to go through it, and I don't want to go to hell." Two of the participants addressed the spiritual question of eternal life with the concrete action of requesting and receiving the Christian rite of baptism. One participant did not use R/S, but rather answered the question, "why me?" with a scientific understanding of genetics and with a philosophy that bad things happen for no reason.

Believing God has a reason

Those using R/S shared a belief that God had a reason. Participants in the first series of interviews did not always have an answer about what the reason was: "Well, I know that He is there and He is helping and there is a reason why I have to go through this." Participants tended to assume it was either a vote of confidence in their strength, a decision to use them in a meaningful way, or a test of faith and, therefore, an opportunity to develop spiritually. One participant succinctly said what several participants echoed: "He chose me 'cause I'm strong. I understand what I have to go through."

Using faith practices

Participants reported using practices such as prayer, Bible reading, speaking with youth ministers and with other spiritual support people, and listening to Christian music. These practices provided several participants with tangible comfort and encouragement. One participant said, "I pray when it just seems really bad, like I pray during my radiation treatments to get me through it." Another said, "And just when I'm in pain and I pray for peace that I won't, you know, let…that side effects won't be too bad and that I will be healed from that and not feel the pain." Being unable to attend church services or youth group because of immunosuppression was a reality for all who attended and a loss voiced by several participants.

Benefiting from spiritual support people

Several participants reported significant support from people from their congregations; 1 participant said, "My pastor's wife is 1 of the biggest helps because she's a pastor but she talks to me like I'm normal." Other people had spiritually supportive family members such as aunts, a godmother, or a grandfather. The content of the support varied based on the relationship; 1 participant's support person was quite forceful: "'(Name), you are acting as if you're not a part of this family, that you're not a child of God. He said you're standing on the outside and He said come near.' And just that once you realize that everything will be OK, but you have to accept that. It was true for me."

Participants reported being encouraged and inspired by those who were formally or informally spiritual support people.

Second set of interviews

Review of the second set of interviews (n = 6), completed 1 year after HSCT, resulted in 4 themes identified by the participants: believing God chose me, affirming that my life has a purpose, receiving spiritual encouragement, and experiencing strengthened faith.

Believing God chose me

One participant gave language to this theme in this way: "It's just, it made me realize that God is using me in a big way and he's just using me to touch a lot of lives. Also, that he is also giving me another chance at life so… I plan on him working through me for the rest of my life."

Participants came to understand that God had chosen them, which seemed, in several cases, to lead to sense of being special to God. This category relates to the theme identified in the first set of interviews that

God had a reason for allowing them to be ill enough to need to receive HSCT. Believing they were chosen by God also led some participants to have a sense of responsibility for understanding what God wanted them to learn from the experience of serious illness and receiving HSCT.

Affirming that my life has a purpose

This theme related to the theme from the first interview series of believing that God has a reason. One participant noted that trusting God's plan did not equate with knowledge of the actual plan: "I trust God's plan more (pause), and I know that He's got a reason even if it takes forever to figure out." Other participants reported that God was or would be using them in a significant way to help others: "I feel my heart just transformed and God really was speaking to me… He gave me my life to honor Him and that I should do all that I can to do that." The experience of illness and receiving HSCT led most participants to question their life path and re-evaluate their values and behaviors.

Receiving spiritual encouragement

This spiritual encouragement was sometimes experienced as coming directly from God and other times was mediated by spiritually supportive people. One participant offered this story of the youth minister's visit:

> Our heads were just kind of like bobbing around, not really knowing what's going on and the youth pastor came in and he just really kind of put us back in the…kind of relaxed mode and not really having many worries and just kind of putting us back on our feet and getting us back to the ground, and I think that really helped us get through it.

Prayers were sometime crying out to God with anger and fear. Some participants felt it would demonstrate a lack of faith to speak to God about fear of death. One participant who felt freedom to voice anger in her prayers had support from her pastor who openly acknowledged that he too would be angry with God. Many participants found conversations with spiritually supportive friend/family/clergy to be very helpful. The participants' descriptions varied in terms of the content of conversation from spiritual support people but they shared appreciation for these people who bolstered their faith.

Experiencing strengthened faith

All participants reported feeling that their faith had grown stronger in the process of receiving HSCT. In the second set of interviews, participants spoke of their faith in these ways: "I've gotten really close to God. Me and him haven't always been close and me going through this just opened my eyes and showed me that he is a very big part of everybody's life," and "I feel like my faith and my trust in the Lord has increased a lot and that I trust him more... I'm closer to Him." Participants' R/S stood the tests of fear and pain, and, in some cases, doubt.

Several participants who had struggled with what would happen if they died conveyed powerful experiences of God's presence: "And for me, it was do you stop believing just because things are not working out the way you expected? And, no, you don't give up hope, you don't give up faith. And maybe that's what builds it." These participants found a sense of reassurance that they would be safe in God's care whether they lived or died.

Overall, the second set of interviews resulted in some themes similar to those in the first set and some areas of change and growth. Participants had worked to make meaning of a very challenging experience and, in the second interview series, they had answers to some of the questions from the first set. The answers weren't conclusive for some participants; some continued to wrestle with "why me?" and "what will happen to me?" All participants in the second interview series said that their faith had grown stronger in the process of HSCT.

Listening to their language and analyzing their descriptions of faith, we noted an increased belief that God cared for them and many had the experience of actual presence and help in the context of HSCT. Some participants reported that they felt that having gone more deeply into their faith, they would be stronger, no matter what happened, either because of illness or, if they lived through this, in other life challenges.

Discussion

AYA HSCT patients are thinking about and using R/S much more than we suspected. Using the method of interview allowed us to encourage AYA participants to describe their R/S experience. Several voiced appreciation of the interview itself as a time to talk about their faith. The literature suggests that a qualitative interview may serve as a chaplaincy intervention.[16] We did not ask participants in our study to comment on the impact the interview had on them. One study about the impact of qualitative interview on research participants found that "the interview had prompted them to look at things in a different way, often gaining insight" or that they "had a view that had now shifted."[17] This study suggests that our method of qualitative interview might have caused the participants to think more or differently about their R/S than they otherwise would have.

From the first set of interviews, we learned that all participants using R/S to help them understand the world were using R/S to address the questions of "why me?" and "what will happen to me?" R/S was a lens through with our participants made meaning of their illness and their hope for recovery as they received HSCT. The 1 other R/S study of HSCT patients that we are aware of, an adult study by Pereira et al.,[4] explored the relationship between spiritual absence, quality of life, and mortality. Pereira et al. found a relationship between spiritual absence and likelihood of death 1 year after receiving HSCT. Their method, the Millon Behavioral Medicine Diagnostic, provided data about 7 domains; 1 domain, the Stress Moderator scale, assesses the degree to which patients lack religious or spiritual personal resources to cope with medical stressors."[4] Data produced from this type of inquiry differs substantially from our qualitative interview data. Therefore, although we find their results interesting, we cannot compare our results with those of their study. We learned that several of the participants in our study had considerable fear that was based in their faith. Not only did they have the fear of pain and of possible death that most, if not all, HSCT recipients feel. They also had the fear of going to hell. This is certainly not the case for all who use R/S; however, the literature says that sustained spiritual struggle may create significant distress that leads to greater depression and negatively impacts quality of life in adult patients.[3, 18, 19] We do not know whether some AYA patients receiving HSCT have issues of sustained R/S struggle. Those in our sample reported spiritual struggle, but those interviewed a second time had worked through their R/S struggle using the tools of their faith: prayer, religious ritual, such as baptism, and receiving spiritual encouragement from others. Our AYA participants were able to use their faith to respond to fear created by their faith, and thus reported strengthened R/S to the point that some voiced gratitude for having the experience of illness and HSCT.

An overarching finding from our analysis is that participants with faith were able to draw on their faith for tangible help with loneliness and fear. We learned that although AYA were very willing to talk about their R/S beliefs and experience in the context of the interview, several of them had not spoken with others about either the depth of fear they had or their use of R/S in medical decision-making. Although the relationship between medical decision-making and R/S was not a major category in our study, 1 YA participant told about privately relying on R/S to decide when to go home. It is increasingly clear that R/S is used by parents of pediatric patients as they make medical decisions for their children.[20] Seeking to understand how R/S informs medical decision-making for older adolescent patients, young adult patients, and parents of pediatric patients will be important in future studies.

Studies in R/S have examined ways patients use R/S for adherence. Given that AYA struggle with assuming health responsibilities,[21] leveraging R/S to support greater responsibility in the AYA's own health care could serve AYA patients. This idea is supported by Mahoney's (2005) study on "sanctity of the body" beliefs in her study of 289 college students.[22] Our study did not address questions of how AYA patients understood their R/S as encouraging them, or not, to adhere to prescribed medical care. This could be an area for future research with AYA HSCT patients.

The literature has some studies suggesting that adolescents use R/S to cope with illness;[6] this is based in large part on survey responses. Our work provides a longitudinal study of 6 AYA HSCT patients offering in-depth descriptions of their journey from struggling with questions of "why?" to a deeper understanding of how R/S served them. Part of their reported growth in faith may be a result of natural development for AYA; between the ages of 18 to 25,[23] adults continue their identity development.[9, 23] We anticipated that the experience of HSCT might lead to a change in participants' R/S. Each participant affirmed a strengthening of his or her faith. For these participants, God is an active being helping them endure pain and suffering and fear.

The implication for care from our study is that AYA recipients of HSCT should have their R/S resources and concerns assessed and, if indicated, addressed as a routine part of their care. We recommend having a well-informed chaplain on the HSCT health care team as an essential support for the AYAs' R/S and to translate R/S concerns/beliefs to the interdisciplinary team. Meeting the R/S needs of patients and families will provide better care and result in greater satisfaction with care.[24] Religious beliefs and faith communities sometimes work at cross purposes from the medical team, especially at the end of life. Having a professional chaplain on the team will provide a liaison who understands the culture of both the R/S world and the health care world. Professional chaplains are academically and clinically educated to understand multiple faith traditions and to provide R/S resources appropriate to the patient's belief system. One study reported that in some end-of-life care situations, religious patients required "more aggressive medical care" than the medical team thought appropriate.[24] Balboni et al. speculated that some religious people see the medical team as God's method of providing a miracle. In this situation, the chaplain may provide a bridge of conversation between the religious community of the patient and the health care team. In an earlier study, Balboni et al. found that "patients ratings of support of their religious/spiritual needs are significantly associated with receiving pastoral care visits...suggesting that pastoral care is a key aspect of spiritual care."[25] From this, we conclude that having a chaplain as a member of the interdisciplinary team addressing the R/S concerns is preferable to relying solely on R/S support from the patients' congregational clergy.

Limitations of our study include our extremely small sample size. Although appropriate for a grounded theory study, we affirm that our results are not to be generalized but rather may be used to create hypotheses. For instance, we would like to explore whether using interview-style questions might form the useful basis for spiritual assessment that could both improved R/S care for patients and also provide meaningful insight for the health care team. Another limitation of our study is the lack of faith traditions beyond Christianity in our sample. Our finding of the importance of R/S to the AYA participants in this study supports findings in adult R/S studies of patients facing life-threatening illnesses that quality of life is increased among patients receiving spiritual support from chaplains or from members of the medical team.[26, 27, 28] We affirm the findings of adult R/S studies suggesting that members of the medical team may assess interest and/or need by patients for R/S care, but that certified chaplains are the only members of the health care team educated and certified to provide in-depth spiritual assessments and R/S interventions.[25, 29] On the basis of our study and the adult R/S literature cited, we suggest that chaplains consider being more proactive in assessing and responding to R/S needs of AYA patients. Two members of our research team have been chaplains with pediatric HSCT patients; neither had heard in routine pastoral care of the depth of religious experience that participants conveyed, in the context of responding to interview questions. This may be a failure of skill on the part of the chaplains or a result of chaplains' seeking to provide emotional support and neutralize faith differences[30] or for some reason yet to be determined. Very few studies have been done on the efficacy of chaplaincy care.[31] Our study suggests that more assertive exploration of how AYA patients understand and use their faith will be meaningful for the patients and helpful for the health care team.

Acknowledgments
Conflict of interest statement
There are no conflicts of interest to report.

Financial disclosure
The authors have nothing to disclose.

References

1. Saleh US, Brockopp DY. Hope among patients with cancer hospitalized for bone marrow transplantation: a phenomenologic study. *Cancer Nurs.* 2001;24:308–314.
2. Evan EE, Zeltzer LK. Psychosocial dimensions of cancer in adolescents and young adults. *Cancer.* 2006;107:1663–1671.
3. King SW, Fitchett G, Berry D. Screening for religious/spiritual struggle in blood and marrow transplant patients. *Support Care Cancer.* 2013;21:993–1001.
4. Pereira DB, Christian LM, Patidar S, et al. Spiritual absence and 1-year mortality after hematopoietic stem cell transplant. *Biol Blood Marrow Transplant.* 2010;16:1171–1179.
5. Pearce M, Coan A, Herndon J, et al. Unmet spiritual care needs impact emotional and spiritual well-being in advanced cancer patients. *Support Care Cancer.* 2012;20:2269–2276.
6. Cotton SS, Grossoehme DH, Tsevat J. Religion/spirituality and health in adolescents. In: Plante TG, Thoresen CE, editors. *Spirit, science, and health: how the spiritual mind fuels physical wellness.* Westport, CT: Praeger Publishers;2007. p.143–156.
7. Cotton S, Zebracki K, Rosenthal SL, et al. Religion/spirituality and adolescent health outcomes: a review. *J Adolesc Health.* 2006;38:472–480.
8. Rew L, Wong YJ. A systematic review of associations among religiosity/spirituality and adolescent health attitudes and behaviors. *J Adolesc Health.* 2006;38:433–442.
9. Kirk CM, Lewis RK. The impact of religious behaviours on the health and well-being of emerging adults. *Ment Health Religion Cult.* 2013;16:1030–1043.
10. Haller DM, Sanci LA, Sawyer SM, Patton G. Do young people's illness beliefs affect healthcare? A systematic review. *J Adolesc Health.* 2008;42:436–449.
11. Hill PC, Pargament K II, Hood JRW, et al. Conceptualizing religion and spirituality: points of commonality, points of departure. J Theory Social Behav. 2000;30:51.
12. Grossoehme DH, Ragsdale J, Wooldridge JL, et al. We can handle this: parents' use of religion in the first year following their child's diagnosis with cystic fibrosis. *J Health Care Chaplaincy.* 2010;16:95–108.
13. Pargament KI. *The psychology of religion and coping: theory, research, practice.* New York: Guilford Press;1997.
14. Glaser BG, Strauss AL. *The discovery of grounded theory: strategies for qualitative research.* Chicago: Aldine Pub. Co.;1967.
15. Tschuschke V, Hertenstein B, Arnold R, et al. Associations between coping and survival time of adult leukemia patients receiving allogeneic bone marrow transplantation: Results of a prospective study. *J Psychosom Res.* 2001;50:277–285.
16. Grossoehme DH. Research as a chaplaincy intervention. *J Health Care Chaplaincy.* 2011;17:97–99.
17. Butterfield LD, Borgen WA, Amundson NE. The impact of a qualitative research interview on workers' views of their situation. *Canadian J Counseling/Revue Canadienne de Counseling.* 2009;43:120–130.
18. Trevino KM, Pargament KI, Cotton S, et al. Religious coping and physiological, psychological, social, and spiritual outcomes in patients with HIV/AIDS: cross-sectional and longitudinal findings. *AIDS Behav.* 2010;14:379–389.
19. Exline JJ, Prince-Paul M, Root BL, Peereboom KS. The spiritual struggle of anger toward God: a study with family members of hospice patients. *J Palliative Med.* 2013;16:369–375.
20. Fanning JB. Sharing decision making (without sharing a religion). *GeneWatch.* 2013;26:24–39.

21. Kazak AE, DeRosa BW, Schwartz LA, et al. Psychological outcomes and health beliefs in adolescent and young adult survivors of childhood cancer and controls. *J Clin Oncol.* 2010;28:2002–2007.
22. Mahoney A, Carels RA, Pargament KI, et al. The sanctification of the body and behavioral health patterns of college students. *Int J Psychol Religion.* 2005;15:221–238.
23. Arnett JJ. Emerging adulthood. A theory of development from the late teens through the twenties. *Am Psychol.* 2000;55:469–480.
24. Balboni TA, Balboni M, Enzinger AC, et al. Provision of spiritual support to patients with advanced cancer by religious communities and associations with medical care at the end of life. *JAMA Int Med.* 2013;173:1109–1117.
25. Balboni T, Balboni M, Paulk ME, et al. Support of cancer patients' spiritual needs and associations with medical care costs at the end of life. *Cancer.* 2011;117:5383–5391.
26. Balboni TA, Paulk ME, Balboni MJ, et al. Provision of spiritual care to patients with advanced cancer: associations with medical care and quality of life near death. *J Clin Oncol.* 2010;28:445–452.
27. El Nawawi N. Palliative care and spiritual care. *Curr Opinion Support Palliative Care.* 2012;6:269.
28. Tarakeshwar N, Vanderwerker LC, Paulk E, et al. Religious coping is associated with the quality of life of patients with advanced cancer. *J Palliative Med.* 2006;9:646–657.
29. Puchalski C, Ferrell B, Virani R, et al. Improving the quality of spiritual care as a dimension of palliative care: the report of the Consensus Conference. *J Palliative Med.* 2009;12:885–904.
30. Cadge W, Ecklund EH, Short N. Religion and spirituality: A barrier and a bridge in the everyday professional work of pediatric physicians. *Social Problems.* 2009;56:702–721.
31. Jankowski KRB, Handzo GF, Flannelly KJ. Testing the efficacy of chaplaincy care. *J Health Care Chaplaincy.* 2011;17:100–125.

ARTICLE 9

Adolescents' Spirituality and Cystic Fibrosis Airway Clearance Treatment Adherence: Examining Mediators

Daniel H. Grossoehme,[1] DMin, Rhonda D. Szczesniak,[1,2] PhD, Sylvie Mrug,[3] PhD, Sophia M. Dimitriou,[1] BA, Alec Marshall,[1] and Gary L. McPhail,[1] MD

1 Division of Pulmonary Medicine, 2 Division Biostatistics and Epidemiology, Cincinnati Children's Hospital Medical Center, and 3 Department of Psychology, University of Alabama – Birmingham

All correspondence concerning this article should be addressed to Daniel H. Grossoehme, DMin, Division of Pulmonary Medicine MLC2021, Cincinnati Children's Hospital Medical Center, 3333 Burnet Avenue, Cincinnati, OH 45229, USA. E-mail: daniel.grossoehmc@cchmc.org

Received September 21, 2015; revisions received March 4, 2016; accepted March 5, 2016

Abstract

Objective: Adolescent cystic fibrosis (CF) treatment adherence is a significant multidimensional issue. Using the Theory of Reasoned Action (TRA), this study examined the role of spiritual factors in adherence.

Methods: Forty-five 11–19-year-olds diagnosed with CF completed questionnaires concerning psychosocial, spiritual, and adherence-related constructs and Daily Phone Diaries to calculate treatment adherence. Exploratory Factor Analysis identified two spiritual factors used in subsequent analyses. The mediating roles of attitude toward the treatment's value (utility), subjective behavioral norms (the product of perceived behavioral norms and one's motivation to comply with them), self-efficacy for completing the treatments and treatment intentions in the relationship between spiritual factors and treatment adherence were tested with path analysis.

Results: Lower 'spiritual struggle' and greater 'engaged spirituality' predicted treatment attitude (utility) and subjective behavioral norms, which, together with self-efficacy, predicted treatment intentions. Finally, treatment intentions predicted airway clearance adherence.

Grossoehme, D.H., Szczesniak, R.D., Mrug, S., Dimitriou, S.M., Marshall, A.L., and McPhail, G.L. (2016) "Adolescents' spirituality and cystic fibrosis airway clearance treatment adherence: examining mediators." *Journal of Pediatric Psychology*, 41, 19, 1022–1032.

Conclusions: Findings were consistent with the TRA. Engaged spirituality supports pro-adherence determinants and behavior. Spiritual struggle's negative associations with outcomes warrant screening and intervention.

Key words: adherence, adolescent, cystic fibrosis, Theory of Reasoned Action

Cystic fibrosis (CF) is a genetic, life-shortening disease requiring a significant daily treatment routine (Modi et al., 2006). Adherence to prescribed evidence-based therapies slows disease progression, and yet, adherence remains low and variable (36–90%), depending on modality and data collection methods (Ball et al., 2013; Modi et al., 2006). These rates are consistent with the poorest treatment adherence among adolescents with chronic diseases and point to the need to better understand factors that contribute to treatment adherence in this population of youth. Numerous barriers to treatment adherence have been identified (Modi & Quittner, 2006), some of which occur across disease populations (e.g., forgetting) and some of which are disease specific (e.g., time management in CF).

Overcoming barriers to treatment completion, and the stressor of a chronic disease, requires coping. An important coping method for adolescents with chronic illness is spirituality (Benore, Pargament, & Pendleton, 2008). The role of spirituality in treatment adherence among youth has been addressed by only one study, which found an association between positive spiritual coping and better adherence to antiretroviral medication among pediatric patients with HIV (Park & Nachman, 2010). Two spiritual factors may be related to treatment adherence in youth with CF—spiritual coping and sanctification of the body (Grossoehme, Opipari-Arrigan, VanDyke, Thurmond, & Seid, 2012; Mahoney et al., 2005). Spiritual coping is defined as "a search for significance, in ways related to the sacred, in times of stress" (Pendleton, Cavalli, Pargament, & Nasr, 2002), and represents a unique way of coping distinct from nonreligious coping (Burker, Evon, Sedway, & Egan, 2005). Spiritual coping has several components, including positive and negative spiritual coping (Pargament, 1997). Positive coping styles refer to relying on a secure attachment to God, finding meaning in life, and being spiritually connected to others. Negative coping style refers to a lack of secure attachment to God, spiritual struggles, and difficulties finding meaning in life. The terms "positive" and "negative" reflect the association of these styles of spiritual coping with positive or negative health outcomes, rather than the nature of coping styles themselves (Pargament, 1997).

In addition to negative and positive spiritual coping, Pargament (1997) has identified spiritual coping styles used for problem-solving to gain control of a stressor. These include Collaboration, in which one believes himself/herself to be solving the problem in partnership with the Divine; Passive Deferral, in which resolution of the problem is left to the Divine; Pleading, in which Divine assistance is sought through prayer or other means of communication; Self-Directed Coping, in which responsibility for problem-solving remains with the individual rather than with the Divine; and Active Surrender, in which a person, having reached the limit of those aspects of the stressor he/she can control, leaves its resolution up to the Divine. Collaborative spiritual coping is included as one of the positive coping styles based on prior research (Pargament, Smith, Koenig, & Perez, 1998); the remaining styles of problem-solving coping are typically not included in the positive or negative spiritual coping constructs or scales (Pargament, 1997). In prior research, positive spiritual coping was associated with more stable trajectories of pulmonary function, nutrition status, and fewer hospitalizations among adolescents with CF (Reynolds et al., 2014), possibly reflecting better adherence behaviors. In addition, parents of children with CF who endorsed using negative spiritual coping were among the least adherent to their child's prescribed therapies (Grossoehme et al., 2015). The odds of an adolescent with CF using a form of negative spiritual coping were found to decrease by 24% for every 1% increase in their pulmonary function (FEV_1: forced expiratory volume in 1 s, expressed as a percentage of what is predicted for their age and gender) (Grossoehme, Szczesniak, McPhail, & Seid, 2013).

Sanctification of the body is defined as imbuing one's body with divine significance and has been associated with pro-healthy behaviors among college students (Mahoney et al., 2005). Sanctification of the body is measured with two dimensions, one using concepts common to monotheistic faiths and one more broadly spiritual. Body sanctification has been measured in adolescents with CF, with values similar to those reported by parents of children with CF (Grossoehme, VanDyke, & Seid, 2008). However, no studies have examined the relationship between body sanctification and treatment adherence among adolescents with chronic disease, suggesting it is an underused and underappreciated construct. However, parents of children with CF who sanctified their child's body were among the most adherent to their child's prescribed treatments (Grossoehme et al., 2015). It is possible that adolescents who view their body as having divine significance may also engage in better self-care.

Although spiritual coping and body sanctification have been linked with better health outcomes, and with variables related to treatment adherence, no study has examined a comprehensive theoretical model that would explain how spiritual factors augment treatment adherence. We formulate and test such a model, drawing on a widely used model of health behaviors, the Theory of Reasoned Action (TRA) (Fishbein & Ajzen, 2010). This behavioral model suggests that a health behavior reasonably follows from beliefs a person has about the behavior. According to the TRA, the best predictor of a behavior (in this case, treatment adherence) is one's intention to perform that behavior. In turn, intentions are shaped by three "determinants": one's attitudes toward the value or utility of the behavior; subjective norms (the product between the perceived norms regarding the behavior by influential others and one's motivation to do what those others expect); and by the degree to which one perceives having control over performing the behavior (self-efficacy). These determinants arise from what Fishbein and Ajzen termed "background factors," which may include (but are not limited to) age, gender, ethnicity, education, socioeconomic status, and religious/spiritual factors. The background factors that are important may differ for different behaviors. Based on prior work using the TRA with parents of children with CF (Grossoehme et al., 2012), we proposed that spiritual coping and body sanctification contribute positively to beliefs about treatment utility, subjective norms, and self-efficacy, which lead to intentions to perform treatments and, in turn, treatment adherence. In addition, gender and depression were chosen as additional background factors to be included in the analyses as covariates. Fishbein and Ajzen name these as potentially important influences on behavioral beliefs (Fishbein & Ajzen, 2010); their inclusion in the present study is further supported by research showing that gender differences in the way CF is experienced account for differences in adherence and disease progression among adolescents. The importance of depression for adolescent treatment adherence has also been clearly demonstrated for adolescents with CF (Quittner et al., 2014a, 2014b). The specific aims for this study were (1) to examine how adolescents' spiritual beliefs and coping relate to adherence to their daily CF airway clearance (AC) treatments and (2) to apply the TRA to study factors that mediate the effects of spiritual beliefs and coping on treatment adherence in adolescents with CF. We hypothesized that greater positive and pleading spiritual coping and body sanctification, as well as lower negative and deferring spiritual coping would predict greater utility, subjective norms, and self-efficacy for CF treatments, which in turn would relate to greater treatment intentions and treatment adherence.

Methods

Participants

This study was approved by the institutional review board and was carried out at an accredited CF center within a 525-bed academic pediatric medical center in the Midwest. The Center followed approximately 265 children and youth, of which 90 were aged 11–19 years and 81 of whom met the eligibility criteria for this study: English literacy, confirmed CF diagnosis, prescribed AC, not participating in a treatment adherence study, and, following the age range used by Britto and colleagues, aged 11–19 years (Britto et al., 2004). An eligibility letter and study information sheet were mailed to legal guardians of eligible patients ($N = 81$) <18 years of age and eligible patients aged 18 or 19 years containing contact information for questions about the study or to indicate interest in the study. Eligible patients and legal guardians were also approached by study staff in the outpatient CF clinic. An *a priori* recruitment goal, based on a power analysis, was that 45 participants would be required for 80% power to detect changes in association of adherence determinants and adherence behavior of magnitude ≥0.40. Eligible participants were approached until the recruitment goal of $N = 45$ was achieved (54 approached with 9 declined for an 83% participation rate). Participants were aware that they were enrolling in a study of treatment adherence. Informed consent was obtained from the legal guardians of participants <18 years of age and participants aged 18 or 19 years; assent was obtained from all participants.

Procedure

Participants completed a set of questionnaires at the conclusion of the same clinic appointment when possible. In all cases, questionnaire completion was proctored by study staff. In addition to a demographic questionnaire, the scales described below were completed. The scales measuring TRA constructs were worded to be specific to the behavior of interest, which in this case was adherence to prescribed AC treatments. AC was chosen as the focus because it was a part of the treatment regimen for all youth in the study and is one of the most difficult parts of the treatment regimen to keep. Others have also shown (Modi et al., 2006) that only AC and enzymes were prescribed to all children with CF in their sample (e.g., vs. nebulized medications, which were not), and that AC frequency was more variable than enzymes or vitamins. Two Daily Phone Diary (DPD) calls were scheduled with participants during the 3 weeks following questionnaire completion to obtain adherence information.

The DPD uses cued recall, in which participants recounted all activities lasting >5 min that they had engaged in during the previous 24 hours. In addition to naming the activity, they also reported duration, companions, mood, and whether the activity was recreational or instrumental. An initial prompt is given to report certain activities that may take <5 min (e.g., taking enzymes). By asking about all activities, the participants are "blinded" to the behaviors of interest, decreasing the likelihood of giving socially desirable responses. Each activity was coded across three increasingly detailed levels of behavioral specificity by a study staff member; the coding was subsequently verified by a second study staff member and discrepancies were resolved by consensus. Activity frequency was averaged over the two DPDs. Therapies prescribed at the clinic visit before questionnaire completion were collected by chart review using a query of the electronic medical record. Adherence was then calculated as the ratio of DPD-reported treatment frequency divided by the prescribed treatment frequency.

Spiritual coping

Spiritual coping was measured with the 14-item Brief R-COPE scale (Pargament, Koenig, & Perez, 2000) to which five additional items from the complete R-COPE were added to measure spiritual coping for control by problem-solving (Pargament, 1999). These five additional items were *Collaborative* ("Tried to put my plans into action together with God"), *Deferring* ("Didn't do much, just assumed God would handle it"), *Active surrender* ("Did what I could and put the rest in God's hands"), *Pleading* ("Pleaded with God to make things turn out okay"), and *Self-directed* ("Tried to deal with the situation on my own without God's help"). These problem-solving and control items were added based on prior research (Burker, Evon, Sedway, & Egan, 2004) that concluded that persons with and without CF use religious or spiritual coping for problem-solving and that they differ in their sense of control and agency in coping with their disease stressors. Their study suggested that the use of self-directed religious coping in particular, rather than Deferring, may be attributable to the self-management skills being taught to persons with CF even in their early years. The Brief R-COPE instructions typically include a cue that makes them situation specific; in this study the cue was, "The following items deal with ways you have coped with your CF." Participants indicated how frequently they used each coping style using a four-item Likert-style response format, coded 0–3 ("not at all" to "a great deal"). The measure includes two seven-item subscales, one for positive and one for negative religious coping styles, derived as sums of the items. Positive religious coping items include statements such as, "Looked for a stronger connection with God." Negative religious coping items include statements such as, "Wondered whether God had abandoned me." The Brief R-COPE (or items from it) has been used with 8–19-year-olds and has acceptable psychometric properties with Cronbach alphas ranging from .59 to .95 (Benore et al., 2008; Cotton et al., 2009; Dew et al., 2010; Molock, Puri, Matlin, & Barksdale, 2006; Reynolds et al., 2014; Reynolds, Mrug, Hensler, Guion, & Madan-Swain, 2014; Terreri & Glenwick, 2013; Westers, Rehfuss, Olson, & Wiemann, 2014). Cronbach's alphas in this sample were .80 for the negative subscale and .89 for the positive subscale.

Sanctification of the body

This construct, described as imbuing one's body with divine significance, has two dimensions, which are measured using two subscales of the body sanctification scale presented by Mahoney and colleagues (2005). These subscales measured religious (12 items) and spiritual (10 items) aspects of body sanctification. The monotheistic religious subscale, *Manifestation of God in the body*, contained items such as, "My body is created in God's image." The spiritual subscale, *Sacred qualities of the body*, included descriptive attributes such as, "miraculous" and "spirit-filled." Participants rated items on a seven-point scale (0–6) from "strongly disagree" to "strongly agree" for the Manifestation of God subscale and "doesn't apply" to "applies strongly" for the Sacred qualities subscale. This scale was previously used with 12–20-year-olds with Cronbach alphas reported from .97 to .98 (Grossoehme et al., 2008; Mahoney et al., 2005). Cronbach's alphas for this sample were .98 for the Manifestation of God subscale and .96 for the Sacred qualities subscale.

Treatment attitude (utility)

Four items comprising the *Perceived utility* (benefits/costs) subscale of the Adherence Determinants Questionnaire (DiMatteo et al., 1993) were used to measure participants' attitudes toward the utility of completing their treatments. The scale is composed of items such as, "The benefits of my treatment plan outweigh any difficulty I might have in following it." Respondents indicated their level of agreement with each statement using a five-item Likert-style response format ("strongly disagree" to "strongly agree"). AC treatment-specific wording was used for these items. This scale has been used with 12–17-year-olds with a reported Cronbach alpha of .76 (Fotheringham, 1998). In the present study, Cronbach's alpha was .57.

Subjective norms

The TRA conceptualizes subjective norms as composed of normative beliefs about a behavior (the extent to which the participant believes that completing AC as prescribed would be approved of by an important other kind of person), and the participant's motivation to do what that important other person expects of the participant (here, to complete their AC as prescribed) (Ajzen & Fishbein, 1980). Following Fishbein and Ajzen's point that no single TRA questionnaire exists and that investigators must construct their own measure based on their theoretical model and the example items provided (Fishbein & Ajzen, 2010), pairs of questions were developed to measure subjective norms for each of two important reference groups ("my immediate family" and "my close friends"). Each question pair consisted of an item for perceived behavioral normative beliefs (e.g., "My family makes sure I get my airway clearance done the number of times recommended each day") and one for motivation to comply with that norm for those important other persons (e.g., "I want to do what my family thinks I should do about my daily recommended airway clearance"). These items were developed based on Fishbein and Ajzen's example using behavior-specific wording for AC, and, to verify understandability by the target sample, were used in a cognitive interview discussion with young adult with CF from this CF Center who was ineligible for the study. Participants indicated their level of agreement with each statement using a five-item Likert-style response format ("strongly disagree" to "strongly agree", coded 1–5). As outlined by Fishbein and Ajzen (p.137), perceived behavioral normative beliefs alone do not adequately predict behavioral intentions. Rather, it is the product of these norms and the person's motivation to comply with them which is salient. Therefore, the magnitude of the subjective norm is defined by calculating the product of the normative belief item by the motivation item for each identified important other group (family and close friends, respectively) (Ajzen & Madden, 1986; Fishbein & Ajzen, 2010).

Self-efficacy

Bandura's guide for constructing self-efficacy scales was used to build an AC treatment-specific, 10-item scale to measure self-efficacy for completing AC treatments (Bandura, 2006). This method has been used with CF samples in prior work (Grossoehme et al., 2012). Using a range of 0–100, respondents indicated their confidence for completing their AC treatment for each of 10 given conditions (e.g., "On a typical weekend," "When I'm running late in the morning," "When our family is feeling stressed"). Cronbach's alpha for this scale was .91.

Treatment intentions

The four-item intentions subscale of the Adherence Determinants Questionnaire (DiMatteo et al., 1993) was used with AC treatment-specific wording. An example item is, "I have made a commitment to follow my AC treatment plan." Respondents indicated their level of agreement with each statement using a five-item Likert-style response format ("strongly disagree" to "strongly agree"). Two items are reverse scored, and the sum of the four items gives the score for intentions. This scale has been used with 12–17-year-olds with a reported Cronbach alpha of .84; in the present study, Cronbach's alpha was .89.

Adherence to treatments

The Daily Phone Diary (DPD) was used with all participants to collect data for actual AC treatment adherence. DPD is widely used in CF adherence research and has acceptable psychometric properties (Quittner, Modi, Lemanek, Ievers-Landis, & Rapoff, 2007; Quittner & Opipari, 1994). Strong convergent validity of the DPD has been documented (Quittner et al., 1998; Quittner & Opipari, 1994). Reliable stability coefficients over a 3-week period ($rs = .61–.71$, $p < .01$) and high levels of interrater reliability (>90%) in a CF population have been reported (Quittner et al., 1998). Use of the DPD with adolescents who have CF have shown adherence rates ranging from 36% to nearly 100% (Modi et al., 2010). Compared with self-report data obtained by direct inquiry of parents about their treatment completion, which may well include overreporting of adherence, adherence measured by DPD, while still considered by some to be a form of self-report, was significantly lower (Modi et al., 2006).

Clinical characteristics

Values for the most recent pulmonary function test and the number of pulmonary exacerbations in the prior year were obtained by chart review.

Statistical analyses

Descriptive statistics and bivariate associations among variables were examined. Given the relatively large number of interrelated spiritual variables that were measured, the variables were first reduced to a smaller number of underlying dimensions using Exploratory Factor Analysis. Before the factor analysis, two spiritual variables (Pleading and Deferring) were excluded, which were not significantly associated with any treatment-related variables (treatment utility, perceived behavioral norms, self-efficacy, and intentions). The remaining seven spiritual variables were then subjected to Exploratory Factor Analysis using principal components extraction and varimax rotation, yielding two factor scores (computed from factor score coefficients) that were used in subsequent analyses. As expected by the factor analysis constraints, the two unrotated factors had virtually no correlation (Pearson's $r = .006$). Varimax rotation was used because the correlation of the two factors under oblique rotation was negligible ($r = -.16$). The hypothesized model was then tested with path analysis in Mplus version 7.3 (Muthen & Muthen, 2010). In this model, the two spiritual TRA background factors were modeled as predictors of treatment utility, subjective norms (immediate family and close friends), and self-efficacy, which in turn, following the TRA, predicted intentions. Finally, intentions predicted AC treatment adherence. Treatment utility, subjective norms, and self-efficacy were allowed to correlate. Missing data (1.4% of all values) were handled with Full Information Maximum Likelihood, which preserves the overall sample size and minimizes bias (Wothke, 2000). The significance of all indirect effects was tested simultaneously with bootstrapping using 10,000 bootstrap samples (Preacher & Hayes, 2008). Results corresponding to $p < .05$ were considered statistically significant.

Results

Preliminary analyses

Descriptive characteristics of the sample are presented in Table I. No associations were found between the study variables and the clinical measures of pulmonary exacerbations and pulmonary function (FEV_1), with correlations ranging from -0.15 to 0.17 ($p > .29$). Mean adherence rates for AC were relatively high as a percentage of prescribed treatments completed. However, only 20% of youth had perfect (100%) adherence for AC over the 3-week period in which adherence data were collected by DPD. The sample overall was relatively healthy, with mild pulmonary disease based on pulmonary function testing, and relatively few pulmonary exacerbations. Compared with eligible patients who were not enrolled, participants did not differ significantly from non-participants in terms of gender, number of pulmonary exacerbations, or pulmonary function (FEV$_1$) (all $p > .30$). There was a significant difference in mean age between the groups ($t = -2.64$; $df = 87.8$; $p = .010$) with participants being younger, on average ($M = 13.9$ years, $SD = 2.3$) than non-participants ($M = 15.3$, $SD = 2.6$).

Table I: Descriptive summary of demographic and clinical characteristics of study participants

Characteristics	N (%)	M (SD)
Female, n (%)	27 (60)	
Age, years		13.8±2.2
Religious affiliation, n (%)		
• Nondenominational Christian	19 (42)	
• Protestant	10 (22)	
• Roman Catholic	6 (13)	
• None	6 (13)	
• Other	3 (7)	
• Did not disclose	1 (2)	
FEV$_1$ % predicted		85.7±20.8
PEx in prior year		1.38±1.79
Adherence to AC treatment frequency, % of prescribed treatment	83[a] (67–100)	
Complete adherence to AC treatment frequency, n (%)	20 (44)	

Note. $N = 45$; FEV$_1$ = forced expiratory volume in 1 s, as a measure of lung function; PEx = pulmonary exacerbation; AC = airway clearance.
[a]Values are median (interquartile range).

Examinations of correlations among variables indicated that pleading and deferring spiritual coping were not associated with any variables related to treatment adherence (Pearson correlation coefficient r's ranged from $-.19$ to $.18$, $p > .232$). Principal component analysis of the seven remaining spiritual variables indicated the presence of two factors based on parallel analysis and Velicer's test, and Kaiser criterion (two eigenvalues were >1). A summary of the individual measures and results from the factor analysis are provided in Table II. The first factor was termed 'engaged spirituality'; it included high positive loadings from positive spiritual coping, collaboration with God, active surrender, and both body sanctification subscales (manifestation of God in the body and sacred qualities of the body). The second factor was termed 'spiritual struggle', and included high loadings from negative religious coping and self-directed coping (see Table II).

Table II: Loadings of spiritual variables

Spiritual variables	M (SD)	Range	Engaged spirituality	Spiritual struggle
Positive spiritual coping	11.11 (6.01)	0–21	**.94**	.04
Collaborative coping	1.41 (1.21)	0–3	**.83**	.17
Active surrender coping	1.62 (1.07)	0–3	**.70**	−.35
Manifestation of God in the body	66.93 (17.22)	12–84	**.89**	−.27
Sacred qualities of the body	53.40 (14.10)	13–70	**.89**	−.25
Negative spiritual coping	2.55 (3.27)	0–16	.13	**.91**
Self-directed coping	1.09 (1.02)	0–3	−.38	**.60**
Eigenvalue			3.95	1.31
% variance			54%	21%

Note. Bold font indicates which factor each spiritual variable loaded on.

Descriptive statistics and correlations of all variables used in the path model are presented in Table III. Engaged spirituality was related to more supportive friend norms, whereas spiritual struggle was associated with lower perceptions of treatment utility. Utility was related to more supportive norms from both friends and family, as well as stronger intentions to perform treatment. Family and friend norms were positively correlated and related to stronger intentions. Self-efficacy was related to stronger intentions and intentions were related to adherence. Gender and age were not related to any variables and were not included in the main model. The zero correlation of the two spiritual variables reflects the forced independence of the factor scores derived from the factor score coefficients after using an orthogonal rotation (Henson & Roberts, 2006).

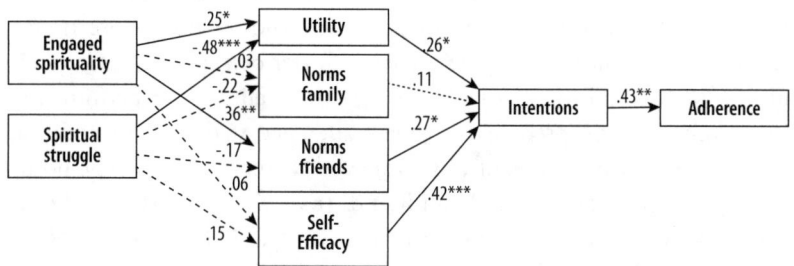

Figure 1: Path analysis model linking spiritual factors with adherence through utility, norms, self-efficacy, and intentions. Note: Path coefficients are standardized. Dashed paths are not significant. $^*p < .05$, $^{**}p < .01$, $^{***}p < .001$

Table III: Correlation matrix of path model variables

	M (SD)	1	2	3	4	5	6	7
1. Engaged spirituality	0.00 (1.00)	–						
2. Spiritual struggle	0.00 (1.00)	.00[a]	–					
3. Utility	34.36 (3.56)	.25	–.48**	–				
4. Family norms	2.93 (2.02)	.03	–.22	.45**	–			
5. Friend norms	5.29 (4.27)	.36*	–.17	.56***	.53***	–		
6. Self-efficacy	75.11 (20.22)	.06	.15	.18	-0.5	–0.5	–	
7. Intentions	17.36 (2.60)	.08	–.02	.51***	–.33*	–.34*	.51***	–
8. Adherence	0.86 (0.30)	.07	–.10	.15	–.20	–.08	.22	.34*

*$p < .05$; **$p < .01$, ***$p < .001$.
[a]Estimated Pearson correlation coefficient between factor scores after rotation; before rotation, Pearson's $r = .006$.

Main analyses

Good model fit for path analytic models is indicated by Comparative Fit Index (CFI) > 0.95, Root Mean Square Error of Approximation (RMSEA) < 0.06, and Standardized Root Mean Square Residual (SRMR) < 0.08 (Hu & Bentler, 1998). Using these guidelines, the path model had excellent fit to the data (χ^2 (10) = 6.91, $p = .734$; CFI = 1.00; RMSEA = 0.00; SRMR = 0.08). Engaged spirituality predicted greater perceived utility of treatment and treatment-supporting norms from close friends (see Figure 1). Spiritual struggle predicted lower perceptions of treatment utility. Neither spiritual variable predicted self-efficacy to perform AC. Intentions, in turn, predicted greater adherence with AC. In addition, perceived utility of treatment was correlated with more supportive norms from family ($r = .38$, $p < .01$) and friends ($r = .47$, $p < .001$), and norms from family and friends were correlated ($r = .53$, $p < .001$). Testing of indirect effects with bootstrapping yielded significant effects from engaged spirituality through friend norms and intentions to adherence (indirect effect $b = 0.012$, $p < .05$; 95% CI = 0.002 to 0.050), as well as from spiritual struggle through utility and intentions to adherence (b –0.017, $p < .05$; 95% CI –0.064 to 0.001). The indirect effects from engaged spirituality through utility and intentions and from self-efficacy through intentions to adherence did not reach statistical significance ($p > .05$).

Discussion

This study applied a theoretical model, the TRA, to better understand how spiritual factors may relate to treatment adherence among youth with CF. As hypothesized, engaged spirituality (involving positive spiritual coping, collaborative and active surrender coping, and body sanctification) was related to greater perceived utility of AC and more supportive norms for doing the treatment from close friends, both of which were associated with stronger intentions to perform the treatment, and in turn greater treatment adherence. Additionally, spiritual struggle (involving negative spiritual coping and self-directed coping) was related to lower perceived utility of AC, which in turn related to weaker intentions to perform AC and lower treatment adherence. Finally, self-efficacy was related to treatment intentions, although it was not associated with the spiritual factors.

Certain forms of spiritual coping are termed "negative" because they are associated with poorer health outcomes. These include not only the styles of constructed meaning of disease as divine punishment or diabolical act, but also spiritual coping for control that is self-directed. It was therefore not surprising that self-directed spiritual coping loaded on the same factor (termed spiritual struggle) as negative spiritual coping in the principal components analysis. Spiritual struggle's association with poorer outcomes is consistent with substantial prior research (Fitchett et al., 2004; Ramirez et al., 2012; Thune-Bolye, Stygall, Keshtgar, Davidson, & Newman, 2011, 2013). Spiritual struggle has been associated with depression (Thune-Bolye et al., 2013), which in turn has been related to poorer adherence (DiMatteo, Lepper, & Croghan, 2000; Smith et al., 2006). It may be that poor treatment adherence among youth who struggle spiritually may be owing to their less positive attitudes toward the value of their treatments (e.g., beliefs that treatments are not useful), and subsequently diminished intentions to complete these treatments. The relationship of spiritual struggles to low perceived utility, intentions, and adherence to AC is consistent with previously reported associations between negative spiritual coping and decline in adolescents' pulmonary function. However, it is also possible that attitudes about treatment utility and treatment intentions may affect spiritual factors, and these alternatives should be evaluated in future longitudinal studies.

The engaged spirituality factor reflected multiple facets of helpful spiritual engagement, including positive spiritual coping (e.g., turning to God for strength), collaboration with God to solve problems, turning problems to God after doing one's best (Active Surrender), and viewing one's body as sacred and a reflection of God. The daily treatments to slow CF disease progression require time and effort—engagement—to provide maximum benefit, and persons with CF are taught disease self-management skills from an early age. It may be that greater positive spiritual engagement promotes greater engagement with one's disease and its treatment.

Engaged spirituality was also associated with perceived behavioral norms by one's friends, but not the perceived norms by one's family. This may be explained by homophily (associating with peers with similar values, beliefs, and behaviors) (Valente, 2010) and peer influence during adolescence. The influence of spirituality and friendship on each other has been described (Schwartz, Bukowski, & Aoki, 2006). Not only may spirituality and its practices influence one's choice of friends and activities with them, so friends can also modify one's spirituality. The greater role of close friends' norms compared with family norms may reflect increasingly greater importance of peer influence compared with that of parents during adolescence (Levenson, Aldwin, & D'Mello, 2006). The role of peer influence, in addition to family influence, may be an important construct to integrate into the design, prototype, and development of interventions aimed at adolescents with CF.

Self-efficacy for completing AC was unrelated to spiritual factors. This may be because it was related to other factors, such as the extent to which the youth have assumed responsibility for completing their AC treatments, or the existence of, and ability to create, routines which include AC (Fiese & Wamboldt, 2000) and family emotional dynamics (Fiese, Wamboldt, & Anbar, 2005). This finding is also consistent with findings from parents of children with CF, for whom self-efficacy was associated with treatment intentions but not spiritual, demographic, or psychosocial factors (Grossoehme et al., 2013).

The present findings suggest the following practice implications. First, screening youth with CF for spiritual struggle may be helpful to identify patients who may be less adherent with their therapies. Methods to screen for spiritual struggle for use by nonchaplain clinicians have been published (Fitchett & Risk, 2009). Interventions exist with demonstrated efficacy in helping adolescents (Oemig Dworsky et al., 2013) and adults decrease spiritual struggles and improve psychological outcomes (Cole, 2005). For instance, spiritually focused cognitive therapy may be used to help youth develop more positive and engaged spirituality and reduce spiritual struggle, while strengthening their perceptions of treatment utility and peer norms for conducting treatments. This would focus attention on the more proximal determinants of treatment adherence rather than interventions aimed at the more distal outcomes such as intentions or adherence behaviors. Second, youth who are spiritually engaged may benefit from an approach that draws parallels between their engagement with faith and engagement with disease self-management.

This study has the following limitations. The relatively small sample size had limited statistical power to detect smaller-sized effects. Specifically, the sample size provided sufficient power (≥ 0.80) to detect only indirect effects consisting of large effects ($\beta = .59$) (Fritz & MacKinnon, 2007); thus the power was limited for the obtained effects ($\beta s< = \leq.048$). In addition, the small sample size relative to the number of free parameters in the model may have resulted in unstable estimates (Bentler & Chou, 1987); replication with a larger sample size would be important. All participants were from a single center, with potential selection bias. Participants had a lower mean age than eligible nonparticipants, so the results may not generalize to older youth with CF. The limited sample size also did not permit comparison of the model across age-groups, which means that possible developmental differences in the results could not be addressed. However, one study found no age differences in the relationship between spiritual coping and internalizing and externalizing problems (Reynolds, Mrug, & Guion, 2013). Adherence rates, as a percentage of prescribed treatments, were relatively high compared with other studies (Ball et al., 2013; Zindani, Streetman, Streetman, & Nasr, 2006). This study was primarily carried out during the school year, when adherence rates tend to be highest (Ball et al., 2013). There also may have been a treatment effect of participation in the study itself; Modi and colleagues have shown that treatment adherence rates are higher when participants are enrolled in trials (Modi et al., 2010). The number of prescribed therapies was based on chart review; it may be that some youth were told orally by their pulmonologist how many treatments to do without that having been reflected in their chart note, which was used to calculate adherence. These factors may explain the relatively higher adherence rates in this study than in some previously published studies. Most of the data obtained in this study came from self-report. This opens the possibility for common method bias, although there is limited consensus on the extent to which it may inflate observed relationships between variables (Siemsen, Roth, & Oliveira, 2010). The utility subscale had a low reliability as measured by Cronbach's alpha. Finally, the cross-sectional design of the study does not allow causal interpretations, although adherence was assessed after the other variables. Future research should replicate the results using longitudinal designs, as cross-sectional studies often yield biased estimates of prospective mediation effects (Maxwell & Cole, 2007).

In conclusion, this study offers novel insights into psychological processes through which spiritual factors may contribute to treatment adherence. It suggests that spiritual factors may promote or hinder perceptions of treatment utility and social norms for completing treatments, which in turn contribute to treatment intentions and adherence. Future research implications include the inclusion of spiritual, together with other psychosocial constructs, to gain a broader understanding of adherence and self-management in adolescence. The role of peers and their influence on treatment adherence, especially during preadolescence and early adolescence (11–13 years old), should be explored. The results also show that TRA is a useful theoretical model for understanding treatment adherence among youth with CF.

Acknowledgments

The authors acknowledge with appreciation the contributions of Elizabeth Lind, Colin Lozier, Sarah Lohbeck, Alaina McCracken, Michael Price, Emily Smith, Matthew Veerkamp, Yu Wang, and Vasilios Zois who conducted DPDs and performed data entry and preliminary analyses for this study. The authors are grateful to medical writer Denise Wetzel for critical review of the manuscript.

Funding

This work was supported by a Places Outcomes Research Awards from the James M. Anderson Center for Health Service Excellence.

Conflicts of interest

Coauthor Gary McPhail served on the national advisory board during 2014 for Vertex Pharmaceuticals, and for Gilead Pharmaceuticals. No other coauthors have any potential or real conflicts of interest.

References

Ajzen, I., & Fishbein, M. (1980). *Understanding attitudes and predicting social behavior.* Englewood Cliffs, NJ: Prentice-Hall.

Ajzen, I., & Madden, T. J. (1986). Prediction of goal-directed behavior: Attitudes, intentions, and perceived behavioural control. *Journal of Experimental Social Psychology, 22,* 453–474.

Ball, R., Southern, K. W., McCormack, P., Duff, A. J. A., Brownlee, K. G., & McNamara, P. S. (2013). Adherence to nebulised therapies in adolescents with cystic fibrosis is best on week-days during school term-time. *Journal of Cystic Fibrosis, 12*, 440–444. doi: 10.1016/j.jcf.2012/12/012

Bandura, A. (2006). Guide for creating self-efficacy scales. In F. Pajares & T. Urdan (Eds.), *Self-efficacy beliefs of adolescents* (p.367). Greenwich, CT: Information Age Publishing.

Benore, E., Pargament, K. I., & Pendleton, S. M. (2008). An initial examination of religious coping in children with asthma. *International Journal for the Psychology of Religion, 18*, 267–290. doi: 10.1080/10508610802229197

Bentler, P. M., & Chou, C.-P. (1987). Practical issues in structural modeling. *Sociological Methods and Research, 16*, 78–117.

Britto, M. T., DeVellis, R. F., Hornung, R. W., DeFriese, G. H., Atherton, H. D., & Slap, G. B. (2004). Health care preferences and priorities of adolescents with chronic illnesses. *Pediatrics, 114*, 1272–1280.

Burker, E. J., Evon, D. M., Sedway, J. A., & Egan, T. (2004). Religious coping, psychological distress and disability among patients with end-stage pulmonary disease. *Journal of Clinical Psychology in Medical Settings, 11*, 179–193.

Burker, E. J., Evon, D. M., Sedway, J. A., & Egan, T. (2005). Religious and non-religious coping in lung transplant candidates: Does adding God to the picture tell us more? *Journal of Behavioral Medicine, 28*, 513–526.

Cole, B. (2005). Spiritually-focused psychotherapy for people diagnosed with cancer: A pilot outcomes study. *Mental Health, Religion and Culture, 8*, 217–226.

Cotton, S., Grossoehme, D. H., Rosenthal, S. L., McGrady, M. E., Roberts, Y. H., Hines, J., … Tsevat, J. (2009). Religious/spiritual coping in adolescents with sickle cell disease: A pilot study. *Journal of Pediatric Hematology Oncology, 31*, 313–318. doi: 10.1097/MPH.0b013e31819e40e3

Dew, R. E., Daniel, S. S., Goldston, D. B., McCall, W. V., Kuchibhatla, M., Schleifer, C., … Koenig, H. G. (2010). A prospective study of religion/spirituality and depressive symptoms among adolescent psychiatric patients. *Journal of Affective Disorders, 120*, 149–157.

DiMatteo, M. R., Hays, R. D., Gritz, E. R., Bastani, R., Crane, L., Elashoff, R., … Marcus, A. (1993). Patient adherence to cancer control regimens: Scale development and initial validation. *Psychological Assessment, 5*, 102–112.

DiMatteo, M. R., Lepper, H. S., & Croghan, T. W. (2000). Depression is a risk factor for noncompliance with medical treatment. *Archives of Internal Medicine, 160*, 2101–2107.

Fiese, B. H., & Wamboldt, F. S. (2000). Family routines, rituals and asthma management: A proposal for family-based strategies to increase treatment adherence. *Families, Systems and Health, 18*, 405.

Fiese, B. H., Wamboldt, F. S., & Anbar, R. D. (2005). Family asthma management routines: Connections to medical adherence and quality of life. *Journal of Pediatrics, 146*, 171–176. doi: 10.1016/j.jpeds.2004.08.083

Fishbein, M., & Ajzen, I. (2010). *Predicting and changing behavior*. New York, NY: Taylor & Francis.

Fitchett, G., Murphy, P. E., Kim, J., Gibbons, J. L., Cameron, J. R., & Davis, J. A. (2004). Religious struggle: Prevalence, correlates and mental health risks in diabetic, congestive heart failure, and oncology patients. *International Journal of Psychiatry in Medicine, 34*, 179–196. doi: 10.2190/UCJ9-DP4M-9C0X-835M

Fitchett, G., & Risk, J. L. (2009). Screening for spiritual struggle. *Journal of Pastoral Care and Counseling, 63*, 1–12.

Fotheringham, M. J. (1998). Adolescents' adherence to chronic medical regimens: Parent–adolescent conflict and adolescent autonomy in relation to adherence to insulin dependent diabetes treatment regimens (doctoral dissertation). Department of Psychiatry, University of Adelaide, Adelaide, Australia.

Fritz, M. S., & MacKinnon, D. P. (2007). Required sample size to detect the mediated effect. *Psychological Science, 18*, 233–239.

Grossoehme, D. H., Opipari-Arrigan, L., VanDyke, R., Thurmond, S., & Seid, M. (2012). Relationship of adherence determinants and parental spirituality in cystic fibrosis. *Pediatric Pulmonology, 47*, 558–566. doi: 10.1002/ppul.21614

Grossoehme, D. H., Szczesniak, R., Dimitriou, S., Dodd, C., Britton, L., Chini, B., & Seid, M. (2013). Parental adherence: Spiritual, religious and psychosocial influences. *Pediatric Pulmonology, S36*, 429.

Grossoehme, D. H., Szczesniak, R., McPhail, G., & Seid, M. (2013). Is adolescents' religious coping with cystic fibrosis associated with the rate of decline in pulmonary function – a preliminary study. *Journal of Health Care Chaplaincy, 19*, 33–42. doi: 10.1080/08854726.2013/767083

Grossoehme, D. H., Szczesniak, R. D., Britton, L. L., Siracusa, C. M., Quittner, A. L., Chini, B. A. ... Seif, M. (2015). Adherence determinants in CF: Cluster analysis of parental psychosocial and religious/spiritual factors. *Annals of the American Thoracic Society, 12*, 838–846. doi: 10.1513/AnnalsATS.201408-379OC

Grossoehme, D. H., VanDyke, R., & Seid, M. (2008). Spirituality's role in chronic disease self-management: Sanctification of the body in families dealing with cystic fibrosis. *Journal of Healthcare Chaplaincy, 15*, 149–158. doi: 10.1080/08854720903163312

Henson, R. K., & Roberts, J. K. (2006). Use of exploratory factor analysis in published research common errors and some comment on improved practice. *Educational and Psychological Measurement, 66*, 393–416.

Hu, L.-t., & Bentler, P. M. (1998). Fit indices in covariance structure modeling: Sensitivity to underparameterized model misspecification. *Psychological Methods, 3*, 424.

Levenson, M. R., Aldwin, C. M., & D'Mello, M. (2006). Religious development from adolescence to middle adulthood. In R. F. Paloutzian & C. L. Park (Eds.), *Handbook of the psychology of religion and spirituality* (pp. 144–161). New York, NY: Guilford Press.

Mahoney, A., Carels, R. A., Pargament, K. I., Wachholtz, A., Leeper, L. E., Kaplar, M. & Frutchey, R. (2005). The sanctification of the body and behavioral health patterns of college students. *International Journal for the Psychology of Religion, 15*, 221–238.

Maxwell, S. E., & Cole, D. A. (2007). Bias in cross-sectional analyses of longitudinal mediation. *Psychological Methods, 12*, 23.

Modi, A. C., Cassedy, A. E., Quittner, A. L., Accurso, F., Sontag, M., Koenig, J. M., & Ittenbach, R F. (2010). Trajectories of adherence to airway clearance therapy for patients with cystic fibrosis. *Journal of Pediatric Psychology, 35*, 1028–1037. doi: 10.1093/jpepsy/jsq015

Modi, A. C., Lim, C. S., Yu, N., Geller, D., Wagner, M. H., & Quittner, A. L. (2006). A multi-method assessment of treatment adherence for children with cystic fibrosis. *Journal of Cystic Fibrosis, 5*, 177–185. doi: 10.1016/j.jcf.2006.03.002

Modi, A. C., & Quittner, A. L. (2006). Barriers to treatment adherence for children with cystic fibrosis and asthma: What gets in the way? *Journal of Pediatric Psychology, 31*, 846–858. doi: 10.1093/jpepsy/jsj096

Molock, S. D., Puri, R., Matlin, S., & Barksdale, C. (2006). Relationship between religious coping and suicidal behaviors among African–American adolescents. *Journal of Black Psychology, 32*, 366–389.

Muthen, L. K., & Muthen, B. O. (2010). *Mplus User's Guide* (7th ed.). Los Angeles, CA: Muthen & Muthen.

Oemig Dworsky, C. K., Pargament, K. I., Reist Gibbel, M., Krumrei, E. J., FAigin, C. A., Haugen, M. R. G., ... Warner, H. L. (2013). Winding road: Preliminary support for a spritually integrated intervention addressing college students' spiritual struggles. *Research in the Social Scientific Study of Religion, 24*, 309–339.

Pargament, K. I. (1997). *Psychology of religious coping*. New York, NY: Guilford Press.

Pargament, K. I. (1999). *Religious/spiritual coping* (pp. 43–56). Kalamazoo, MI: Fetzer Institute, National Institute on Aging Working Group.

Pargament, K. I., Koenig, H. G., & Perez, L. M. (2000). The many methods of religious coping: Development and initial validation of the RCOPE. *Journal of Clinical Psychology, 56,* 519–543. doi: 10.1002/(SICI)1097-4679

Pargament, K. I., Smith, B. W., Koenig, H. G., & Perez, L. (1998). Patterns of positive and negative religious coping with major life stressors. *Journal for the Scientific Study of Religion, 37,* 710–724.

Park, J., & Nachman, S. (2010). The link between religion and HAART adherence in pediatric HIV patients. *AIDS Care, 22,* 556–561. doi: 10.1080/09540120903254013

Pendleton, S. M., Cavalli, K. S., Pargament, K. I., & Nasr, S. Z. (2002). Religious/spiritual coping in childhood cystic fibrosis: A qualitative study. *Pediatrics, 109,* E8.

Preacher, K. J., & Hayes, A. F. (2008). Asymptotic and resampling strategies for assessing and comparing indirect effects in multiple mediator models. *Behavior Research Methods, 40,* 879–891.

Quittner, A. L., Abbott, J., Georgiopoulos, A. M, Goldbeck, L., Smith, B., Hempstead, S E., ... Elborn, S. (2014a). the International Committee on Mental Health (2016). International Committee on Mental Health in cystic fibrosis: Cystic Fibrosis Foundation and European Cystic Fibrosis Society consensus statements for screening and treating depression and anxiety. *Thorax,* online publication (October, 2015, doi: 10.1136/thoraxjnl-2015-207488. International%20Guidelines.pdf. Retrieved 14 May 2015.

Quittner, A. L., Espelage, D. L., Opipari, L. C., Carter, B., Eid, N., & Eigen, H. (1998). Role strain in couples with and without a child with a chronic illness: Associations with marital satisfaction, intimacy, and daily mood. *Health Psychology, 17,* 112.

Quittner, A. L., Goldbeck, L., Abbott, J., Duff, A. J., Lambrecht, P., Sole, A. ... Barker, D. (2014b). Prevalence of depression and anxiety in patients with cystic fibrosis and parent caregivers: Results of The International Depression Epidemiological Study across nine countries. *Thorax, 69,* 1090–1097. doi: 10.1136/thoraxjnl-2014-205983

Quittner, A. L., Modi, A. C., Lemanek, K. L., Ievers-Landis, C. E., & Rapoff, M. A. (2007). Evidence-based assessment of adherence to medical treatments in pediatric psychology. *Journal of Pediatric Psychology, 33,* 916–936. doi: 10.1093/iPePS//jsm064

Quittner, A. L., & Opipari, L. C. (1994). Differential treatment of siblings: Interview and diary analyses comparing two family contexts. *Child Development, 65,* 800–814. doi: 10.1111/1467-8624.ep9408220881

Ramirez, S. P., Macedo, D. S., Sales, P. M. G., Figueiredo, S. M., Daher, E. F., Araujo, S. M., ... Carvalho, A. F. (2012). The relationship between religious coping, psychological distress and quality of life in hemodialysis patients. *Journal of Psychosomatic Research, 72,* 129–135. doi: 10.1016/j.jpsychores.2011.11.012

Reynolds, N., Mrug, S., Britton, L., Guion, K., Wolfe, K., & Gutierrez, H. (2014). Spiritual coping predicts 5-year health outcomes in adolescents with cystic fibrosis. *Journal of Cystic Fibrosis, 13,* 593–600. doi: 10.1016/j.jcf.2014.01.013

Reynolds, N., Mrug, S., & Guion, K. (2013). Spiritual coping and psychosocial adjustment of adolescents with chronic illness: The role of cognitive attributions, age, and disease group. *Journal of Adolescent Health, 52,* 559–565. doi: 10.1016/j.jadohealth.2012.09.007

Reynolds, N., Mrug, S., Hensler, M., Guion, K., & Madan-Swain, A. (2014). Spiritual coping and adjustment in adolescents with chronic illness: A 2-year prospective study. *Journal of Pediatric Psychology, 39,* 542–551. doi: 10.1093/jpepsy/jsu011

Schwartz, K. D., Bukowski, W. M., & Aoki, W. T. (2006). Mentors, friends, and gurus: Peer and nonparent influences on spiritual development. In E. C. Roehlkepartain, P. E. King, L. Wagener, & P. L. Benson (Eds.), *Handbook of spiritual development in childhood and adolescence* (pp.310–323). Thousand Oaks, CA: Sage Publications.

Siemsen, E., Roth, A., & Oliveira, P. (2010). Common method bias in regression models with linear, quadratic, and interaction effects. *Organizational Research Methods, 13,* 456–476.

Smith, A., Krishnan, J. A., Bilderback, A., Riekert, K. A., Rand, C. S., & Bartlett, S. J. (2006). Depressive symptoms and adherence to asthma therapy after hospital discharge. *CHEST Journal, 130,* 1034–1038.

Terreri, C. J., & Glenwick, D. S. (2013). The relationship of religious and general coping to psychological adjustment and distress in urban adolescents. *Journal of Religion and Health, 52,* 1188–1202. doi: 10.1007/s10943-011-9555-8

Thune-Bolye, I. C., Stygall, J., Keshtgar, M. R. S., Davidson, T. I., & Newman, S. P. (2011). Religious coping strategies in patients diagnosed with breast cancer in the UK. *Psycho-Oncology, 20,* 771–782. doi: 10.1002/pon.1784

Thune-Bolye, I. C., Stygall, J., Keshtgar, M. R. S., Davidson, T. I., & Newman, S. P. (2013). Religious/spiritual coping resources and their relationship with adjustment in patients newly diagnosed with breast cancer in the UK. *Psycho-Oncology.* doi: 10.1002/pon.3048

Valente, T. W. (2010). *Social networks and health.* New York, NY: Oxford University Press.

Westers, N. J., Rehfuss, M., Olson, L., & Wiemann, C. M. (2014). An exploration of adolescent nonsuicidal self-injury and religious coping. *International Journal of Adolescent Medicine and Health, 26,* 345–349. doi: 10.1515/ijamh-2013-0314

Wothke, W. (2000). Longitudinal and multigroup modeling with missing data. In T. D. Little, K. U. Schnable and J. Baumert (Eds.) *Modeling longitudinal and multilevel data: Practical issues, applied approaches, and specific examples* (pp.219–240, 269–281). Mahwah, NJ: Lawrence Erlbaum Associates Publishers.

Zindani, G. N., Streetman, D. D., Streetman, D. S., & Nasr, S. Z. (2006). Adherence to treatment in children and adolescent patients with cystic fibrosis. *Journal of Adolescent Health, 38,* 13–17. doi: 10.1016/j.jadohealth.2004.09/013

ARTICLE 10

Hospital Chaplains: Through the Eyes of Parents of Hospitalized Children

Pamela K. Donohue, ScD,[1,2] *Matt Norvell, MDiv, MS,*[3]
Renee D. Boss, MD, MHS,[1,4] *Jennifer Shepard, CRNP,*[1]
Karen Frank, DNP,[5] *Christina Patron, BS,*[1]
and Thomas Y. Crowe, II, MDiv[3]

1 Department of Pediatrics, Johns Hopkins School of Medicine, Baltimore, Maryland

2 Department of Population Family and Reproductive Health, Johns Hopkins School of Public Health, Baltimore, Maryland

3 Department of Spiritual Care and Chaplaincy, Johns Hopkins Hospital, Baltimore, Maryland.

4 Berman Institute of Bioethics, Baltimore, Maryland

5 Department of Acute and Chronic Care, Johns Hopkins University School of Nursing, Baltimore, Maryland

Address correspondence to: Pamela K. Donohue, ScD, Johns Hopkins Hospital, Charlotte R. Bloomberg Children's Center, 1800 Orleans Street, Room 8527, Baltimore, MD 21287

E-mail: pdonohu2@jhmi.edu

Accepted May 17, 2017

Abstract

Background: Chaplain services are available in 68% of hospitals, but hospital chaplains are not yet incorporated into routine patient care.

Objectives: To describe how families of hospitalized children view and utilize hospital chaplains.

Design: Telephone survey with 40 questions: Likert, yes/no, and short-answer responses.

Subjects: Parents visited by a hospital chaplain during their child's hospitalization in a tertiary care center.

Measurements: Descriptive statistics were used to characterize the sample. Nonparametrics were used to compare religious versus nonreligious parents. Regression was used to identify independent predictors of a chaplain visit positively influencing satisfaction with hospital care.

Results: Seventy-four parents were interviewed; most were 25–50 years old, and 75% felt their child was very sick. Children ranged from newborn to adolescence. Forty-two percent of parents requested a chaplain visit; of the 58% with an unsolicited visit, 11% would have preferred giving prior approval. Parents felt that chaplains provided religious and secular services, including family support and comfort, help with decision making, medical terminology, and advocacy. Chaplains helped most parents maintain hope and reduce stress. Seventy-five percent of parents viewed chaplains as a member of the healthcare team; 38% reported that chaplains helped medical personnel understand their preferences for care and communication. Most parents (66%) felt that hospital chaplaincy increased their satisfaction with hospital care.

Conclusion: Families play a fundamental role in the recovery of hospitalized children. Parents view hospital chaplains as members of the healthcare team and report that they play an important role in the well-being of the family during childhood hospitalization. Chaplains positively influence satisfaction with hospital care.

Key words: hospital chaplain, parents, pediatrics, spirituality

Introduction

More than 50% of Americans pray daily[1] and 49% pray about health concerns.[2] Patients and families report that religious/spiritual beliefs provide comfort in healthcare settings beyond other coping strategies.[3,4] Across sites of medical care, patients incorporate their religious/spiritual views into high-risk decision making.[5,6] We have previously shown that women with a high-risk pregnancy make healthcare decisions for their fetus based on gut feelings and religious views over medical information.[7] Yet, few physicians routinely ask about patient spirituality.[8,9,10]

Attending to the religious and spiritual needs of patients and families is endorsed by the Joint Commission,[11] hospital administrators and leadership,[12,13] and national palliative care organizations.[14] Sixty-eight percent of U.S. hospitals now have chaplain services,[15] but physicians infrequently refer patients to hospital chaplains.[10,16,17,18] Although they appreciate the relevance of religion and spirituality to patients' well-being, physicians are hesitant to engage with patients around these issues due to lack of training and fear of damaging the physician–patient relationship.[10,19] Physicians may feel comfortable involving chaplain support for end-of-life care,[8,10] but integration of the hospital chaplain into the culture of day-to-day patient care is not routine.

There is scant information on how families perceive hospital chaplains in pediatric care, but some literature exists on how chaplains perceive their role. Feudtner et al.[20] reported a large unmet need for spiritual care of pediatric patients and families as judged by hospital chaplains in 115 U.S. pediatric hospitals. Perceived barriers to quality spiritual care were physicians' lack of training to recognize spiritual suffering and referrals made too late in the course of an illness for chaplains to provide all the care that families needed.

We were interested in how families of hospitalized children view and utilize hospital chaplains. Specifically, we wondered whether parents perceive the hospital chaplain to be separate from or part of the medical team, their understanding of the role of the chaplain, and their experience of solicited versus unsolicited interactions with hospital chaplains. We hypothesized that most families view a chaplain's visit as supportive, but those without religious affiliation might find it intrusive, and some might find it frightening if perceived as associated with end-of-life care. The goal of this research is to help guide the hospital chaplain practice as it relates to children and families.

Methods

Parents who were visited by a hospital chaplain in 2013 during their child's hospitalization at our tertiary care hospital were eligible for the survey study. Eligible parents were identified by linking a list of patients visited by hospital staff chaplains, including Clinical Pastoral Education residents and interns, with hospital admission records. Parents were sent a letter explaining the study and asking permission to contact them by telephone about study participation. An opt-out postcard allowed parents to decline further contact. Parents who did not opt out were contacted for verbal consent and telephone interview. The Institutional Review Board approved the study.

The survey instrument was developed by the investigators and consisted of 40 questions with Likert, yes/no, and short-answer responses. Questions concerning specific chaplain interventions were adapted from Flannelly et al.[21] The survey targeted parents' perception of hospital chaplain visits, including provision of spiritual/religious and psychosocial support, integration into the healthcare team, and feelings about unsolicited visits that were initiated by the chaplain without prior request. The survey was piloted with members of the Department of Spiritual

Care and Chaplaincy and four parents of children currently hospitalized for authenticity and clarity. Adjustments were made based on feedback on the pilot survey. Interviewers (J.S., K.F., and C.P.) were trained with the instrument and have experience interacting with parents of children in the context of acute and intensive care. Any parent considered by the interviewer to be distressed by the survey was referred, with permission, to a hospital social worker for evaluation and referral to mental health services if warranted.

Descriptive statistics were used to characterize the sample. Parents who identified that their spiritual/religious values always/usually guide the way they live (deemed religious) were compared, by nonparametric methods for categorical and continuous variables, with those who indicated that spiritual/religious values never/sometimes guide their lives or that they have no religious tradition that they follow (deemed nonreligious). A multiple logistic regression model was built to identify independent predictors of a chaplain visit positively influencing satisfaction with hospital care (a lot/some = 1, none = 0). Parent responses to the final question "Is there anything else you want us to know about hospital chaplains?" were categorized and counted. IBM SPSS 24 was used for statistical analyses.

Results

Two hundred fifty-seven families visited by a hospital chaplain had current addresses or working telephone numbers at the time of the study; parents of 74 (29%) children were interviewed. Of those not interviewed, 21 opted out, and three declined participation after telephone contact; the remainder did not answer several attempts to reach them by phone or return voicemail messages.

Demographic data for survey respondents and the hospitalized child are shown in Table 1. All respondents reported that they were the primary person with the child during the hospitalization. The majority of respondents considered themselves a spiritual/religious person and reported that their spiritual/religious values always guide the way they live. Eighty-one percent of respondents were visited more than once by the hospital chaplain. Nearly three-quarters of respondents considered their child very sick during the hospitalization.

About half of the parents (59.6%) knew a hospital chaplain was available to them; 42.3% of parents requested a chaplain visit. Sixty-two percent of parents understood that the role of a hospital chaplain included providing religious and secular services: prayer and sacraments, family support, and comfort. The remaining 38% of parents reported that chaplains help patients/parents with decision making, medical terminology, advocacy, and by just being there.

Among the 57.7% of parents who had unsolicited chaplain visits, 26% reported that a staff member suggested and arranged the visit (the staff member was usually a nurse, 73%). More than half (54%) of the respondents receiving an unsolicited visit reported being grateful and appreciative of the sincerity and caring behavior demonstrated to the whole family. Only five respondents would have preferred giving prior approval before the chaplain visit. For three of these respondents, the unsolicited visit was viewed as surprising, awkward, or frightening. Two parents reported that they feared the staff called the chaplain because bad news was going to be delivered or that doctors had been withholding information about the seriousness of the child's condition. In all five of these cases, respondents reported that once they understood the purpose of the chaplain's visit, they appreciated the support and welcomed additional visits.

Table 2 indicates how parents perceive the relationship between chaplains and the healthcare team. About 75% of parents agreed with the statement, "during the hospital stay, I viewed the chaplain as part of my child's healthcare team," and 38% reported that chaplains helped healthcare providers understand parents' preferences for care at least some of the time. Just over half of the parents reported some conflict or tension with the healthcare team; for 21.6% of these parents, a chaplain helped resolve the conflict.

The frequency of interventions performed by chaplains and parents' perceptions of chaplain empathy are shown in Table 3. Almost all parents felt the chaplain provided emotional support (87%) and caring (95%).

Table 1: Demographic characteristics of participants and children

Participant	N (%)
Relationship to child	
• Parent	70 (94.6)
• Grandparent	2 (2.7)
• Other	2 (2.7)
Race/ethnicity	
• Caucasian	49 (66.2)
• African American	11 (14.9)
• Hispanic	6 (8.1)
• Asian	5 (6.8)
• Native Hawaiian/Pacific Islander	2 (2.8)
• Other	1 (1.4)

cont.

Participant	N (%)
Age, years	
• 16–24	2 (2.7)
• 25–35	25 (33.8)
• 36–50	36 (48.6)
• >50	11 (14.9)
Do you consider yourself a spiritual/religious person?	
• Yes	67 (90.5)
• No	7 (9.5)
Do you have a specific religious tradition that you follow?	
• Yes	60 (81.1)
• No	14 (18.9)
Would you say your spiritual/religious values guide how you live? ($n = 60$; only asked of those who responded yes to previous question)	
• Always	35 (47.3)
• Usually	16 (21.6)
• Sometimes	9 (12.2)
• Never	1 (1.7)
No. of visits by the hospital chaplain	
• 0	3 (4.0)
• 1	11 (14.9)
• 2	20 (27.0)
• 3 or more	40 (54.1)
Child	
Age at hospitalization, years	
• <1	26 (35.1)
• 1–5	20 (27.0)
• 6–12	13 (17.6)
• 13 or more	15 (20.3)
Why hospitalized	
• Problems immediately after birth	18 (24.3)
• Acute illness	11 (14.9)
• Chronic condition	28 (37.8)
• Cancer	4 (5.4)
• Trauma/injury	8 (10.8)
• Other	5 (6.8)
Parent perception of child's condition	
• Very sick	54 (73.0)
• Sick	8 (10.8)
• Somewhat sick	7 (9.5)
• Not very sick	5 (6.8)

Site of hospital care[a]	
• Neonatal Intensive Care Unit	19 (25.7)
• Pediatric Intensive Care Unit	40 (54.1)
• Floor	48 (64.9)
Duration of hospitalization, days	
• 1–7	18 (24.3)
• 8–14	8 (10.8)
• 15–28	9 (12.2)
• >28	38 (51.4)
• No answer	1 (1.4)

a   Categories are overlapping as children were often transferred from intensive care to the floor before discharge.

Table 2: Parent perception of the chaplains' relationship with the healthcare team

Participant	N (%)
I viewed the chaplain as a part of my child's healthcare team.	
• Always	20 (28.2)
• Usually	11 (15.5)
• Sometimes	21 (29.6)
• Never	18 (25.4)
The chaplain helped the healthcare team understand my preferences for care (for example: my goals for medical care for my child, making decisions, or acknowledging the way I wanted to be treated as a person).	
• Always	10 (14.1)
• Usually	11 (15.5)
• Sometimes	6 (8.5)
• Never	43 (60.6)
The chaplain asked me about my child's pain and responded to my concerns.	
• Always	29 (40.8)
• Usually	10 (14.1)
• Sometimes	12 (16.9)
• Never	19 (26.8)
I experienced conflict or tension with the healthcare team.	
• Always	5 (7.0)
• Usually	2 (2.8)
• Sometimes	30 (42.3)
• Never	33 (46.5)

cont.

Participant	N (%)
Did the chaplain help you resolve conflicts with the healthcare team?[a]	
• Yes	9 (24.3)
• No	28 (75.7)

n = 70, only includes parents for whom complete data are available.

[a] n = 37; only asked of those who answered always, usually, or sometimes to the item "I experienced conflict or tension with the healthcare team."

For the majority of parents, hospital chaplains helped meet their religious/spiritual needs, reduced stress, and helped them maintain hope throughout their child's hospitalization, Table 4. Two-thirds of parents reported that hospital chaplaincy positively influenced their satisfaction with overall hospital care. None of the child or parent demographic variables or the number of chaplain visits were independent predictors of a chaplain visit influencing satisfaction with hospital care in a regression model (data not shown, but available).

When asked what else they wanted to tell us about hospital chaplains, 50 parents responded. Illustrative quotations are presented for each category of response. Numbers after quotes are participant's unique identifiers.

The majority of parents (38/50, 76%) felt the chaplain services were beneficial to the family:

> It's nice to have [a chaplain visit] because you feel a burden to others with your problems, but chaplains are there for just this type of thing. (229)

> Multiple chaplains were very helpful and the ability to go to mass [in the hospital] truly provided a community for us. Johns Hopkins did this very well. (224)

> Single patient rooms are nice but isolate parents from the support of other parents; chaplains are key. (256)

> The chaplain was very helpful, and I hope they will continue to be there for other families like they were there for me. (40)

Six percent of parents (3/50) were uninformed of the availability of a chaplain:

> No one initiated a visit with the chaplain. We have been in many hospitals and a chaplain usually visits, I was disappointed with Johns Hopkins. (339)

A few parents (3/50, 6%) did not feel adequate spiritual care was available:

> We would have liked more visits when having conflict with healthcare team, to reduce stress. (309)
>
> We are grateful for the care…but would have liked continuous care with just one chaplain. (80)

Some parents (6/50, 12%) took the opportunity to comment on other hospital services:

> The [chaplain] service was important, but we also needed to be prepared for how our whole world would change after discharge. (220)

An analysis of religious parents compared with nonreligious parents revealed few differences with regard to perception of hospital chaplains, Table 5. When asked if there were any additional comments they wanted to make, nonreligious respondents were overwhelmingly positive about the role of the hospital chaplain:

> A chaplain visit is part of a holistic approach to care, which is very helpful. (257)
>
> Even though we are not religious, the chaplain was very supportive during a long hospitalization. If asked, we would have turned down a chaplain visit….[but] chaplains should visit all patients and families. (3)
>
> A very worthwhile service. The chaplain did not push religion or read from the bible; was kind and thoughtful. I placed my faith in science and the doctors and nurses. (71)

Table 3: Parent perception of chaplain interventions

The hospital chaplain	n (%)
Cared about me	
• Yes	67 (95.7)
• No	3 (4.3)
Sat down and talked with me	
• Yes	61 (85.9)
• No	9 (12.7)
Listened to my concerns	
• Yes	63 (90)
• No	7 (10)
Provided emotional support	
• Yes	61 (87.1)
• No	9 (12.9)
Resolved conflict within my own family	

cont.

The hospital chaplain	n (%)
• Yes	15 (21.4)
• No	54 (77.1)
Prayed with me	
• Yes	58 (81.7)
• No	12 (16.9)
Provided a ritual or sacrament	
• Yes	33 (46.5)
• No	37 (52.1)
Helped coordinate support within my own faith community	
• Yes	17 (23.9)
• No	53 (74.6)
Helped me find meaning in illness	
• Yes	36 (50.7)
• No	34 (47.9)

Table 4: Parents' perception of hospital chaplain effectiveness and the relationship to satisfaction with hospital care

	n (%)
The hospital chaplain was helpful in meeting my spiritual/religious needs.	
• Always	38 (54.3)
• Usually	10 (14.3)
• Sometimes	13 (18.6)
• Never	4 (5.7)
• No needs	5 (7.1)
Do you feel the chaplain helped you cope with the stress related to having a hospitalized child?	
• Yes	58 (82.9)
• No	12 (17.1)
Do you feel the chaplain helped you maintain hope during your child's hospitalization?	
• Yes	58 (82.9)
• No	12 (17.1)
How would you rate the importance of a visit from the hospital chaplain?	
• Very important	46 (65.7)
• Somewhat important	13 (18.6)
• Neutral	11 (15.7)
• Not important	0
When talking with another family, would you recommend they ask for a visit from the hospital chaplain?	

• Yes	62 (88.6)
• No	7 (10.0)
• No answer	1 (1.4)
How would you rate the quality of care your child received in the hospital? Would you say it was…	
• Excellent	54 (77.1)
• Very good	10 (14.3)
• Good	3 (4.3)
• Fair	3 (4.3)
• Poor	0
Did your visit with the chaplain influence your overall rating of the hospital?	
• A lot	10 (14.3)
• Some	36 (51.4)
• Not at all	24 (34.3)

Table 5: Comparison of religious versus nonreligious parents for secular questions

	Religious ($n = 50$), N (%)	Nonreligious ($n = 20$), N (%)
Did you know a chaplain was available?		
• Yes	29 (58)	15 (75)
• No	21 (42)	5 (25)
Did you request a chaplain visit?		
• Yes	24 (48)	6 (30)
• No	26 (52)	14 (70)
Would you have liked more visits from the chaplain?		
• Yes	14 (28)	2 (10)
• No	36 (72)	18 (90)
I viewed the chaplain as a part of my child's healthcare team.		
• Always	16 (32)	4 (20)
• Usually	7 (14)	4 (20)
• Sometimes	13 (26)	8 (40)
• Never	14 (28)	4 (20)
The chaplain helped the healthcare team understand my preferences for care (for example: my goals for medical care for my child, making decisions, or acknowledging the way I wanted to be treated as a person).		
• Always	8 (16)	2 (10)
• Usually	7 (14)	4 (20)
• Sometimes	3 (6)	3 (15)
• Never	32 (64)	11 (55)

cont.

	Religious (n = 50), N (%)	Nonreligious (n = 20), N (%)
I experienced conflict or tension with the healthcare team.		
• Always	3 (6)	2 (10)
• Usually	2 (4)	0
• Sometimes	23 (46)	7 (35)
• Never	22 (44)	11 (55)
Did the chaplain help you resolve conflicts with the healthcare team? (Among those with conflict)		
• Yes	7 (25)	2 (22.2)
• No	21 (75)	7 (77.8)
[The chaplain] helped me find meaning in illness		
• Yes	25 (50)	9 (45)
• No	25 (50)	11 (55)
Do you feel the chaplain helped you cope with the stress related to having a hospitalized child?		
• Yes	42 (84)	16 (80)
• No	8 (16)	4 (20)
Do you feel the chaplain helped you maintain hope during your child's hospitalization?		
• Yes	43 (86)	15 (75)
• No	7 (14)	5 (25)
How would you rate the importance of a visit from the hospital chaplain?[a]		
• Very important	36 (72)	10 (50)
• Somewhat important	10 (20)	3 (15)
• Neutral	4 (8)	7 (35)
• Not important	0	0
Did your visit with the chaplain influence your overall rating of the hospital?		
• A lot	7 (14)	3 (15)
• Some	27 (54)	9 (45)
• Not at all	16 (32)	8 (40)

[a] $\chi2$ 7.87 (2) $p = 0.02$; no other significant differences between groups.

Discussion

Hospital chaplains are described as working on the margins of medicine[22] or between the worlds of doctors and patients,[23] with little data to support the efficacy of their work.[24] In this study, we quantify satisfaction with the day-to-day routine care provided by hospital chaplains from the viewpoint of recipients of that care, the families of hospitalized children. Most families viewed a chaplain visit, whether solicited or not, as a positive and helpful component of the care provided during a child's hospitalization. This was true of religious/spiritual parents and those who did not identify themselves as religious or spiritual. Remarkably, 66% of parents reported that as few as one or two visits from a hospital chaplain positively influenced their satisfaction with hospital care.

Our findings are consistent with a systematic review that indicates that providing for patients' emotional and spiritual needs is highly correlated with satisfaction with the hospital experience.[25] Most parents in our study reported feeling personally cared for by hospital chaplains and that chaplains provide families with what one parent described as much-needed respite from medical talk by focusing on parent well-being. Piderman[26] and others[27] have shown that adult patients find a chaplain visit particularly important during times of anxiety or uncertainty. These emotional states may apply to our sample as many parents experienced an intensive care hospitalization with their child. As in our study, research with adult patients has documented that religiousness plays little part in the benefit patients perceive from a chaplain visit.[28]

Caregivers of children with chronic conditions, such as HIV,[29] bronchopulmonary dysplasia,[30] and disabilities such as autism,[31,32] use prayer as a coping mechanism. In our inpatient study, prayer was a frequently used intervention by chaplains (for 82% of parents) and may have helped parents cope with childhood illness or injury. Data from both inpatient and outpatient samples illustrate the benefit of supporting a family's spiritual coping strategies around childhood illness.

Hospital chaplains increasingly provide for more than the explicit religious/spiritual needs of patients and families (prayers, religious ritual); they also address implicit needs such as values clarification or the search for meaning in illness.[27,33] In our study, more than 50% of parents reported that hospital chaplains helped them explore the meaning of their child's illness, and more than 80% reported that chaplains helped them maintain hope during the hospitalization. Families and pediatricians acknowledge hope as an important strategy in coping with serious childhood illness.[34] Hospital chaplains are specifically trained to support and guide individuals as they explore existential questions and so are the logical team members to provide this service.[33] Physicians may be less likely to avoid asking about these important topics if there is a chaplain available to devote time to parents as they explore these issues.

Half of the parents in our study experienced conflict with the healthcare team, a similar percentage as reported by others.[35] We did not ask the nature of this conflict, but disagreement concerning the benefit of continued medical interventions is a known source of conflict between families and physicians.[36] Inexpert communication during difficult conversations can also lead to conflict[35,37] and has prompted medical schools and professional organizations to increase communication training.[38,39,40] In our study, chaplains assisted in resolving interpersonal conflict for 25% of parents who reported discord with providers; others have reported that adult patients value a chaplain's assistance with communicating with physicians.[27] As neutral and respected professionals, chaplains can serve as valuable mediators when conflict arises.

Three-quarters of parents in our study felt the chaplain was part of their child's healthcare team at least some of the time. This perception is different from that reported by healthcare providers.[27] Chaplains in our pediatric hospital are a visible presence, particularly in the ICU; they routinely attend family meetings and participate in rounds. Participation in these activities may increase parents' perception that chaplains are part of the medical team. Physicians and nurses also utilize hospital chaplains for staff debriefings, support, and counseling during times of high moral distress, increasing their familiarity with chaplains, which they openly display to parents. There are differing opinions as to whether chaplains are, or should be, part of the medical team.[41,42,43] Physicians may utilize chaplains more frequently if they are perceived as members of the medical team, but their role as patient advocates could be diminished. As a bona fide member of the medical team, patients and families may view chaplains as representing the medical system or hospital, which could adversely affect trust for some. Chaplains' vision of themselves as apart may also facilitate their effectiveness in mediating physician–family conflict, which could be lost if they are an integrated member of the team.

Our study has limitations. Only 29% of parents who were located could be contacted and participated in the study; their views may not be representative of all parents of hospitalized children. We do not know if parents who opted out of the study had unsolicited chaplain visits. The prolonged hospitalization of many of the children in our sample and the perceived seriousness of their condition may have influenced parents' appreciation of hospital chaplains; about 80% of the children in our sample spent some time in intensive care, legitimizing parents' perception of illness severity. Because the acuity in our hospital is high, and our chaplain staffing low, chaplains are preferentially staffed to respond to emergencies and cover ICU admission and so may be more available to these parents than to parents of children hospitalized on the general medical–surgical floors. Prolonged hospitalization may have contributed to the high proportion of parents who reported conflict with the healthcare team. Information from hospitalized children on their perception of the role of the hospital chaplain is missing from our study. Most of our respondents were mothers; fathers' views may differ. Although 90.5% of our sample identified themselves as religious, the proportion is not appreciatively different from the 89% of a representative sample of Americans who reported they believe in God.[1]

A primary tenet of pediatric patient- and family-centered care is the acknowledgement that families play a fundamental role in the health of children. Hospital chaplains honor the responsibility and role parents play in their child's recovery by providing them with the psychosocial and spiritual support they need during a hospitalization. Our study highlights the important role chaplains play in the overall well-being of the family through a routine presence, support, counseling, and conflict mediation. Chaplains contribute to the quality of day-to-day care of the religious and nonreligious families of hospitalized children and positively influence satisfaction with hospital care.

Acknowledgment

P.D. was supported by the Thomas Wilson Sanitarium for the Children of Baltimore City for this work.

Author disclosure statement

No competing financial interests exist.

References

1. Pew Research Center. U.S. Public Becoming Less Religious. 2015. www.pewforum.org/2015/11/03/u-s-public-becoming-less-religious (Last accessed February 11, 2016).
2. Wachholtz A, Sambamoorthi U: National trends in prayer use as a coping mechanism for health concerns: Changes from 2002 to 2007. Psycholog Relig Spiritual 2011;3:67–77.
3. VandeCreek L, Pargament K, Belavich T, et al.: The unique benefits of religious support during cardiac bypass surgery. J Pastoral Care Counsel 1999;53:19–30.
4. Kristeller JL, Sheets V, Johnson T, Frank B: Understanding religious and spiritual influences on adjustment to cancer: Individual patterns and differences. J Behave Med 2011;34:550–561.
5. Ehman JW, Ott BB, Short TH, et al.: Do patients want physicians to inquire about their spiritual or religious beliefs if they become gravely ill? Arch Intern Med 1999;159:1803–1806.
6. Hexem KR, Mollen CJ, Carroll K, et al.: How do parents of children receiving pediatric palliative care use religion, spirituality or life philosophy in tough times. J Palliat Med 2011;14:39–44.
7. Boss RD, Hutton N, Sulpar LJ, et al.: The values parents apply to decision-making about delivery room resuscitation for high risk newborns. Pediatrics 2008;122:583–589.

8. Armbruster CA, Chibnall JT, Legett S: Pediatrician beliefs about spirituality and religion in medicine: Associations with clinical practice. Pediatrics 2003;111:e227–e235.
9. Grossoehme DH, Ragsdale JR, McHenry CL, et al.: Pediatrician characteristics associated with attention to spirituality and religion in clinical practice. Pediatrics 2007;119:e117–e123.
10. King SD, Dimmers MA, Langer S, Murphy PE: Doctors' attentiveness to the spirituality/religion of their patients in pediatric and oncology settings in the Northwest USA. J Health Care Chaplain 2013;19:140–164.
11. Hodge DR: A template for spiritual assessment: A review of the JCAHO requirements and guidelines for implementation. Soc Work 2006;51:317–326.
12. Flannelly KJ, Galek K, Bucchino J, et al.: Department directors' perceptions of the roles and functions of hospital chaplains: A national survey. Hosp Top 2005;83:19–28.
13. Flannelly KJ, Weaver AJ, Handzo GF, Smith WJ: A national survey of health care administrators' views on the importance of various chaplain roles. J Pastoral Care Counsel 2005;59:87–96.
14. National Consensus Project for Quality Palliative Care: Clinical Practice Guidelines for Quality Palliative Care, 3rd ed. 2013. www.nationalconsensusproject.org (Last accessed June 16, 2016).
15. Jankowski KRB, Handzo GF, Flannelly KJ: Testing the efficacy of chaplaincy care. J Health Care Chaplain 2011;17:100–125.
16. Flannelly KJ, Weaver AJ, Handzoa GF: Three-year study of chaplains' professional activities at Memorial Sloan-Kettering Cancer Center in New York city. Psycho-oncology 2003;12:760–768.
17. Flannelly KJ, Galek K, Handzo GF: To what extent are the spiritual needs of hospital patients being met? Int J Psychiatry Med 2005;35:319–323.
18. Galek K, Flannelly K J, Koenig HG, Fogg SL: Referrals to chaplains: The role of religion and spirituality in healthcare settings. Ment Health Relig Cult 2007;10:363–377.
19. Curlin FA, Sellergren SA, Lantos JD, Chin MH: Physicians' observations and interpretations of the influence of religion and spirituality on health. Arch Intern Med 2007;167:649–654.
20. Feudtner C, Haney J, Dimmer MA: Spiritual care needs of hospitalized children and their families: A national survey of pastoral care providers' perceptions. Pediatrics 2003;111:e67–e72.
21. Flannelly KJ, Galek K, Tannenbaum HP, Handzo GF: A preliminary proposal for a scale to measure the effectiveness of pastoral care with family members of hospitalized patients. J Pastoral Care Counsel 2007;61:19–29.
22. Norwood F: The ambivalent chaplain: Negotiating structural and ideological difference on the margins of modern-day hospital medicine. Med Anthropol 2006;25:1–29.
23. Vries R, Berlinger N, Cadge W: Lost in translation: The chaplain's role in health care. Hastings Cent Rep 2008;38: 23–27.
24. Proserpio T, Piccinelli C, Clerici CA: Pastoral care in hospitals: A literature review. Tumori 2011;97:666–671.
25. Clark PA, Drain M, Malone MP: Addressing patients' emotional and spiritual needs. Jt Comm J Qual Saf 2003;29:659–670.
26. Piderman KM, Marek DV, Jenkins SM, et al.: Patients' expectations of hospital chaplains. Mayo Clin Proc 2008;83:58–65.
27. Bryant C: Role clarification: A quality improvement survey of hospital chaplain customers. J Healthc Qual 1993;15:18–20.
28. Handzo GF, Flannelly KJ, Kudler T, et al.: What do chaplains really do? II. Interventions in the New York chaplaincy study. J Health Care Chaplain 2008;14:39–56.
29. Richards TA, Wrubel J, Grant J, Folkman S: Subjective experiences of prayer among women who care for children with HIV. J Relig Health 2003;42:201–219.

30. Wilson SM, Miles MS: Spirituality in African-American mothers coping with a seriously ill infant. J Spec Pediatr Nurs 2001;6:116–122.
31. Ekas NV, Whitman TL, Shivers C: Religiosity, spirituality, and socioemotional functioning in mothers of children with autism spectrum disorder. J Autism Dev Disord 2009;39:706–719.
32. Benson PR: Coping, distress, and well-being in mothers of children with autism. Res Autism Spectr Disord 2010;4: 217–228.
33. Hodge DR: Implicit spiritual assessment: An alternative approach for assessing client spirituality. Soc Work 2013;58:223–230.
34. Reder EA, Serwint JR: Until the last breath: Exploring the concept of hope for parents and health care professionals during a child's serious illness. Arch Pediatr Adolesc Med 2009;163:653–657.
35. Abbott KH, Sago JG, Breen CM, et al.: Families looking back: One year after discussion of withdrawal or withholding of life-sustaining support. Crit Care Med 2001;29:197–201.
36. Widera EW, Rosenfeld KE, Fromme EK, et al.: Approaching patients and family members who hope for a miracle. J Pain Symptom Manage 2011;42:119–125.
37. Studdert DM, Mello MM, Burns JP, et al.: Conflict in the care of patients with prolonged stay in the ICU: Types, sources, and predictors. Intensive Care Med 2003;29:1489–1497.
38. Boss RD, Urban A, Barnett MD, Arnold RM: Neonatal critical care communication (NC3): Training NICU physicians and nurse practitioners. J Perinatol 2013;33:642–646.
39. Serwint JR: The use of standardized patients in pediatric residency training in palliative care: Anatomy of a standardized patient case scenario. J Palliat Med 2002;5:146–153.
40. Bell SK, Pascucci R, Fancy K, et al.: The educational value of improvisational actors to teach communication and relational skills: Perspectives of interprofessional learners, faculty, and actors. Patient Educ Couns 2014;96:381–388.
41. VandeCreek L, Burton L (eds): Professional chaplaincy: Its role and importance in healthcare. J Pastoral Care 2001;55: 81–97.
42. Tovino SA: Hospital chaplaincy under the HIPAA privacy rule: Health care or "Just Visiting the Sick." Indiana Health Law Rev 2005;2:51.
43. Loewy RS, Loewy EH: Healthcare and the Hospital Chaplain. Med Gen Med 2007;9–53

ARTICLE 11

Service User Views of Spiritual and Pastoral Care (Chaplaincy) in NHS Mental Health Services: A Co-Produced Constructivist Grounded Theory Investigation

Julian Raffay*,1, Emily Wood[2] and Andrew Todd[2]

* Correspondence: julian.raffay@merseycare.nhs.uk

1 Spiritual and Pastoral Care, Mersey Care NHS Foundation Trust, Indigo Building, Ashworth Hospital Parkbourn, Liverpool L31 1HW, England

2 Cardiff Centre of Chaplaincy Studies, St Michael's College, 54 Cardiff Road, Llandaff, Cardiff CF5 2YJ, Wales

Abstract

Background: Within the UK National Health Service (NHS), Spiritual and Pastoral Care (SPC) Services (chaplaincies) have not traditionally embraced research due to the intangible nature of their work. However, small teams like SPC can lead the way towards services across the NHS becoming patient-centred and patient-led. Using co-production principles within research can ensure it, and the resulting services, are truly patient-led.

Methods: A series of interviews were conducted with service users across directorates of a large NHS mental health trust. Their views on the quality of SPC services and desired changes were elicited. Grounded theory was used with a constant comparative approach to the interviews and analysis.

Results: Initial analysis explored views on spirituality and religion in health. Participants' concerns included what chaplains should do, who they should see, and how soon after admission. Theoretical analysis suggested incorporating an overarching spiritual element into the bio-psycho-social model of mental healthcare.

Conclusions: Service users' spirituality should not be sidelined. To service users with strong spiritual beliefs, supporting their spiritual resilience is central to their care and well-being. Failure will lead to non-holistic care unlikely to engage or motivate.

Raffay, J., Wood, E., and Todd, A. (2016) "Service user views of spiritual and pastoral (chaplaincy) in NHS mental health services: a co-produced constructivist grounded theory investigation." *BMC Psychiatry*, 16, 200.

Key words: chaplaincy, co-production, spiritual and pastoral care, service user perspectives, participation, grounded theory, qualitative research

Background

Public spending is under intense scrutiny. NHS services need to justify their funding. Spiritual and Pastoral Care (SPC) services (also called chaplaincies) have traditionally stayed away from standard outcome measures as they do not fit with the ethos of the service. This must change as organisations including the National Secular Society have campaigned to have NHS funding removed from SPC.[1] If SPC is to survive and modernise, research and outcome measures are unavoidable.[2] Developing suitable and reliable measurement within the field is vital.

SPC departments have traditionally lacked other NHS departments' protocols or guidance. Recent guidelines[3,4] have been more about recommended staffing numbers and training than the day-to-day activities conducted by chaplains. The impact of such voluntary competencies is unclear.[5] The lack of clarity about what chaplains should be doing makes outcome measures difficult to design.[2]

Chaplains have been likened to advocates, providing cultural advice and support[6] but they also support spiritual and religious observance. A collaborative (as opposed to a dependent) religious coping style (working with God rather than waiting for God to fix things) correlates with a positive impact on mental health and recovery.[7, 8] Table 1 presents the working definitions of key words used in this paper, recognising the literature has not reached consensus and concepts overlap.

Chaplains can work with service users and carers to build resilience. Resilience and spirituality have numerous links including finding meaning in life and having a sense of hope.[9] These concepts also overlap with the Recovery Model's recovery processes: connectedness, hope, identity, meaning in life and empowerment (CHIME)[10] which have a spiritual component. Although Leamy and colleagues associated spirituality with meaning in life,[10] there may be greater association. Many people experience connectedness to others of faith, to humanity, nature, or the Universe as a whole as part of their spirituality.

Co-designing and co-evaluating services can make them truly patient-centred. Co-production recognises that everyone has a vital contribution to make and brings people who use mental health services, carers, and staff together on equal terms.[11] It creates opportunities to understand each other's concerns and builds on recovery approaches by facilitating empowerment.[12] In this research, the research team comprising service users, carers, and staff, explored what service users value in their spiritual and pastoral care and what changes they want.

Table 1: Key definitions: chaplaincy, spirituality, religion, pastoral, and resilience

Term	Definition
Chaplaincy	Modern healthcare chaplaincy is a service and profession working within the NHS that is focused on ensuring that all people, be they religious or not, have the opportunity to access pastoral, spiritual or religious support when they need it[4]
Spirituality	A phenomenon unique to the individual and has been defined as the 'breath' that animates life or a sense of connection to oneself, others, and that which is beyond self and others, spirituality is an individual construct, denoting a personal relationship with the transcendent[42]
Religion	Religion is an organised system of beliefs, practices, rituals and symbols designed a) to facilitate closeness to the sacred or transcendent (God, higher power, or ultimate truth/reality) and b) to foster an understanding of one's relationship and responsibility to others in living together in a community[43]
Pastoral care	Pastoral care is rooted in non-judgemental listening and attentiveness to service-users, carers and staff. It pays supportive and enabling attention to a range of human needs and aspirations, in the context of healthcare, being especially alert to questions of identity and belief (whether presented as religious, spiritual or neither of those)
Resilience	Resilience is the ability of an individual to respond to stress in a way that is healthy and adaptive and allows personal goals to be achieved with the minimum psychological and physical cost[44]

Method

Co-production is a key philosophy of the research team. The patient and public involvement panel (Panel) was recruited from the start and contributed throughout. It comprised NHS service users and carers. Contributions (in keeping with INVOLVE recommendations[13]) included writing the interview schedule, piloting interviews, deciding which service user groups to target, and insights for the analysis.[14] To explore service user perceptions, grounded theory with its origins in the symbolic interactionist approach of Mead offered the most promising approach.[15] Constructivist grounded theory was chosen as the researchers were already immersed in the participant's context prior to the study.[16] Comparing interviews using the constant comparative method allowed deep penetration into the lived experience of mental health service users on psychiatric wards. This was in part based on Kara's insight that research team members may hold multiple roles and 'mutable identities'.[17] Interpreting findings with the Panel ensured fidelity to the data and mitigated the impact of the researchers' predetermined expectations.[18]

Semi-structured interviews were conducted at a place and time convenient to participants. Potential participants were given at least 24 hours to consider joining the research. Before the interview commenced, participants were told the research's purpose and aims. They received guidance about how they could withdraw consent at any point. All participants had capacity to consent and gave informed consent to be in the research and for their data to be used in the write up. Topics that appeared important to earlier participants were included in later interviews to elaborate on the issues. Thus interview schedules were altered in keeping with the constant comparative method.[18] Theoretical saturation was considered to have been reached.

Audio recorded interviews with participants were undertaken by one of two researchers (JR and EW). EW transcribed verbatim, checking for accuracy, and removing names and identifiers. Participants were invited to review their transcripts. Four asked to do this without reporting errors. To support reflective practice and enable constant comparison,[19] transcriptions, coding, and analysis were completed as soon as possible after each interview.

Initial line-by-line coding was completed by EW, to explore meanings and actions, but remaining close to the data.[19] Focused coding re-evaluated the initial codes, combining some before grouping codes into categories. JR and AT cross-checked the coding and analysis. The whole team had extensive discussions in person and by email to decide on the final categories. The final step involved conceptualising what had been said and generating a theory grounded in the data.[20] The Panel provided feedback on the results. The data was managed using NVivo software.

Reflexivity

The researchers are a Christian chaplain (JR), and an academic (AT) with constructivist backgrounds, and a mental health nurse (EW) with a critical realist background, identifying as 'spiritual but not religious'. This diversity allowed the team to challenge assumptions and discuss preconceptions. Some of the participants knew JR in his capacity as chaplain prior to the commencement of interviews. EW was new to the Trust and did not establish a relationship with participants prior to the interviews. AT had no direct contact with participants (other than meeting the Panel). Participants were informed of the research team's motivation for studying this area but not the motivations of individuals. Information about individual researchers was limited to their name, professional background, and how to make contact later if they wished to complain/comment further. Service user volunteers from Mersey Care NHS Foundation Trust's adult acute, medium and high secure services were recruited, mainly by a chaplain attending routine ward meetings. These wards were chosen to reflect a variety of inpatient experience, SPC use, treatment, and demographics. Theoretical sampling was attempted within each ward but reliance on psychiatric inpatient volunteers and a small population curtailed the possibilities. Mersey Care covers the North Merseyside region of North West England. According to the 2011 census, Merseyside is more religious, more Christian and more socially and economically deprived than the UK average.[21, 22]

Five pilot interviews were undertaken in January and February 2015 to ensure processes were safe for participants and researchers alike and valid for the purposes of the research. Pilot participants came from the Panel. They recommended changes to the wording of the standard consent form around access to patient records. This was resubmitted and the ethics committee approved the revision.

Between April 2015 and August 2015, a further seventeen service users were interviewed in private rooms on the participant's ward or unit. In most cases only the participant and interviewer were present. For two interviews a student nurse observed; explicit consent was sought for this. Participants were only interviewed once; interviews lasted from seven minutes to one hour. The participant demographics are shown in Table 2. The age data is incomplete due to missing data.

Table 2: Participant demographics

Demographic	Type	Number of participants
Gender	Male	17
	Female	5
Age	Under 40	5
	40–59	8
	60 and over	6
Relationship to the Trust	Open acute ward service user	10
	Secure^ ward service user	7
	Community service user	2
	Carer	3
Faith group	Atheist	1
	Did not identify	2
	Multiple	1
	Christian (no denomination)	1
	Church of England	5
	Roman Catholic	8
	Pentecostal	2
	United Reform	1
	Born-Again	1

^Secure in this context refers to high and medium secure mental health units. It does not include psychiatric intensive care (PICU), low secure units, or prison inreach services.

Service User Views of Spiritual and Pastoral Care (Chaplaincy) in NHS Mental Health Services 229

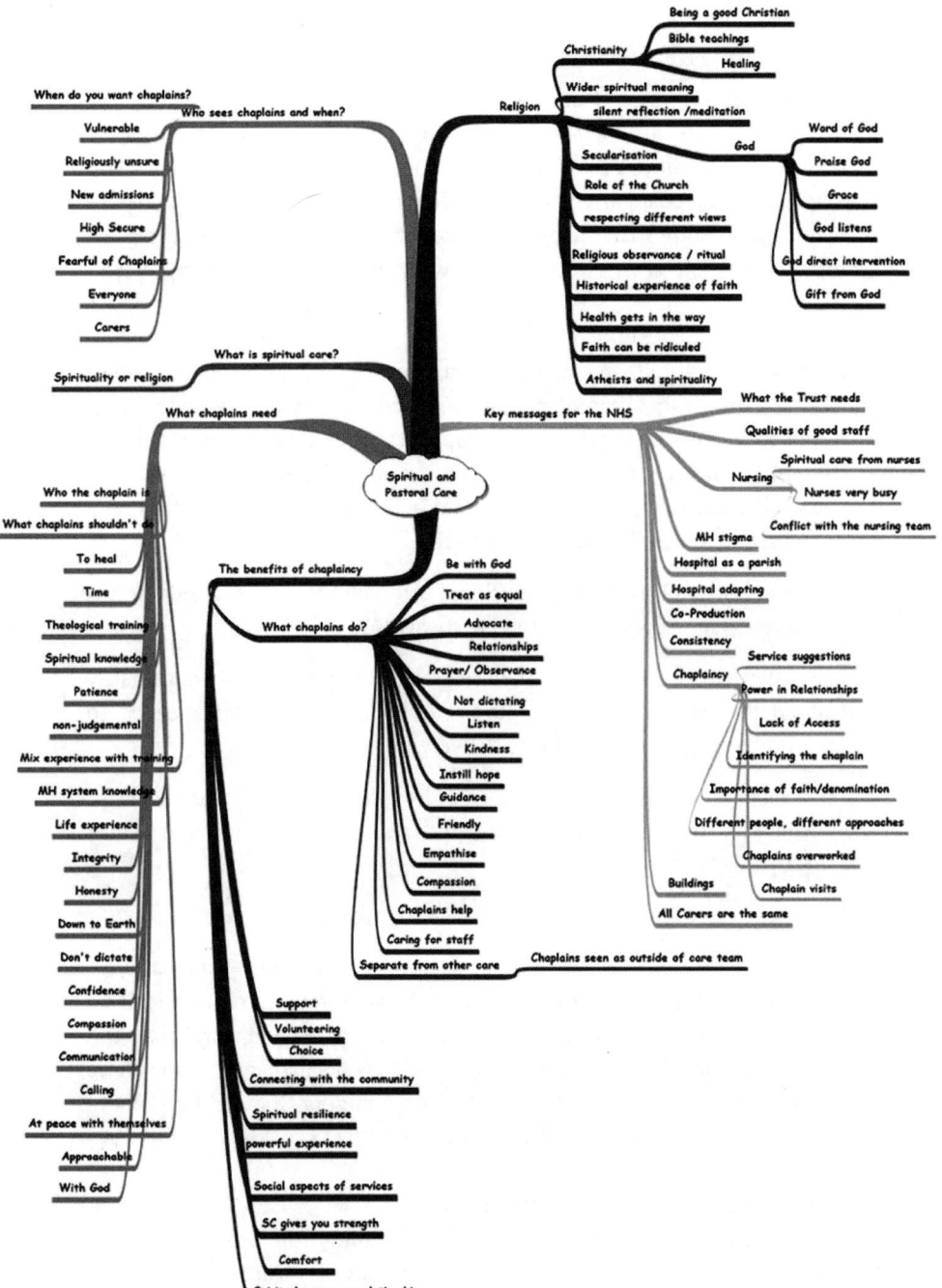

Fig. 1: A category map illustrating the breadth of views elicited in the interviews

Results

Categories

Six categories emerged from the interviews. These were: (1) the meaning of spiritual care, (2) benefits of the SPC department, (3) the role of religion, (4) qualities of a 'good' chaplain, (5) who talks to chaplains and when, and (6) chaplains and the multidisciplinary team. The category map (Fig. 1) shows the range of themes within the categories and what topics arose. The arms of the map show the breadth of views expressed.

THE MEANING OF SPIRITUAL CARE

As previously noted, spiritual care is a poorly defined concept, meaning different things to different people. The participants were asked what it meant to them. Although religious support was a key element, it was not the only thing mentioned. Participants communicated a wider view of spirituality involving pastoral care and a holistic view of healthcare in which spiritual care has an important role.

> 'I think it's not just a religious thing, is it really, the pastoral side of it is more to talk to people and to help them.' (67)

Most participants described themselves as religious. Their spirituality was interwoven with their religion. For them, spiritual care needed to incorporate religion. It might be delivered by:

> 'Someone who is from a religious order who prays with you and helps you with spiritual questions and helps you understand your faith better.' (20)

Some described the chaplains' work as a key part of their healthcare.

> '[spiritual care's] very very important for mental health; sometimes it's the only thing that seems, that can maybe get through to someone. It's a different sort of level of understanding, that goes beyond words that goes beyond, something you can touch, it goes beyond all that and I do believe in the power of Grace. I do believe in the Almighty God and I do believe that Jesus was the best healer that this world had ever known.' (21)

THE BENEFITS OF THE SPC DEPARTMENT

The participants listed many SPC services, ranging from providing formal religious services, to the more pastoral *'having someone to talk to'*, as helpful. Table 3 shows the specific SPC services participants valued (at least two participants mentioned each service in the table).

Table 3: Helpful services provided by SPC staff

Religious provision	Pastoral provision
Formal religious service	Listening
Prayer	The social side of religious services
Spiritual advice/guidance	Providing an emotional connection
Holy Communion*	Providing hope/self-worth
Confession^	A critical friend
Normalising faith	A bridge between community and ward
	'Tending the good in someone'

*Holy Communion, shared between Christians, involves breaking bread and wine to commemorate Jesus' life, death, and resurrection. It is usually a communal ceremony.
^Confession, a mainly Roman Catholic practice, involves sharing perceived wrongdoings with a priest in the anticipation of divine forgiveness.

Health professionals are generally less religious than service users.[23] This has caused some service users difficulty in expressing religious ideas for fear of being considered psychotic.[24] The presence of a chaplain on the ward was seen as 'normalising faith', meaning faith was seen as a normal occurrence. This gave service users confidence to speak about faith or look for support in accessing it without feeling their request would be considered pathological.

Pentecostal participants and those from secure services (from several Christian denominations) emphasised the social side of services and the fellowship that it provided. Feeling part of a community, valued, and loved was important.

> 'Having fellowship is important.' (21)

Participants found involvement in planning and delivering formal religious services helpful as was the social side of services. Pentecostal and Anglican participants suggested Bible study groups. The Roman Catholics highlighted strength received from God to help in recovery. The Born-Again Christian participant spoke of the benefit of accessing an evangelical faith healer, though no one else mentioned it. This may be specific to certain Evangelical denominations and not a regular request.

One frequent comment was that chaplains helped service users find hope. This spiritual resilience was important to many.

> 'I find it helps me, you know, it helps me no end, you know in all sorts of ways. Sometimes I might have been having a particularly you know, particularly bad week, overwhelming, Sister [—] comes and I have communion and I sit and reflect and you know, it means so much to me and it brings me back up.' (32)

The role of religion

Many noted access to church or chaplains helped them in various ways included feeling at one with God, expecting God would directly intervene or providing hope and strength.

> 'It wasn't like I needed to speak to the priest or anything special. It was just to be part of that Christian service, and have the chance to pray and things and just feel that I was part of that service and part of prayer opportunity and to sort of I don't know maybe feel I was squaring something with God or something. Because I felt angry about the situation and somehow it seemed to work for me, I felt there was a certain resolution in my own mind about what had happened by just being there.' (68)

Some participants understood God as the primary agent of healing and source of hope for recovery. Supporting (and sometimes moderating) this belief could benefit therapeutic relationships with other professions.

> 'I think healing is a miracle from God.' (21)

For most, their faith provided strength, hope, and self-worth rather than God providing any direct intervention. These are key aspects of resilience and mental well-being, essential for mental health recovery.

Participants wanted religious activities one might find in an ordinary parish, including prayer, confession, communion, and Bible study. Christian and atheist participants showed clear respect for other religions.

> 'I just treat every religion the same.' (33)

Although participants respected other faith leaders, they preferred a chaplain of their own faith. For some Roman Catholics and the Born-Again Christian, denomination was important.

Even in Liverpool, which is more religious than the United Kingdom average, some people reported stigma associated with being religious.

> 'You don't want people laughing in front of us while we're praying and that.' (23)

> 'I find it difficult when people put me down for my faith. Again going back to "oh are you going God bothering" and people don't understand me I think.' (31)

Qualities of a 'good' chaplain

All participants felt 'good' staff, regardless of their profession, were distinguished by human qualities such as listening and compassion rather than by technical skill. 'Good' staff were empathetic and kind. Participants felt 'bad' staff were those they saw as overworked. They stressed it was the hospital management's responsibility to prevent overworking as it impacted negatively on patients. This mirrors research showing a link between burnout in staff and lower levels of patient satisfaction.[25] Table 4 shows some of the characteristics participants said they looked for in a good chaplain. The human or pastoral qualities were those you would look for in any health professional, the ability to represent God distinguishing the chaplain.

Younger participants tended to focus more on the need for the chaplain to be an ordained minister. Older participants were more concerned that the chaplain had life experience.

The list of human qualities was similar across all demographics.[26] Roman Catholics more often reported wanting an ordained priest than other groups. Participants differed around the importance attached to ordination. Many said they were unconcerned about a chaplain's qualifications, preferring life experience as a quality, but then listed services often requiring a highly-trained individual. These included: Mass, confession, teaching scripture, and the meaning of the Bible, linking scripture with modern events, communion, and church services.

Table 4: Participants' views on what made a 'good chaplain'

Human qualities	'Man of God'
Non-judgemental	Be a 'man of God'
Honest	Church leader/spiritual training (whether this necessitates ordination varies)
Approachable	
Trustworthy	Walk with God
Genuine	Have a prayerful life
Kind	Have a genuine relationship with God
Friendly	Bring the word of God
Confidence	The ability to represent multiple faiths
Empathetic	Channel the Grace of God
Critical friend	
Have time	
Good communication	
Life experience	
Down to Earth	
Knowledge of the mental health system	

Who talks to chaplains and when

The general feeling was that everyone, regardless of faith background, would need pastoral care. Although people of other faiths were well respected, people of no faith were generally considered to be '*unawakened*' and in need of conversion. Many respondents felt bringing non-believers into the fold was one of a chaplain's roles.

> 'It would be nice to say the non-religious to try to get them to change their minds and that there is a God, because those are the ones that need the help, not the religious ones.' (19)

Whilst NHS staff are prohibited from evangelising, it was a commonly expressed wish from the service user participants.

There was a feeling that SPC services do not reach widely enough and chaplains should serve carers and community patients. Some suggested chaplains acting as a bridge between community and ward.[27, 28]

> 'I would say if they have been a member of a church before, that might not be too difficult but if they have never been there needs to be some sort of cooperation between the chaplaincy and the people…who are the pastors in the community.' (21)

On the ward it was acknowledged that people would benefit from seeing a chaplain at different times. This links to themes about advertising so patients know what services are available and how to access them when they need them. Several participants suggested need could be unanticipated and wanted an on-call chaplain. They recommended a regular presence on the ward so patients could expect someone coming round at a certain time on a certain day. This would mean that they could make sure they did not go out on leave and miss the chaplains. This was especially important on wards without an onsite chaplain.

Secure service participants suggested following the prison model, where someone admitted would see a chaplain within 24 hours. This was valued because it welcomes the patient, lets them know what services are available and shows a friendly face at a distressing time. Waiting until someone can leave the ward, perhaps months or years into their stay, before the chaplains made contact was considered inadequate.

> 'I feel like when new patients arrive in the hospital, someone from the spiritual care should go and see them, straight away. To make them aware that there is a church service going on every week and they, what it's about and making people feel welcome and accepted into the church.' (19)

The participants were generally positive about current SPC services; however, they had many suggestions for improvements. Universally, participants felt that chaplains were under time pressure. They wanted to see chaplains more often and have more available. They wanted an increase in services (especially on Sundays), Bible study groups, and hymn practices, as well as more informal association.

> 'like a Bible study but prepare for the Sunday coming so that the patients together with the staff are designing the service' (62)

CHAPLAINS AND THE MULTIDISCIPLINARY TEAM

Although the interview questions asked specifically about the SPC department, participants also made many comments about wider issues. Common statements considered differences between chaplains and other professionals and chaplains' role in the multidisciplinary team. Most reported a good relationship with the nursing staff but found chaplains easier to talk to.

> 'But the psychologist inevitably has an alternate agenda... Yeah the chaplain just listens and doesn't necessarily have an opinion on it or an ulterior motive.' (95)

There was a sense other professionals spent much time monitoring service users, trying to find out about them, or seeking to change them. Chaplains were seen differently, as having no agenda or goal other than listening.

Chaplains' integration into the multidisciplinary team (including access to patient notes, being part of ward rounds and care planning activities) divided opinion around personal preference rather than demographics. Those in favour suggested it would normalise faith and facilitate accessing SPC. They said it would improve communication between different services. Those wanting a separate SPC felt it would make talking to chaplains harder without the 'confidentiality of the confessional'. There is a sense that chaplains offer a fundamentally different type of service to other hospital staff.

> 'I prefer to keep my spiritual needs to one side and my nursing team to another side because it's a different approach it is a different sort of mind set.' (31)

Those mentioning confidentiality accepted chaplains were NHS staff and had to pass on risk information but preferred they didn't pass on anything else.

Some religious participants were uninterested in SPC religious services, preferring the local church on a Sunday morning rather than the hospital chapel.

> 'I'd like to go to Mass on a weekend.' (66)

Most could not do this as they would need staff escorts. Most wards run on fewer staff at the weekend, meaning escorted leave was harder to grant.

> 'There is a Catholic Church only round the corner only they won't let me go there, they won't take people who want to go to church because they haven't got the staff.' (67)

This lack of provision was criticised. One participant felt ward staffing should be highest on a Sunday morning to allow large scale church attendance.

Grounded theory

Most NHS mental health services use the bio-psycho-social model[29] (Fig. 2). This revolves around separate but interacting biological, psychological, and social dimensions of health, illness, and well-being. NHS treatments (including social care) focus on one or more of these dimensions.

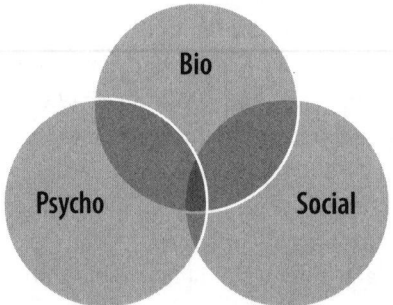

Fig. 2: A representation of the bio-psycho-social model

Some participants felt this model was missing a key component – the spiritual. They specified why spirituality was important. One participant spoke of how her belief in God had helped motivate her to work with a psychotherapist. Another said she disliked taking tablets but felt God had revealed this knowledge so it was okay to take them. These explanations and motivations may not suit everyone but, for these service users, they were key to engaging with treatment. Others spoke of the importance of fellowship, feeling loved and being part of a community, and how that helped combat the isolation of mental illness. Others talked of the peace and calming nature of prayer and attending religious services. All these aspects are clearly important in mental health recovery[10] but not easily contained within the bio-psycho-social model. Adding spirituality to the bio-psycho-social model has been suggested before[30] although usually as an additional but equal element, represented by a fourth identical circle in the diagram (Fig. 3). This reinterpretation identifies four distinct but interacting dimensions of a person's well-being, none of which can be removed from the whole.[30]

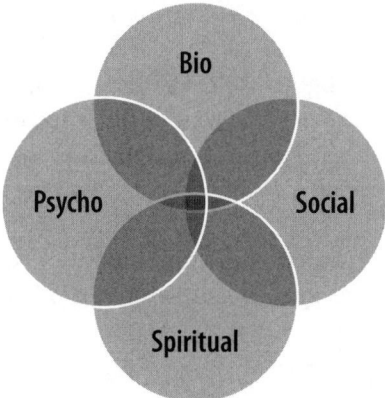

Fig. 3: The traditional view of the bio-psycho-social-spiritual model

This study's findings suggest spirituality interacts with the other dimensions and yet also transcends them. A revised model is therefore proposed (Fig. 4) with the participants' views more accurately representing the place of spirituality in healthcare. They identified it as crucial to engaging the other dimensions. For example, if services had failed to respect the beliefs of the participant who took medication because she saw it as God-given, she may have refused it. Engaging in psychotherapy is often a very challenging experience for service users. If they gain motivation by believing God is helping them, it should not be ignored as a source of strength and resilience. A service user without hope has a poor prognosis and many people draw hope from religious belief. Religious communities, formal and informal, within NHS services and in the wider community can provide a sense of belonging, of fellowship, and of being part of a greater whole.

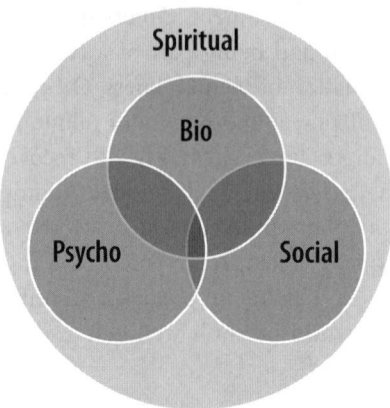

Fig. 4: A revised bio-psycho-social-spiritual model of care

The model can use a lighter colour where the spiritual dimension is less salient in a person's experience. For some service users, the yellow (spiritual) will be pale, perhaps transparent, and insignificant for them either in terms of providing resilience or meeting needs. For most of our participants, it was their motivation. Ignoring this motivation will alienate them and fail to engage them in their care. The dotted lines reinforce our finding that all concepts interact and affect each other.

Discussion

This study's findings are generated by the confluence of the researchers' commitment to co-production (of both SPC and research) and a constructivist grounded theory methodology. They force a rethink of the bio-psycho-social model of mental health, suggesting modification to recognise spirituality and spiritual care. Seeing the spiritual as a wider dimension interacting with some, all, or none, of the bio-psycho-social dimensions explains discrepancies. It explains why our participants see spiritual care as an essential part of care whereas others disregard it.

If the bio-psycho-social model is considered in more fluid terms, as the interaction of influences and social processes, a different picture emerges. Spirituality may then be considered in significant part to be a mechanism used by service users to retain their sense of self in response to being treated according to the bio-psycho-social model. It may be a defence against perceived (or actual) totalising influences, whether directly attributable to treatment or broader aspects of institutionalisation. For most of the participants, it expressed itself in overtly religious terms but this need not necessarily be the case. This interpretation of spirituality resembles understandings of patient experience.[31] It is not intrinsically hostile to treatment (the example of the woman who saw medication as God-given was very supportive). It warrants sensitive exploration to build therapeutic relationship and address anxieties. Ignoring spirituality is likely to compromise effectiveness. The spiritual, thus understood, helps make sense of some instances of frustration and aggression. The authors' opinion is that health service professionals should engage with this element regardless of whether a person presents as spiritual, religious, or otherwise. Differences need to be acknowledged, respected, and considered when planning care.[32, 33] Whilst advocating this understanding, it is also important not to subordinate all spiritual expression to a response to treatment or institutionalisation. Many service users ordinarily engage in spiritual practices that they would value being able to continue when hospitalised.

This study aimed to learn what SPC users wanted from the service. All participants valued the SPC department and felt that seeing a chaplain had helped their recovery. Most could see ways of improving SPC; none found it unhelpful. Further work on how chaplains can best support the spiritual needs of those without faith is required.[34] Some participants in this study felt one role of chaplains should be to convert those with no faith, however, support, not proselytising, is the role of NHS chaplains.

The role of the chaplain included a variety of human or pastoral roles as well as a faith representation. It was viewed as clearly differentiated from the role of other professionals, though how closely chaplains should work with those other professionals was contested. Spiritual care services appear to be more aligned with the recovery processes of connectedness, hope, identity, meaning in life and empowerment (CHIME) than in traditional healthcare approaches of the medical model, although it can certainly work with those approaches where necessary.

Our six categories reflect other research on the domains of spiritual care. Burkhart and Hogan (2008) ran focus groups with American nurses to study their role in spiritual care. Their grounded theory research reported nurses saying that spiritual care came in the three categories: promoting patient self-reflection, promoting connectedness between the patient and the family and promoting connectedness between the patient and God.[35] The self-reflection theme closely resembles the pastoral care that chaplains provide; listening and philosophical discussion. Promoting connectedness between the patient and God closely resembles the religious aspects that our participants expected from chaplains. There was little mention in our interviews about promoting connectedness between patient and family. Some people suggested chaplains for carers but distinct from the patient.

The USA is a more overtly religious society than the UK, with average church attendance around 50%[36] as opposed to 15% in the UK.[37] Reflecting these cultural differences, Burkhart and Hogan's nurses regularly prayed with their patients, though only if initiated by the patient. As in the UK, the American nurses highlighted that their nurse training did not prepare them for delivering spiritual care.[35]

Koslander and Arvidsson (2007), again using grounded theory, explored patient perspectives on spiritual care in Swedish mental health settings. They identified three main categories: (1) it was important to patients that spiritual needs were met, (2) patients felt it was up to them to be proactive in making sure they received spiritual care, and (3) patients lacked confidence in talking to nurses about spiritual care.[38] This generally reflected the responses from participants in our study although Koslander and Arvidsson made no reference to chaplains. The Swedish patients were keen to talk to their nurses about spirituality. Though our participants were less likely to want this, they still thought nurses should know about the issue, be willing to discuss spiritual care, and know about available SPC services.

The present study's findings are also consistent with Rosmarin and colleagues' (2015) observation that it is important to offer suitable spiritual care to mental health service users. Simply recording a service users' religious affiliation is inadequate[40]. Rosmarin used a survey to gauge service user attitudes to spiritual care in a Massachusetts hospital. Although mainly asking about spiritually integrated psychotherapy rather than SPC, well over half of the respondents were keen to have a spiritual dimension to their care.[40] Walsh reported that proper consideration of the spiritual dimension could not be presumed upon in the NHS.[39]

Co-producing the research was felt to be a valuable experience, with deep respect developing between the members of the Panel. Involving people with lived experience of using mental health services from the outset and sharing experience throughout the research cycle significantly improved the fidelity of the research and facilitated recruitment into the study. Overall, most participants revealed profound insight into their experience and many of their stories were deeply moving. Being part of this research project has felt a privilege in every way and the researchers hope the expectation would be that all future UK-based research would be co-produced by default.

Limitations of the study

This has been a small qualitative study in a more religious and more Christian than average part of the UK. Participants' opinions may not represent the UK as a whole, or mental health service users in other countries. Nonetheless, they are helpful for service design in this part of the country; and the service user view that spirituality is an important part of their holistic treatment is supported by studies from other countries.[40, 41]

Almost all the participants were inpatients from open acute or secure wards. Older adults with dementia and smaller services (including brain injury, drug and alcohol services, and learning disability) were excluded. Our sample was disproportionately male and older than the average inpatient. Although everyone on the included wards was invited, those without interest in SPC may have declined to be interviewed.

Both the Panel and participants reflected a wide spread of demographics and educational attainment but the findings' generalisability may be questioned at two levels. The first concerns the details regarding aspects of SPC that were valued. Different findings might have been generated elsewhere or at different times or by different researchers. More challenging is the implication that co-production would be desirable worldwide. There is real risk of dogmatically imposing a seemingly benign Euro-centric model on cultures where it may be inappropriate or actually harmful. Authentic co-production would allow for genuine consultation but is predicated on profound respect and considerable skill in communication. Superficial or coercive pseudo co-production would not only be paternalistic but could potentially be more damaging than its displaced alternative.

The initial coding was undertaken by EW who is not theologically trained. Although the coding frame was cross-checked and discussed in depth with researchers who are, it may have been done differently by a chaplain.

Conclusions

In common with other recent studies,[35, 38, 40] this study shows mental health service users are keen to have spiritual and religious elements to their care. Many regard this as essential to the healing process. NHS services should consider a bio-psycho-social-spiritual model in their aim to provide holistic, patient-centred care to their patients. Co-producing the research has proved invaluable.

Abbreviations
NHS, National Health Service, SPC, Spiritual and Pastoral Care

Acknowledgements
The authors thank all the staff who helped recruit service users and members of the patient and public involvement panel.

Funding
This research was funded by a grant from Mersey Care NHS Foundation Trust.

Availability of data and materials
Supporting data will not be made available as it contains indirect identifiers and releasing it could breach the confidentiality of our participants.

Authors' contributions
JR conceived the study and led on the co-production, interviewing, and study design. EW undertook some interviews, transcribed the interviews, analysed the data, and drafted the manuscript. AT shared in designing the study, cross-checking data coding and analysis. All authors read and approved the final manuscript.

Competing interests
The authors declare that they have no competing interests.

Consent for publication
Participants gave consent for their data to be used in the manuscript.

Ethics approval and consent to participate
Ethical approval for the data collection was granted by the Haydock NHS Research Ethics Committee (14/NW/1040). Potential participants were given at least 24 hours to consider joining the research. Before the interview commenced, participants were told the research's purpose and aims. They received guidance about how they could withdraw consent

at any point. All participants had capacity to consent and gave informed consent to be in the research and for their data to be used in the write up. Consent forms were signed in the presence of a researcher, countersigned and kept in the main study site file.

References

1. NSS. Hospital Chaplaincy. London: The National Secular Society; 2012.
2. Handzo GF, Cobb M, Holmes C, Kelly E, Sinclair S. Outcomes for professional health care chaplaincy: An international call to action. J Health Care Chaplain. 2014;20(2):43–53.
3. UKBHC. Standards for Healthcare Chaplaincy Services. Cambridge: UK Board of Healthcare Chaplaincy; 2009.
4. Swift C. NHS Chaplaincy Guidelines 2015: Promoting Excellence in Pastoral, Spiritual and Religious Care. London: NHS England; 2015.
5. UKBHC. Spiritual and Religious Care Capabilities and Competences for Healthcare Chaplains. Cambridge: UK Board of Healthcare Chaplaincy; 2015.
6. Morgan G. Independent Advocacy and the "Rise of Spirituality": Views from Advocates, Service Users and Chaplains. Ment Health Relig Cult. 2010;13(6):625–36.
7. Cornah D. The impact of spirituality on mental health: A review of the literature. London: Mental Health Foundation; 2006.
8. Koenig HG. Research on religion, spirituality, and mental health: A review. Can J Psychiatr. 2009;54(5):283.
9. Vanistendael S. Resilience and spirituality. Resilience in Palliative Care: Achievement in Adversity 2007:115–135.
10. Leamy M, Bird V, Le Boutillier C, Williams J, Slade M. Conceptual framework for personal recovery in mental health: systematic review and narrative synthesis. Br J Psychiatry. 2011;199(6):445–52.
11. Slay J, Stephens L. Co-production in mental health: A literature review. London: New Economics Foundation; 2013.
12. Slade M, Amering M, Farkas M, Hamilton B, O'Hagan M, Panther G, Perkins R, Shepherd G, Tse S, Whitley R. Uses and abuses of recovery: implementing recovery-oriented practices in mental health systems. World Psychiatry. 2014; 13(1):12–20.
13. National Institute for Health Research. Patient and Public Involvement in Health and Social Care Research: A Handbook for Researchers. In. London: National Institute for Health Research; no date.
14. Wood E, Raffay J, Todd A. How Could Co-production Principles Improve Mental Health Spiritual and Pastoral Care (Chaplaincy) Services? Journal of Health and Social Care Chaplaincy. 2016;4(1).
15. Mead GH, Morris CW. Mind, Self and Society from the Standpoint of a Social Behaviorist. Chicago; London: University of Chicago Press; 1934
16. Charmaz K. Constructing Grounded Theory. 2nd ed. London: Sage; 2014.
17. Kara H. Mental health service user involvement in research: where have we come from, where are we going? J Public Mental Health. 2013;12(3):122–35.
18. Charmaz K. Constructionism and the Grounded Theory Method. Handbook of Constructionist Research 2013:397.
19. Charmaz K. Constructing Grounded Theory: A Practical Guide Through Qualitative Analysis. London: Sage Publications Ltd; 2006.
20. Glaser BG. Conceptualization: On Theory and Theorizing Using Grounded Theory. Int J Qualitative Methods. 2002;1:2.
21. ONS. 2011 Census: Quick statistics for England and Wales. London: Office of National Statistics; 2013.

22. Attwood M. 2011 Census: Liverpool Summary. Liverpool: Liverpool City Council; 2013.
23. Moreira-Almeida A, Lotufo Neto F, Koenig HG. Religiousness and mental health: a review. Rev Bras Psiquiatr. 2006;28(3):242–50.
24. Huguelet P, Mohr S, Borras L, Gillieron C, Brandt P-Y. Spirituality and religious practices among outpatients with schizophrenia and their clinicians. Psychiatric Services 2006.
25. Vahey DC, Aiken LH, Sloane DM, Clarke SP, Vargas D. Nurse burnout and patient satisfaction. Medical Care. 2004;42(2 Suppl):II57.
26. Forrest S, Risk I, Masters H, Brown N. Mental health service user involvement in nurse education: exploring the issues. JPMHN. 2000;7(1):51–7.
27. Wood E, Watson R, Hayter M. To what extent are the Christian clergy acting as frontline mental health workers? A study from the North of England. Ment Health Relig Cult. 2011;14(8):769–83.
28. Wonders S. The experiences of those providing pastoral care in the Christian church community: Supporting people with their mental health and interacting with health professionals. Unpublished doctoral thesis, University of Sheffield; 2011 [Embargoed until October 2016].
29. Engel GL. The clinical application of the biopsychosocial model. Am J Psychiatry. 1980;137(5):535–44.
30. Sulmasy DP. A biopsychosocial-spiritual model for the care of patients at the end of life. The Gerontologist. 2002;42 suppl 3:24–33.
31. Doyle C, Lennox L, Bell D. A systematic review of evidence on the links between patient experience and clinical safety and effectiveness. BMJ Open. 2013;3(1):1–18.
32. McDaid S. An equality of condition framework for user involvement in mental health policy and planning: Evidence from participatory action research. Disabil Soc. 2009;24(4):461–74.
33. Staniszewska S, Mockford C, Gibson A, Herron-Marx S, Putz R. Moving Forward: Understanding the Negative Experiences and Impacts of Patient and Public Involvement in Health Service Planning, Development, and Evaluation. In: Critical Perspectives on User Involvement. Edited by Barnes M, Cotterell P. Bristol: Policy; 2012: 129–141.
34. Hayward RD, Krause N, Ironson G, Hill PC, Emmons R. Health and Well-Being Among the Non-religious: Atheists, Agnostics, and No Preference Compared with Religious Group Members. J Relig Health. 2016:1–14.
35. Burkhart L, Hogan N. An experiential theory of spiritual care in nursing practice. Qual Health Res. 2008;18(7):928–38.
36. Smith G, Cooperman A, Hamar-Martinez J, Podrebarac-Sciupac E, Hackett C, Mohamed B, Alper B, Gecewicz C, Esarza-Ochoa J. U.S. Public Becoming Less Religious. Washington DC: Pew Research Center; 2015.
37. Tearfund. Churchgoing in the UK: A research report from the Tearfund on church attendance in the UK. Middlesex, UK: Tearfund; 2007.
38. Koslander T, Arvidsson B. Patients' conceptions of how the spiritual dimension is addressed in mental health care: a qualitative study. J Adv Nurs. 2007;57(6):597–604.
39. Walsh J, McSherry W, Kevern P. The representation of service users' religious and spiritual concerns in care plans. J Public Mental Health. 2013; 12(3):153–64.
40. Rosmarin DH, Forester BP, Shassian DM, Webb CA, Björgvinsson T. Interest in Spiritually Integrated Psychotherapy Among Acute Psychiatric Patients. J Consult Clin Psychol. 2015. (Advance online publication.)
41. Ho RTH, Chan CKP, Lo PHY, Wong PH, Chan CLW, Leung PYP, Chen EYH. Understandings of spirituality and its role in illness recovery in persons with schizophrenia and mental-health professionals: a qualitative study. BMC Psychiatry. 2016;16(1):1–11.
42. Dyson J, Cobb M, Forman D. The meaning of spirituality: A literature review. J Adv Nurs. 1997;26(6):1183–8.
43. King MB, Koenig HG. Conceptualising spirituality for medical research and health service provision. BMC Health Serv Res. 2009;9(1):116.
44. Epstein RM, Krasner MS. Physician resilience: what it means, why it matters, and how to promote it. Acad Med. 2013;88(3):301–3.

ARTICLE 12

Cultural Differences in Spiritual Care: Findings of an Israeli Oncologic Questionnaire Examining Patient Interest in Spiritual Care

Michael Schultz[1]*, Doron Lulav-Grinwald[1] and Gil Bar-Sela[2]

* Correspondence: m_schultz@rambam.health.gov.il

1 Division of Oncology, Rambam-Health Care Campus, Technion-Israel Institute of Technology, POB 9602, Haifa 31096, Israel

2 Faculty of Medicine, Technion-Israel Institute of Technology, POB 9602, Haifa 31096, Israel

Abstract

Background: As professional spiritual care (chaplaincy) is introduced to new cultures worldwide, it bears examining which elements of screening and care are universal and, for those elements showing cultural difference, to study them in each culture. No quantitative spiritual care patient study had previously been done in Israel. Our objectives were twofold: 1) to examine who wants spiritual care in Israel, including demographic and clinical variables, and to compare against other results worldwide to further develop universal screening protocols; 2) to see what patients want from spiritual care specifically in the Israeli setting.

Methods: Self-administered patient questionnaire examining spirituality/religiosity, interest in spiritual care (subdivided by type of care), and key demographic, social, and clinical data. The study setting was an Israeli oncology center at which spiritual care had been recently introduced.

Results: Data from 364 oncology patient questionnaires found 41% interest in spiritual care, as compared to 35%–54% in American studies. Having previously been visited by a spiritual caregiver predicted patient interest in further spiritual care (AOR 2.4, 95% CI 1.2–4.6), suggesting that the new service is being well received. Multivariate stepwise logistic regression analysis identified additional predictors of openness to receiving spiritual care: self-describing as somewhat/very spiritual vs. not

---

Schultz, M., Lulav-Grinwald, D., and Bar-Sela, G. (2014) "Cultural differences in spiritual care: findings of an Israeli oncologic questionnaire examining patient interest in spiritual care." *B Palliative Care*, 13, 1, 19–29.

spiritual (adjusted odds ratio [AOR] 3.9 and 6.3, 95% CI 1.8–8.6 and 2.6–15.1) or traditional/religious vs. secular (AOR 2.2 and 2.1, 95% CI 1.3–3.6 and 1.1–4.0); and receiving one visit a week or less from family and friends (AOR 5.6, 95% CI 2.1–15.1). These findings are in line with previous American studies, suggesting universality across cultures that could be utilized in screening. Differences in demographic data and medical condition were not significant predictors of patient interest, suggesting a cultural difference, where age and education were predictors in the American context. Levels of interest in explicitly religious or spiritual support such as prayer or addressing religious/spiritual questions were much lower than in other cultures.

Conclusions: Results illustrate the demand for and satisfaction with the new Israeli service. The cross-cultural comparison found both culture-dependent and possibly universal predictors of patient interest, and found lower interest in Israel for explicitly religious/spiritual types of support.

Key words: spiritual care, oncology, chaplaincy, spiritual screening, patient education, international, pastoral care

Background

Spiritual care addresses a key patient need[1, 2] in a manner that has significant benefits, such as improved quality of life[1, 3, 4] well-being,[5] and reduced anxiety, despair, or depression[6, 7, 8] that have been demonstrated cross-culturally.[9] Spiritual care has become an integral part of palliative care[10, 11] and should be seen as an element of providing care for the whole person.[12]

Professional spiritual care has been introduced to more and more countries worldwide. While spirituality is a universal phenomenon, spiritual care in a particular setting may have unique culture-specific aspects due to the specific religions and spiritual approaches to be found there. One area where we expect to find cross-cultural difference is in patients' spiritual needs. For example, in Taiwan, where the culture is heavily influenced by Taoism, Confucianism, and Buddhism, a key spiritual need expressed is facing death peacefully;[13] and in Tanzania, addressing concerns about witchcraft, devils, and curses are important spiritual needs.[14, 15] Some aspects of spiritual needs are universal while others find a culture-specific expression – "spirituality is embedded within culture."[16] For this reason, there is an ongoing effort either to develop tools that are valid for a particular cultural setting (for example, Spain, Iran, or for African–Americans[17, 18, 19]) or to establish cross-cultural validity for instruments that presumably are limited to universal needs.[16, 20]

The introduction of spiritual care to any new setting needs to be accompanied by research establishing the local parameters for care provision, including examining the spiritual needs of the local population. This will help address all their needs, whether they are likely to be cross-culturally universal or not. One question of particular interest in the Israeli setting is the place of religious care within spiritual care. In some countries, such as Japan[21] and Korea,[9] studies of spiritual care reveal a close link between religious care and spiritual care. But in Israel, our profession has been very concerned to distinguish between the two, following the broader definition of spirituality that has increasingly become accepted in the field in the West.[11] One qualitative study examining key Israeli stakeholders' attitudes towards spiritual care highlights the tension among Jews in Israel, "where the religious and secular publics are polarized and the secular shy away from anything that may be interpreted as religious coercion."[22] As one nursing institution director said, "'I don't want it to appear as if the spiritual support provider has anything to do with things such as organ donations or religion.'" Out of awareness of this concern regarding the relationship between spiritual care and religion, spiritual care in Israel has intentionally been built not on a religious framework, in contrast with some other parts of the world.[23] Our study in part examines this concern from a quantitative perspective, measuring patients' expressed spiritual needs. In another more secular society, Australia, researchers found that patients' desire to speak about their spirituality was similar to that found in the United States, a religious society, suggesting that it is important to test these assumptions.[24] One article looking at the spiritual care needs of Muslims in Israel, though not research based, suggests that this religious/secular tension is less relevant for spiritual care provision to Israeli Muslims.[25]

By contrast, it is not clear to what extent appropriate screening methods need to reflect cultural differences. Numerous studies have found that patients are not receiving as much spiritual care as they would like,[26] either because of a shortage of resources or because their spiritual distress remained unidentified. In the EAPC Spiritual Care Taskforce's recent large international survey of clinicians and researchers determining key research priorities, improving the means of patient screening was one of three priority areas identified.[27] There are at least two elements of screening: measuring spiritual distress and determining which patients would express a desire to receive spiritual care. The former requires demonstrating the cultural fit of the measurement tool, as has recently been done in Brazil,[28] and that remains the subject of future study in Israel. The latter is one of the focal areas of the present study.

Who wants to receive spiritual care, and can those results be generalizable? In any cultural setting, researching the key demographic traits that significantly predict patient interest in spiritual care would help to streamline the process of screening. However, it bears consideration whether some of these factors are cross-cultural and possibly do not require renewed study in each particular setting.

Several studies provide data regarding which types of patients (distinguished by demographic, cultural, sociological, or disease-related difference) are most likely to be interested in spiritual care.[29, 30, 31, 32] Older age was a significant factor in three studies,[29, 30, 31] though not in the fourth.[32] Educational level was a significant factor in every study, but it was inconsistent, with lower educational level predicting higher interest in three studies but higher educational level in the fourth.[32] Gender, marital status, ethnicity, and religion were consistently insignificant factors. Most measures of illness were insignificant predictors of patient interest, though three studies found some limited relationship.[29, 30, 31] Increased experience in receiving spiritual care predicted more positive attitudes towards spiritual care in the two studies that examined that factor.[31, 32] Spirituality, religiosity, or religious practice were significant predictors in at least three of the studies.[29, 30, 31] However, all of these studies were carried out in the United States. As a result, even items that seem to be nearly always either significant or insignificant predictors of interest in spiritual care, which in theory could be integrated into a screening protocol, might not be reliably significant or insignificant in other cultural settings. This study will examine the factors predicting Israeli patient interest in spiritual care in order to compare it with the American results.

Regarding the level of interest in spiritual care, a number of American studies surveying patients in a variety of different departments found interest ranging from 35% to 54%. [26, 29, 30, 33] However, it may not be possible to infer interest levels from a country with an established spiritual care service, like the US, to one where spiritual care is new and not well-known,[22] like Israel.

There have been qualitative studies examining the challenges and accomplishments in introducing professional spiritual care in Israel over the past decade.[22, 23, 34] However, there have not been any quantitative studies in Israel nor studies of any kind of the question of patient interest in spiritual care prior to the present study.

Rambam is the tertiary care medical center for Haifa and its environs as well as for all of northern Israel. Haifa proper is 82% Jewish and 14% Christian, while northern Israel is 44% Jewish, 38% Muslim, 8% Druze, and 7% Christian.

Method
This study is a patient survey, completed independently.

Sample and procedure

A questionnaire with 61 items to be completed independently and anonymously was distributed to patients who were in the hospital's chemotherapy or radiation outpatient treatment rooms or who were hospitalized in the Division of Oncology at Rambam Health Care Campus in Haifa, Israel. Questionnaires were not distributed in each patient area every day. On those days randomly selected for questionnaire distribution in a particular patient area, questionnaires were distributed to all patients present at the time of distribution. Distribution was done by staff not already part of the patient's care team, to limit desirability bias. Questionnaires were available in Hebrew, Arabic, Russian, and English, thereby ensuring that the vast majority of our patient population would not be excluded for reasons of language. The questionnaire was written in English and translated to Hebrew. Next it was translated to Arabic and Russian by staff in a process of translation–reverse translation to check for consistency. The study was approved by the Rambam institutional ethics review board (ref. #2999), and as per their guidelines, patient consent to self-complete the anonymous questionnaire was granted verbally.

The questionnaire

The questionnaire contained three sections: Spiritual identity (self-defined spirituality and religiosity); Types of support provided by spiritual care, rated by importance assigned to them; and Demographic and clinical details. The cover page described spirituality and spiritual care. The full questionnaire can be viewed in the Additional file 1.*

Measures

SPIRITUALITY/RELIGIOSITY AND SPIRITUAL RESOURCES

Self-defined spirituality and religiosity were selected in two items from among the options: Not spiritual/Somewhat spiritual/Very spiritual and Secular/Traditional/Religious. The religious terminology chosen followed previous Israeli studies.[35] These three options are the standard terms used across the various religions represented, where "religious"

---

* Please see the original publication of this article for the link to the additional file.

connotes stricter observance of the religion's commandments while "traditional" connotes strong affiliation and belief without full religious observance. A fourth option from other studies, "ultra-Orthodox," was excluded since it applies to Judaism but not to the other Israeli religions.

TYPES OF SUPPORT THE SPIRITUAL CAREGIVER COULD PROVIDE

Our goal was to assess the extent to which patients valued different aspects of spiritual care. Because we were researching a new cultural setting, we wanted to ensure that we examined a substantially broad range of descriptors of spiritual care, including both "secular" and "religious" descriptors. Because the questionnaire would be completed while receiving or waiting for treatment, it needed to be shorter than existing measures. Since our goal was to establish a baseline data set for Israeli spiritual care needs and desires, we did not consider instruments designed for spiritual assessment or spiritual history taking.

This section of our questionnaire was a composite of four previously reported instruments itemizing spiritual needs that can be addressed by pastoral care. Galek et al.[36] analyzed a large cohort of studies of patient spiritual needs. Content analysis discerned seven representative constructs, from which they designed a 29-item patient survey of spiritual needs, all of which could potentially be addressed by pastoral care. Their literature review (articles from 1990–2004) was not geographically limited, but predates most of the recent efforts to verify cross-cultural validation of spiritual care instruments used.[16] Kernohan et al.'s semi-structured questionnaire, based on the standards of the Association for Hospice and Palliative Care Chaplains, was conducted in an Irish hospice and asked patients about the importance for them of defined spiritual needs which the pastoral care team could help address.[37] VandeCreek's large study[31] of 1440 patients used a shortened version of the Patient Satisfaction Instrument – Chaplaincy (PSI-C), developed in Canada, to assess patient satisfaction with various aspects of the support provided by the chaplain. Flannelly et al.[38] conducted a meta-analysis of the literature (not geographically limited) reporting key items determining patient/family satisfaction, then combined it with VandeCreek's instrument in order to create a survey measure of the effectiveness of pastoral care.

Galek, Flannelly, and Vandecreek identify, with some variation, thematic areas for the care provided by chaplains, grouped together below. We assigned the items in all four measures[31, 36, 37, 38] to these thematic areas. Following the approach of Fitchett,[29] we synthesized our 15-item instrument from the four instruments enumerated above,[31, 36, 37, 38] thereby ensuring that our questionnaire examined elements of each of these thematic areas, as follows:

Sensitivity/caring/support/love: Two items from Flannelly ("Listen to your concerns and show care for you"; "Show care for your family").

Information/decision-making/coordination: Two items from Flannelly ("Help you make difficult decisions"; "Help you obtain information or help in communicating with staff").

Reflecting/finding meaning: Three items from Flannelly, Kernohan, and Galek ("Help you reflect on your experience"; "Help you find meaning in your situation"; "Address spiritual or religious questions").

Coping/peace/hope/dignity: Five items from Flannelly, VandeCreek, and Galek ("Help you face your situation with calmness and dignity"; "Help you find hope or encouragement"; "Help you cope with your sense of loss"; "Help you cope with and adjust to the whole situation"; "Help you find strength to continue").

Spiritual experiential: Two items from Galek and Flannelly ("Pray with you"; "Bring a sense of spirituality into the room").

Activities/rituals: Appropriate to our cultural context, in which spiritual caregivers are not religious figures, in place of a question about religious rituals we added one item about common Israeli spiritual practices, such as meditation, guided imagery, music, and relaxation.[39]

Patients were asked to indicate the level of importance they ascribed to each way in which the spiritual caregiver could support them. Level of importance was rated on a seven-point Likert-type scale. For our analysis, responses of 1–3 indicated the item was not important to patients, 4 was neutral, and 5–7 indicated importance.

Demographic and clinical details

Demographic variables collected were age, marital status, number of children, education, religion, gender, and country of birth. Sociological/behavioral characteristics assessed were level of support in living situation, level of support from family and community, level of support during hospitalization, and attendance at religious services. Clinical measures, as self-reported by respondents, were cancer diagnosis, stage of treatment, time since primary diagnosis, whether cancer had recurred, and whether cancer had metastasized. One question asked patients how worrisome their cancer is. The questions and response categories may be viewed in the article Additional file 1.[*]

ATTITUDE TOWARD SPIRITUAL CARE

Respondents were asked four questions relating to their experience with and disposition toward spiritual care: 1) Have you ever had a visit from a spiritual caregiver? 2) Do you think you have a good understanding of what a spiritual caregiver is or does? 3) How important do you think it is that the oncology institute includes spiritual care in its services? 4) How open do you think you would be to a visit from the spiritual caregiver? That final question formed the primary basis for our analysis of patient interest in spiritual care.

STATISTICAL ANALYSES

Statistical analyses were performed using SPSS (Statistics Products Solutions Services) 18.0 software for Windows. Binary logistic regression was used for the calculation of the odds ratios (OR) with 95% confidence intervals (CI) and P-values in bivariate analysis. Multivariable stepwise logistic regression analysis was performed to assess the relationship between the patient demographic or social data and patient interest in a visit from the spiritual caregiver. The area under the receiver operating characteristic (ROC) curve was used as a measure of model discrimination. The Hosmer-Lemeshow goodness-of-fit statistic was calculated.

Comparisons between patient interest in a visit from the spiritual caregiver and interest in specific types of support were performed using the χ^2 test. Two-tailed P-values of 0.05 or less were considered statistically significant.

Results

We received 364 sufficiently complete questionnaires, a large majority of which were completed in the outpatient clinics. Questionnaires were distributed from March through August 2010 and again from April through mid-May 2011. Completion of questionnaires was voluntary. The most common reason volunteered by patients for non-completion was physical distress.

Fifty-five percent of respondents were female, and 52% were over the age of 60. Ethnic and religious orientation, as shown in Table 1, was largely in keeping with regional demographic patterns, though the

---

[*] Please see the original publication of this article for the link to the additional file.

Arab population may be slightly under-represented, composing 16% of respondents but approximately 25% of the regional population.

In response to the question, "How important do you think it is that the oncology institute includes spiritual care in its services?", 60% of patients felt it was important for spiritual care to be offered, regardless of their own personal interest in the service.

In response to the question, "How open do you think you would be to a visit from the spiritual caregiver?", 41% of patients were positively predisposed to such a visit (25% definitely interested; 16% possibly interested). Bivariate analysis of the other items in relation to this question determined the significant predictors of interest in spiritual care.

As shown in Table 1, none of the demographic or clinical items predicted a particular degree of openness to spiritual care. However, items describing one's own level of spirituality or religiosity were strongly significant in our bivariate analysis. Patients self-describing as "somewhat spiritual" or "very spiritual" were 4.2 and 8.4 times as likely (odds ratio [OR]) to be interested in spiritual care as those who were "not spiritual" (95% CI, 1.94–8.94 and 3.58–19.47; $P < 0.001$), while those who were "traditional" or "religious" were 1.8 and 2.4 times as likely, respectively (OR), to be interested as those who were "secular" (95% CI, 1.10–2.90 and 1.31–4.43; $P = 0.019$ and 0.005, respectively).

Certain experiential factors were significant predictors of an interest in spiritual care in our bivariate analysis, as listed in Table 2. Hospitalized patients receiving one visit a week or less from family or friends were more likely to want a spiritual care visit than those visited almost daily (OR, 3.9; 95% CI, 1.54–9.63; $P = 0.004$). Patients who had been visited previously by spiritual caregivers were more likely to want another visit, compared to those who had never experienced spiritual care (OR, 3.9; 95% CI, 2.0–7.8; $P < 0.001$). Those who felt they had a good understanding of what spiritual care is were more likely to be open to a visit than those who felt they did not understand it (OR, 2.9; 95% CI, 1.8–4.8; $P < 0.001$). The other sociological or experiential factors examined (living alone; supportive community; family nearby; attending religious services) were not significant predictors.

We attempted to construct a model of the patient most likely to be open to receiving spiritual care, using multivariate logistic regression. Because we found co-linearity between religiosity and spirituality ($P < 0.001$), we could not use the same model for both variables. Table 3 presents two possible models side-by-side, one including religiosity and excluding spirituality, and the other including spirituality and excluding religiosity. The other predictors previously identified (frequency of friend/family visits; previous visit from spiritual caregiver; understanding of what spiritual care is) retained their statistical significance in the multivariate analysis in both models.

The importance attached to particular ways that spiritual care can be supportive significantly predicted a patient's interest in personally receiving spiritual care in every case – the higher the patient interest in a particular kind of support, the greater the interest in personally receiving spiritual care, as shown in Table 4. Among those interested in receiving spiritual care, "Help you face your situation with calmness and dignity" (74.8%) and "Show care for your family" (71.5%) were the types of support most often rated as important, while "Address spiritual or religious concerns" (47.7%), "Bring a sense of spirituality into the room" (45.7%) and "Pray with you" (30.5%) rated lowest. Even among those indifferent to a visit from the spiritual caregiver, over half the respondents rated as important 10 out of 15 types of support.

Table 1: Associations between patient demographic, spiritual, and clinical data and patient openness to receiving a spiritual care visit (bivariate analysis)

	No. of patients (%)	No. interested in spiritual care (%)	Odds ratio	Confidence interval (95%)	p value
Gender					
• Male	151 (41)	59 (39)	1.00	Ref.	
• Female	186 (51)	84 (45)	1.26	0.81–1.94	0.305
• Non-response	27 (7)				
Age					
• Under 40	33 (9)	16 (48)	1.00	Ref.	
• 40–50	47 (13)	24 (51)	1.11	0.46–2.70	0.820
• 50–60	90 (25)	33 (37)	0.62	0.28–1.38	0.237
• 60–65	62 (17)	27 (44)	0.82	0.35–1.91	0.646
• 66–70	43 (12)	15 (35)	0.57	0.23–1.44	0.233
• Over 70	79 (22)	31 (39)	0.69	0.30–1.56	0.367
• Non-response	10 (3)				
Marital status					
• Single	19 (5)	7 (37)	1.00	Ref.	
• Married	264 (73)	108 (41)	1.17	0.45–3.06	0.752
• Divorced	40 (11)	19 (48)	1.56	0.51–4.75	0.442
• Widowed	33 (9)	14 (42)	1.26	0.40–4.03	0.693
• Non-response	8 (2)				
Educational level					
• Primary school	49 (13)	22 (45)	1.00	Ref.	

• High school	115 (32)	48 (42)	0.88	0.45–1.73	0.708
• More than high school	184 (51)	74 (40)	0.83	0.44–1.56	0.554
• Non-response	16 (4)				
Religion					
• Jewish	276 (76)	119 (43)	1.00	Ref.	
• Muslim	34 (9)	16 (47)	1.19	0.58–2.43	0.633
• Druze	11 (3)	3 (27)	0.50	0.13–1.93	0.317
• Arab Christian	12 (3)	5 (42)	0.96	0.30–3.09	0.941
• Other Christian	8 (2)	3 (38)	0.80	0.19–3.43	0.767
• Other	8 (2)	2 (25)	0.45	0.09–2.25	0.328
• Non-response	15 (4)				
Place of birth					
• Israel	168 (46)	77 (46)	1.00	Ref.	
• FSU	70 (19)	27 (39)	0.72	0.40–1.30	0.277
• Europe	47 (13)	15 (32)	0.54	0.27–1.09	0.084
• Middle East/N. Africa	51 (14)	22 (43)	0.87	0.45–1.67	0.677
• Other	14 (4)	5 (36)	0.64	0.20–2.01	0.441
• Non-response	14 (4)				
Spirituality					
• Not spiritual	58 (16)	9 (16)	1.00	Ref.	
• Somewhat spiritual	203 (56)	87 (43)	4.17	1.94–8.94	<0.001*
• Very spiritual	76 (21)	46 (61)	8.35	3.58–19.47	<0.001*
• Non-response	27 (7)				
Religiousness					
• Secular	146 (40)	48 (33)	1.00	Ref.	
• Traditional	135 (37)	63 (47)	1.79	1.10–2.90	0.019*
• Religious	61 (17)	33 (54)	2.41	1.31–4.43	0.005*
• Non-response	22 (6)				
Time since primary diagnosis					
• <4 weeks	25 (7)	11 (44)	1.00	Ref.	
• 1–3 months	59 (16)	21 (36)	0.70	0.27–1.82	0.469
• 3–6 months	76 (21)	33 (43)	0.98	0.39–2.43	0.960
• >6 months	176 (48)	79 (45)	1.04	0.45–2.41	0.934
• Non-response	28 (8)				

*p <0.05.
Data not showing significant correlation not included in table: disease recurrence, metastatic disease, status of oncology treatment.

Table 2: Significant associations between experiential factors and patient openness to receiving a spiritual care visit, bivariate analysis

	No. of patients (%)	Interested in spiritual care (%)	Odds ratio	Confidence interval (95%)	p value
Frequency of visitors (if hospitalized)					
• Almost every day	174 (48)	71 (41)	1.00	Ref.	
• Few times a week	22 (6)	10 (45)	1.18	0.48–2.88	0.715
• Once a week or less	26 (7)	19 (73)	3.85	1.54–9.63	0.004*
• Not hospitalized	99 (27)	41 (41)	1.00	0.61–1.65	0.996
• Non-response	43 (12)				
Previous visit from spiritual caregiver?					
• No	312 (86)	115 (37)	1.00	Ref.	
• Not sure	9 (2)	5 (56)	2.1	0.6–8.0	0.272
• Yes	43 (12)	30 (70)	3.9	2.0–7.8	<0.001*
Understanding of what a spiritual caregiver is/does					
• No	102 (28)	27 (26)	1.00	Ref.	
• Unsure	37 (10)	12 (32)	1.4	0.6–3.2	0.418
• Yes	225 (62)	113 (50)	2.9	1.8–4.8	<0.001*

*p <0.05.

Table 3: Prediction of openness to spiritual care visit, multivariate logistic regression model

Variable	Response	Coefficients	p value	Adjusted OR	Confidence interval
Religiosity	Secular		0.004	1.00	
	Traditional	0.79	0.002	2.2	1.3–3.6
	Religious	0.74	0.024	2.1	1.1–4.0
Frequency of visits	Once/wk or less	1.73	0.001	5.6	2.1–15.1
Previous visit from spiritual caregiver	Yes	0.86	0.011	2.4	1.2–4.6
Understanding of spiritual care	Yes	1.04	<0.001	2.8	1.7–4.7
Constant	Constant	−1.69	<0.001	0.19	
Spirituality	Not spiritual		<0.001	1.0	
	Somewhat spiritual	1.37	0.001	3.9	1.8–8.6
	Very spiritual	1.83	<0.001	6.3	2.6–15.1

Frequency of visits	Once/wk or less	1.57	0.004	4.8	1.7–13.9
Previous visit from spiritual caregiver	Yes	0.75	0.034	2.1	1.1–4.2
Understanding of spiritual care	Yes	0.81	0.002	2.3	1.3–3.8
Constant	Constant	−2.348	<0.001	0.10	

Table 4: Importance of specific types of support the spiritual caregiver can provide associated with openness to spiritual care visit, bivariate analysis

Variable	% of those not open to visit (N=120)	% of those unsure about visit (N=93)	% of those interested in visit (N=151)	p value
Help you face your situation with calmness and dignity	34.2	65.6	74.8	<0.001
Show care for your family	37.5	52.7	71.5	<0.001
Help you find strength to continue	33.3	67.7	70.9	<0.001
Help you find meaning in your situation	26.7	55.9	68.9	<0.001
Help you find hope or encouragement	30.8	66.7	68.9	<0.001
Help you obtain information or help in communicating with staff	34.2	50.5	68.2	<0.001
Listen to your concerns and show care for you	34.2	53.8	67.5	<0.001
Help you cope with and adjust to the whole situation	30.0	57.0	66.9	<0.001
Help you make difficult decisions	34.2	52.7	64.2	<0.001
Help you reflect on your experience	25.0	45.2	62.3	<0.001
Help you cope with your sense of loss	23.3	44.1	61.6	<0.001
Offer you supportive techniques like relaxation, meditation, music, and guided imagery	23.3	51.6	58.9	<0.001
Address spiritual or religious questions	15.8	37.6	47.7	<0.001
Bring a sense of spirituality into the room	15.8	38.7	45.7	<0.001
Pray with you	14.2	35.5	30.5	0.001

Note: "Important" defined as 5–7 on the 7-point Likert scale.

Discussion

Despite the relatively recent introduction of professional spiritual care in Israel, the percentage of patients interested in the service (41%) or valuing its inclusion in the hospital's services (60%) indicates a significant positive disposition towards hospital-based spiritual care. Previous studies in hospitals where spiritual care was better established found a range of patient interest in spiritual care: 54% (rehabilitation),[33] 41% (internal medicine),[30] and 35% (medical/surgical).[29] Despite the newness of the Israeli spiritual care service, levels of patient interest were within the range found in those more established settings. As can be seen in Table 4, the value given to addressing spiritual needs correlates with a desire for spiritual care, suggesting that patients already look positively at this service as a means of helping them with their spiritual needs. Patients' sense of understanding what spiritual care is was a predictor of their interest in the service that persisted in the multivariate analysis. This suggests the importance of education and awareness in determining public interest in the service – the more patients understood what the service has to offer, the greater their interest in receiving the service. That result parallels the finding that lack of knowledge and understanding are key factors in institutions not including spiritual care.[22] The results for patient interest may be expected to change as levels of awareness grow.

Even among those who expressed indifference to a spiritual care visit, between half and two-thirds of such patients found the kinds of support spiritual caregivers provide to be important to them for most items. Increased patient education might shift that indifference into openness, although it also could be the case that those patients' needs are being met elsewhere.

The significance of previous experience in receiving spiritual care as a positive predictor of patient interest in the service supports previous findings.[31, 32] The persistence of this factor even in the multivariate model suggests that it is not just that those who were previously likely to be interested in spiritual care continue to be interested. Rather, this finding supports the positive impact of care and suggests that it is being well received.

To what extent does the significance of demographic, medical, and social/experiential factors vary between Israel and other cultural settings, in predicting patient interest or satisfaction? As described in the Background, we are aware of four studies, all American, that measured this question. In the present study, as in those previous studies, gender, marital status, religion, and ethnicity were not predictive factors[29, 30, 31, 32] (with the exception of "Other" ethnicity in[30]).

Older age was a significant predictor in 3 of 4 studies, but not in the present study. Perhaps its significance was confounded in our results by the fact that younger Israelis show increased spirituality,[40] or it may provide evidence for a cross-cultural difference. Educational level, significant in every prior study though not always in the same direction, was not significant here, perhaps suggesting that it, too, can reflect cultural difference.

Our study was the only one to examine country of origin. Israel is a nation of immigrants from countries with widely differing cultural approaches in caring for illness and spirituality.[39] This item is of particular interest regarding the question of whether we should expect to find cross-cultural difference in patient interest around the world, and the fact that it was an insignificant factor in our study strengthens the above conclusion that variance between countries will not be significant.

As in most other studies, self-defined spirituality,[30, 32] or religiosity[29, 30] were significant predictors of positive perceptions of spiritual care. It seems likely that these are fairly universal factors. Our study did not find significance in public religious practices, such as attendance at worship services; other studies also differed regarding the significance of that item[29, 30, 31]. It should be noted that our results showed co-linearity between spirituality and religiosity even though the questionnaire cover letter, viewable in the Additional file 1,* distinguishes clearly between the two.

In examining the impact of the seriousness of the medical condition on patient interest in spiritual care, the results have not been uniform. Ledbetter's approach to spiritual screening assumes that the likely impact of the medical condition on the patient's life is a major factor.[41] Some studies found significance in average disease length of stay[29] or severity of pain[30], but other medical factors including cancer diagnosis and co-morbidity were found in those studies and elsewhere[32] not to be statistically significant. Our study did not find any of the medical factors, including recurrence, metastasis, and treatment stage, to be significant. However, the fact that respondents had to be physically able to answer the questions, even if at times with the help of family or staff member, excluded those who were in worse condition, perhaps masking the predictive significance of medical condition. In addition, because all respondents were diagnosed with cancer, we could not measure the differential impact of a cancer diagnosis to that of other illnesses.

Lucas' approach to pastoral care emphasizes community, with the expectation that lesser community support increases the need for spiritual

---

* Please see the original publication of this article for the link to the additional file.

care,[42] and community is one of the key areas covered by Puchalski's FICA tool for spiritual history taking.[43] Ledbetter's screening approach considers lack of social support to be a major factor determining low coping resources.[42] One study did not find a significant relationship between social support and patient requests for spiritual care,[29] and some of the social support items we included were insignificant as well. However, Lucas' and Ledbetter's predictions of the significance of community were supported by our persistent finding that lower frequency of visits by friends and family was a predictor of patient interest in spiritual care. Identifying "lonely" patients as more likely candidates for spiritual care helps provide direction to departmental staff members and spiritual caregivers in determining whom to visit in the limit number of available staff hours.

What do these results suggest for the viability of cross-cultural screening protocols? The current data suggest that most demographic factors are consistently irrelevant, though age and education may be significant in certain cultures. The stage or severity of disease is of ambiguous utility for screening regardless of cultural setting. It should be noted that the persistent factors in the present study, including spirituality/religiousness and support from family/friends, largely match the factors identified in the FICA tool, which may prove to be a valuable cross-cultural measure.

In looking at spiritual needs and the kinds of spiritual care support patients most valued, there was a significant cultural difference, as predicted, regarding explicitly religious/spiritual items. There were four such items, and they were the four lowest-rated. Prayer ranked last in our study among kinds of spiritual support desired, at 30% of those interested in spiritual care, whereas in America prayer was the most common intervention expected of spiritual caregivers,[44] desired by 74% of those interested in spiritual care in one study.[29] Other low-ranked items were addressing spiritual/religious questions (35% overall) and bringing a sense of spirituality to the room (46% of those interested in the service), versus 61% of Irish hospice patients[37] and 78% of religious Japanese bereaved family members,[21] respectively. Only 43% of patients overall were interested in relaxation, meditation, music, or guided imagery, which could be generally characterized as spiritual techniques. Although interest in these religious/spiritual items predicted interest in spiritual care, there were many similarly predictive items, not explicitly religious/spiritual, endorsed by a much larger percentage of the population. The spiritual care desired by Israeli patients is not limited or primarily directed to the explicitly religious/spiritual realm.

The main methodological limitation of the study was the population response bias. The questionnaires were offered to all patients currently hospitalized or in the treatment clinic at that moment. However, we did not gather demographic data on those who chose not to complete the survey to compare with those who did, and did not analyze the bias in who chose to participate. We also did not record what percent of patients approached chose not to complete a questionnaire, for physical or other reasons.

The question regarding "Frequency of Visitors (if Hospitalized)" had the final answer option "not hospitalized." However, many respondents did not see that option and left this question blank, although many outpatients did answer this question. Thus, those data should best be looked at as a composite of all patients, rather than distinguishing between in- and outpatients. As a result, we do not have precise data on the breakdown among respondents between outpatient and inpatient, though we can provide a general estimation that at least 80% were outpatient. Finally, the question about types of support was not pilot tested with patients.

Conclusion

This study finds significant patient interest in a new field, Israeli spiritual care, similar to the level of interest found in countries where the service is well-established, and suggests that increased patient education and awareness will increase that interest. We found that receipt of spiritual care was a positive experience, leaving patients wanting future visits from the spiritual caregiver. As expected, what patients wanted from the spiritual caregiver showed cross-cultural difference, with explicitly religious or spiritual support less frequently desired in Israel. This study helps strengthen the formulation of cross-cultural screening tools, supporting the use of a measure of social isolation and contraindicating the use of demographic or medical data beyond self-identified religiosity/spirituality.

Additional file

Additional file 1: Patient Questionnaire.*

Competing interests

The authors declare that they have no competing interests.

---

* Please see the original publication of this article for the link to the additional file.

Authors' contributions

MS prepared the initial study design in light of previous studies, distributed the questionnaires, and drafted the manuscript. DLG helped design and coordinate the study. GBS conceived of the study, coordinated its administration, and helped to draft the manuscript. All authors read and approved the final manuscript.

Authors' information

Gil Bar-Sela, Clinical Assistant Professor, Deputy Director of the Oncology Section and the Director of the Palliative Care Unit at Rambam Health Care Campus. Michael Schultz, Board Certified Chaplain, Rabbi, MA, Director of the Spiritual Care Service of the Oncology Section, Rambam Health Care Campus. Doron Lulav-Grinwald, Clinical Psychologist (MA), Director of the Psychology Service of the Oncology Section, Rambam Health Care Campus.

Acknowledgement

We gratefully thank the UJA/Federation of New York for their ongoing support for the spiritual care program at Rambam Health Care Campus.

Received: 18 December 2013

Accepted: 31 March 2014

Published: 8 April 2014

References

1. Balboni TA, Vanderwerker LC, Block SD, Paulk ME, Lathan CS, Peteet JR, Prigerson HG: Religiousness and spiritual support among advanced cancer patients and associations with end-of-life treatment preferences and quality of life. *J Clin Oncol* 2007, 25:555–560.
2. Sulmasy DP: Spiritual issues in the care of dying patients: "…it's okay between me and god". *JAMA* 2006, 296:1385–1392. Sulmasy DP: Spiritual issues in the care of dying patients: "… it's okay between me and god." *JAMA* 2006, 296:1385–1392.
3. Cohen SR, Mount BM, Tomas JJ, Mount LF: Existential well-being is an important determinant of quality of life. Evidence from the McGill Quality of Life Questionnaire. *Cancer* 1996, 77:576–586.
4. Vallurupalli M, Lauderdale K, Balboni MJ, Phelps AC, Block SD, Ng AK, Kactnic LA, Vanderwede TJ, Balboni TA: The role of spirituality and religious coping in the quality of life of patients with advanced cancer receiving palliative radiation therapy. *J Support Oncol.* 2012, 10(2):81–7.
5. Balboni T, Balboni M, Paulk ME, Phelps A, Wright A, Peteet J, Block S, Lathan C, Vanderwede T, Prigerson H: Support of cancer patients' spiritual needs and associations with medical care costs at the end of life. *Cancer* 2011, 117:5383–5391.

6. McClain CS, Rosenfeld B, Breitbart W: Effect of spiritual well-being on end-of-life despair in terminally-ill cancer patients. *Lancet* 2003, 361:1603–1607.
7. Iler W, Obenshain D, Camac M: The impact of daily visits from chaplains on patients with chronic obstructive pulmonary disease (COPD): a pilot study. *Chaplaincy Today* 2001, 17:5–11.
8. Kristeller JL, Rhodes M, Cripe LD, Sheets V: Oncologist Assisted Spiritual Intervention Study (OASIS): patient acceptability and initial evidence of effects. *Int J Psychiatry Med* 2005, 35(4):329–47.
9. Kang J, Shin DW, Choi JY, Park CH, Baek YJ, Mo HN, Song MO, Park SA, Moon do H, Son KY: Addressing the religious and spiritual needs of dying patients by healthcare staff in Korea: patient perspectives in a multi-religious Asian country. *Psycho-Oncology* 2012, 21(4):374–81.
10. National consensus project: quality palliative care guidelines. www.nationalconsensus project.org/Guideline.pdf. (Last accessed Feb. 27, 2014).
11. Puchalski C, Ferrell B, Virani R, Otis-Green S, Baird P, Bull J, Chochinov H, Handzo G, Nelson-Becker H, Prince-Paul M, Pugliese K, Sulmasy D: Improving the quality of spiritual care as a dimension of palliative care: the report of the Consensus Conference. *J Palliat Med* 2009, 12:885–904.
12. Sulmasy DP: A biopsychosocial–spiritual model for the care of patients at the end of life. *Gerontologist* 2002, 42:24–33.
13. Hsiao SM, Gau ML, Ingleton C, Ryan T, Shih FJ: An exploration of spiritual needs of Taiwanese patients with advanced cancer during the therapeutic processes. *J Clin Nurs* 2011, 20(7–8):950–9.
14. Dhamani KA, Paul P, Olson JK: Tanzanian nurses understanding and practice of spiritual care. *ISRN Nurs* 2011, 2011:534803.
15. Kale SS: Perspectives on spiritual care at Hospice Africa Uganda. *Int J Palliat Nurs* 2011, 17(4):177–82.
16. Selman L, Harding R, Gysels M, Speck P, Higginson IJ: The measurement of spirituality in palliative care and the content of tools validated cross-culturally: a systematic review. *J Pain Symptom Manage* 2011, 41(4):728–53.
17. Benito E, Oliver A, Galiana L, Barreto P, Pascual A, Gomis C, Barbero J: Development and validation of a new tool for the assessment and spiritual care of palliative care patients. *J Pain Symptom Manage* 2013 [Epub ahead of print].
18. Iranmanesh S, Tirgari B, Cheraghi MA: Developing and testing a spiritual care questionnaire in the Iranian context. *J Relig Health* 2012, 51(4):1104–16.
19. Lewis LM: Spiritual assessment in African-Americans: a review of measures of spirituality used in health research. *J Relig Health* 2008, 47(4):458–75.
20. Selman L, Siegert R, Harding R, Gysels M, Speck P, Higginson IJ: A psychometric evaluation of measures of spirituality validated in culturally diverse palliative care populations. *J Pain Symptom Manage* 2011, 42(4):604–22.
21. Ando M, Kawamura R, Morita T, Hirai K, Miyashita M, Okamoto T, Shima Y: Value of religious care for relief of psycho-existential suffering in Japanese terminally ill cancer patients: the perspective of bereaved family members. *Psycho-Oncology* 2010, 19:750–755.
22. Bentur N, Resnitzky S, Sterne A: Attitudes of stakeholders and policymakers in the healthcare system towards the provision of spiritual care in Israel. *Health Policy* 2010, 96:13–19.
23. Bar-Sela G, Bentur N, Schultz M, Corn B: [A profession in formation – spiritual care in hospitals and other health care settings in Israel]. [Article in Hebrew]. *HaRefuah*. in press.
24. Best M, Butow P, Olver I: Spiritual support of cancer patients and the role of the doctor. *Support Care Cancer* 2013 [Epub ahead of print].
25. Baddarni K: [Spiritual care for the Muslim patient] [Article in Hebrew]. *Biton HaSiud HaOncology BiYisrael* 2013, 24(3):26–36.

26. Pearce MJ, Coan AD, Herndon JE 2nd, Koenig HG, Abernethy AP: Unmet spiritual care needs impact emotional and spiritual well-being in advanced cancer patients. *Support Care Cancer* 2012, 20(10):2269–76.
27. Selman L, Young T, Vermandere M, Stirling I, Leged C, on behalf of the EAPC Spiritual Care Taskforce: Research priorities in spiritual care: an international survey of palliative care researchers and clinicians. *J Pain Symptom Manage* 2013. in press.
28. Chaves ECL, Carvalho EC, Beijo LA, Goyatá SLT, Pillon SC: Efficacy of different instruments for the identification of the nursing diagnosis spiritual distress. *Rev Lat Am* 2011, 19:902–910.
29. Fitchett G, Meyer PM, Burton LA: Spiritual care in the hospital: Who requests it? Who needs it? *J Pastoral Care* 2000, 54:173–186.
30. Williams JA, Meltzer D, Arora V, Chung G, Curlin FA: Attention to inpatients' religious and spiritual concerns: predictors and association with patient satisfaction. *J Gen Intern Med* 2011, 26:1265–1271.
31. VandeCreek L: How satisfied are patients with the ministry of chaplains? *J Pastoral Care Counsel* 2004, 58:35–342.
32. Phelps AC, Lauderdale KE, Alcorn S, Dillinger J, Balboni MT, Van West M, Vanderwede TJ, Balboni TA: Addressing spirituality within the care of patients at the end of life: perspectives of patients with advanced cancer, oncologists, and oncology nurses. *J Clin Oncol* 2012, 30:2538–2544.
33. Anderson JM, Anderson LJ, Felsenthal G: Pastoral needs and support within an inpatient rehabilitation unit. *Arch Phys Med Rehabil* 1993, 74:574–578.
34. Bentur N, Resnizky S: Challenges and achievements in the development of spiritual-care training and implementation in Israel. *Palliat Med* 2010, 24(8):771–6.
35. Shalom T, Schiff E, Steiner M, Katz M, Ben-Arye E: [Integrating complementary medicine in oncology supportive care: assessment of patients' needs and expectations during chemotherapy]. [Article in Hebrew]. *Harefuah* 2011, 150(8):642–5–689.
36. Galek K, Flannelly KJ, Vane A, Galek RM: Assessing a patient's spiritual needs: a comprehensive instrument. *Holist Nurs Pract* 2005, 19:62–69.
37. Kernohan WG, Waldron M, McAfee C, Cochrane B, Hasson F: An evidence base for a palliative care chaplaincy service in Northern Ireland. *Palliat Med* 2007, 21:519–525.
38. Flannelly KJ, Galek K, Tannenbaum HP, Handzo GF: A preliminary proposal for a scale to measure the effectiveness of pastoral care with family members of hospitalized patients. *J Pastoral Care Counsel* 2007, 61:19–29.
39. Ben-Arye E, Karkabi S, Shapira C, Schiff E, Lavie O, Keshet Y: Complementary medicine in the primary care setting: results of a survey of gender and cultural patterns in Israel. *Gend Med* 2009, 6:384–397.
40. Ben-Arye E, Schiff E, Vintal H, Agour O, Preis L, Steiner M: Integrating complementary medicine and supportive care: patients' perspectives toward complementary medicine and spirituality. *J Altern Complement Med* 2012, 18:824–831.
41. Ledbetter TJ: Screening for pastoral visitations using the Clinical + Coping Score. *J Pastoral Care Counsel* 2008, 62:367–374.
42. Lucas AM: Introduction to the discipline for pastoral care giving. *J Health Care Chaplain* 2001, 10:1–33.
43. Puchalski C, Romer AL: Taking a spiritual history allows clinicians to understand patients more fully. *J Palliat Med* 2000, 3:129–137.
44. Hover M, Travis JL 3rd, Koenig HG, Bearon LB: Pastoral research in a hospital setting: a case study. *J Pastoral Care* 1991, 46(3):283–90.

doi:10.1186/1472-684X-13-19

Cite this article as: Schultz et al.: Cultural differences in spiritual care: findings of an Israeli oncologic questionnaire examining patient interest in spiritual care. BMC Palliative Care 2014 13:19.

ARTICLE 13

The Frequency and Correlates of Spiritual Distress Among Patients with Advanced Cancer Admitted to an Acute Palliative Care Unit

David Hui, MD[1], Maxine de la Cruz, MD[1], Steve Thorney, MDiv, MA[1], Henrique A. Parsons, MD[1], Marvin Delgado-Guay, MD[1], and Eduardo Bruera, MD[1]

1 Department of Palliative Care and Rehabilitation Medicine, The University of Texas MD Anderson Cancer Center, Houston, TX, USA

Corresponding Author: Eduardo Bruera, Department of Palliative Care and Rehabilitation Medicine, The University of Texas MD Anderson Cancer Center, 1515 Holcombe Blvd, Unit 1414, Houston 77030, TX, USA
Email: ebruera@mdanderson.org

Abstract

Limited research is available on the frequency of spiritual distress and its relationship with physical and emotional distress. We reviewed patients admitted to our acute palliative care unit (APCU) and determined the association between patient characteristics, symptom severity using the Edmonton Symptom Assessment scale (ESAS), and spiritual distress as reported by a chaplain on initial visit. In all, 50 (44%) of 113 patients had spiritual distress. In univariate analysis, patients with spiritual distress were more likely to be younger (odds ratio [OR] = 0.96, $P = .004$), to have pain (OR = 1.2, $P = .010$) and depression (OR = 1.24, $P = .018$) compared to those without spiritual distress. Spiritual distress was associated with age (OR = 0.96, $P = .012$) and depression (OR = 1.27, $P = .020$) in multivariate analysis. Our findings support regular spiritual assessment as part of the interdisciplinary approach to optimize symptom control.

Key words: palliative care, spirituality, distress, advanced cancer, symptoms, depression

---

Hui, D., de la Cruz, M., Thorney, S., Parsons, H.A., Delgado-Guay, M., and Bruera, E. (2011) "The frequency and correlates of spiritual distress among patients with advanced cancer admitted to an acute palliative care unit." *American Journal of Hospice and Palliative Medicine*, 28, 4, 264–270.

Introduction

A diagnosis of cancer or news of recurrent or progressive disease is a very traumatic event that can cause significant spiritual distress. Patients with advanced cancer have to face the fear of suffering, disability, helplessness, isolation, and impending death.[1,2] Spiritual distress has been found to be associated with psychosocial needs, communication issues, death anxiety, hopelessness, and despair.[3,4,5,6] Since quality of life is affected by all domains of personhood, spirituality in the context of overall care needs to be given importance.[7]

Spirituality is a subjective experience that occurs both within and outside the context of religious traditions. It is not defined by a set of beliefs about humanity, divinity, or the ultimate truth[8] but rather as a means by which people understand and live in view of their ultimate meaning and value.[9] Spirituality is characterized by the capacity to love and forgive, to worship, to see beyond the current circumstances, and to transcend suffering.[10] Spiritual concerns are typically awakened at the end of life, and the lack of meaning at that time may have important bearing on the will to live.[11] Lack of spiritual well-being is also associated with depression and lower tolerance to physical symptoms.[12,13] Spiritual pain may manifest itself as symptoms in any area of a person's experience[14,15] and can threaten the intactness of the person as a complex psychological and social entity.[14,16,17] Evidence suggests that spiritual well-being is an important protective factor against psychological distress in patients with terminal disease such as advanced cancer.[18]

In recent years, there has been a growing body of literature on psychosocial and spiritual well-being in patients with terminal illness, as it relates to their quality of life. There have been numerous studies describing the relationship of psychosocial distress such as depression, anxiety, and hopelessness with patients' physical symptoms and well-being.[19] However, there remains limited information on the frequency of spiritual distress and its relationship with physical and psychological symptoms, particularly in patients with advanced cancer. The purpose of this study was to determine the frequency and factors associated with spiritual distress in patients with advanced cancer admitted to the acute palliative care unit (APCU).

Methods

We reviewed the electronic charts of 165 consecutive patients with advanced cancer that were admitted to the APCU at MD Anderson Cancer Center between July 1, 2007 and October 31, 2007. The study protocol was approved by the Institutional Review Board of the University of Texas MD Anderson Cancer Center, with waiver of informed consent. The APCU is a 12-bed unit that provides inpatient palliative care services with the goal of enhancing quality of life.

Demographic data including age, gender, and religion were collected for each patient as well as length of APCU stay and reason for admission. The Edmonton Symptom Assessment scale (ESAS)[20] was collected from the day corresponding to the date of the initial chaplain evaluation. ESAS is a validated tool that assesses 9 different symptoms (pain, fatigue, nausea, depression, anxiety, drowsiness, sleep, appetite, and shortness of breath) and feeling of well-being using numeric rating scale ranging from 0 to 10, where 0 = *no symptom* and 10 = *worst possible*, and is usually completed by the patient independently. However, a family member, physician, or nurse can help the patient complete in the assessment if he is unable to rate all the symptoms. Patients were excluded from the study if they were unresponsive, had delirium or if sedation limited their participation.

As a part of our interdisciplinary approach, all patients that are admitted to the APCU are seen by a chaplain early in the course of their admission, who provides spiritual assessment and support for patients and family members/caregivers. Although a number of questionnaires such as the Functional Assessment of Chronic Illness Therapy-Spiritual Well-Being, Expanded version (FACIT-SpEx)[8] are available for the assessment of spiritual well-being, there is a lack of validated assessment tools to specifically assess spiritual distress. Thus, our chaplains developed an empiric clinical tool based on the work of Roy Nash, a pastoral psychotherapist who has written about spirituality, ethics, and clinical pastoral care. In his work, *Life's Major Spiritual Issues*, Nash described 22 spiritual polarities or domains that people experience throughout the course of their life journey.[21] Examples of such spiritual domains include meaninglessness and fullness of life, brokenness and wholeness, despair and hope, and dread and courage. A person journeys freely at different time points along these domains. For example, difficult life experiences may bring about fear of loss or function or even life, but if life goals are reframed, then one may move toward the opposite end of the pole which is courage. In developing the spiritual assessment tool, Jenkins and Thorney reduced the list to include 7 spiritual distress domains that were felt most relevant to supportive cancer care: hope versus despair, wholeness versus brokenness, courage versus anxiety/dread, connected versus alienated, meaningful versus meaningless, grace/forgiveness versus guilt, and empowered versus helpless. This assessment tool is used by chaplains throughout our institution.

Operational definitions used in the MD Anderson spiritual assessment tool are listed here. Hope is a realistic and adaptive response to extreme stress or crisis that requires a patient to surrender to transcendent forces. In contrast, despair is a more objectless and profound depressed state of being than, for example, grief, which attaches to a specific loss. Wholeness connotes right relationships with the self, others, and a higher power, whereas brokenness is the spiritual unrest stemming from the knowledge that 1 or more of these relationships are conflicted. Anxiety and dread are thought to be an individual's response to the threat of nonbeing, a threat which includes nihilism and death. Courage, however, is the confrontation of this anxiety of nonbeing. Individuals are connected through a variety of relationships to a higher power, self, and others. When these relations are in harmony, there is a sense of connectedness as opposed to alienation when the person isolates or withdraws from 1 or more of those relationships as a response to crisis. The concept of meaningful or meaningless stems from the existentialist's position that a person's finite freedom is distorted by the anxiety it engenders. Guilt is a violation of the laws, norms, and values of the community in which a person is connected. Subjectively, it is a feeling that results when one violates his or her own conscience. Forgiveness is one aspect of remedy for guilt in both the secular and religious worlds. Grace is generally understood from a Christian vantage point as an expression of God's unconditional, forgiving, and empowering love for humanity. In the context of hospital-based spiritual care, empowerment and helplessness address the capacity of an individual to act (empowerment) as well as the attendant necessity to be acted on by others (helpless), ostensibly in the patient's best interest.

There is only one chaplain in our palliative care service, who works closely with other members of the interdisciplinary team and routinely attends the morning patient rounds, as well as weekly interdisciplinary rounds and family conferences. The board-certified APCU chaplain has more than 22 years of experience as pastor of a local congregation in Houston, clinical ethicist, and also as a clinical chaplain working with cancer patients. The chaplain outlines in his progress notes important spiritual distress domains covered during the visit. For this study, the APCU chaplain retrospectively reviewed his initial visit notes for each of the spiritual distress domains. Spiritual distress was considered present if patients had 2 or more of the following distress domains: despair, dread, brokenness, helplessness, alienation, meaningless, and guilt/shame.

We summarized baseline demographics using descriptive statistics, including medians, means, standard deviations, ranges, and frequencies. We conducted univariate logistic regression analysis to determine the association between spiritual distress and various clinical factors. Subsequent multivariate logistic regression analysis was performed using variables with $P < .20$ in univariate analysis. We also assessed factors association with severity of spiritual distress using multivariate nonparametric linear regression analysis. Two-sided P values less than .05 were considered statistically significant. The same statistical analyses were performed for each of the 7 spiritual distress domains. The Statistical Package for the Social Sciences (SPSS version 16.0, SPSS Inc, Chicago, Illinois) software was used for statistical analysis.

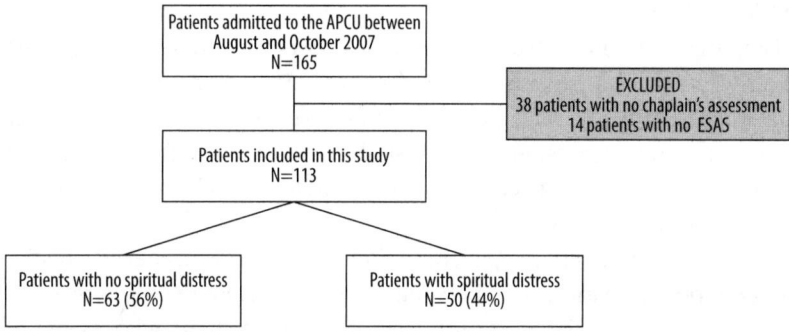

Figure 1: Study flowchart. APCU indicates acute palliative care unit; ESAS, Edmonton Symptom Assessment Scale

Results

Among the 165 consecutive patients reviewed, 52 were excluded because of the absence of either a chaplain assessment or a recorded ESAS (Figure 1). Reasons for lack of chaplain assessment included delirium (N = 38, 73%), actively dying (N = 9, 17%), patient refusal (N = 3, 6%), and chaplain on holiday (N = 3, 6%). Table 1 shows the characteristics of the 113 patients included in the study. A majority were Christians. Spiritual distress was noted to be present in 50 (44%) of 113 patients. The distribution of the number of spiritual distress domains is shown in Figure 2.

In univariate analysis, younger age, pain, and depression were significantly associated with spiritual distress (Table 2). Other demographic and clinical variables tested did not show any significant association with spiritual distress. Multivariate logistic regression analysis showed younger age and depression to be independently associated with spiritual distress (Table 2). Younger age ($P = .009$), pain ($P = .027$), and depression ($P = .021$) were also found to be associated with a greater number of spiritual distress domains in multivariate nonparametric linear regression analysis.

The frequency of each of the 7 spiritual distress domains is shown in Table 3. On the initial chaplain visit, despair was the most common spiritual distress domain expressed by patients in the APCU, followed by dread and brokenness. Multivariate analysis for each of the spiritual distress domains is summarized in Table 4. Younger patients were more likely to report despair, brokenness, helplessness, and meaninglessness. Male patients were more likely to report despair. Patients with pain were more likely to feel alienation.

Discussion

Using the MD Anderson chaplains' clinical assessment tool, we found that nearly half of the patients admitted to the APCU had spiritual distress on initial chaplain visit. Spiritual distress was associated with younger age, pain, and depression. Further studies are required to elucidate the nature of spiritual distress and to identify strategies to better manage this multidimensional construct.

A significant number of patients living with cancer consider spirituality as an important part of their personhood that gains more relevance at the end of life.[22, 23, 24, 25] Patients' spirituality may provide them with a sense of well-being by giving structure and meaning to their difficult experience and serve as a buffer against depression, hopelessness, desire for death, and existential suffering.[4, 26, 27] However, at the end of life, when patients are confronted with complex physical, psychosocial, and existential concerns, spiritual distress can occur. Frequent struggles with fear, anger, physical discomfort, loss of independence, changing self-image, roles and relationships,[28, 29, 30, 31] and failure to find meaning[32] can also contribute to spiritual distress.

Almost half of our patients were found to have spiritual distress, defined here as the presence of at least 2 spiritual distress domains. In a survey of 57 patients with advanced cancer, Mako et al.[33] reported that about 61% of patients had spiritual distress at the time of chaplain visit. The difference in observed frequencies may be related to how spiritual distress was defined and measured.[34] Spiritual distress that is present in the form of depression and hopelessness occur in a substantial minority of patients with advanced cancer.[18, 27, 35] The high prevalence of spiritual distress in the palliative care population highlights the need to develop validated assessment tools and targeted interventions for this construct.

In our study, younger patients were found to have more spiritual distress compared with older patients. When the domains were considered separately, younger age was likewise a risk factor for despair, brokenness, helplessness, and meaningless. For patients in the prime of their lives, the possibility of a life curtailed, of decline in function, and unfulfilled aspirations can be sources of great spiritual and psychosocial distress. A previous study showed that patients older than 50 years were more likely to describe themselves as being at peace than younger patients.[36] Ellis et al.[37] reported that younger patients were referred more to a specialized psychology oncology service for management of both psychosocial and spiritual distress. Younger patients may be less likely to let go, as evident by the higher likelihood of receiving cancer treatments close to the end of life.[38] This, coupled with the lack of resources[39] and self-esteem issues,[40] could potentially exacerbate the sense of spiritual distress.

Pain, which may be a symbol of worsening disease for some patients, was associated with poor spiritual well-being. The term total pain recognizes the interaction of the 3 domains of personhood and how they influence each other. Cicely Saunders defined it as the suffering that encompasses all of a person's physical, psychological, social, spiritual, and practical struggles.[41, 42] Such other forms of pain may often be manifested and interpreted as physical pain without consideration of the psychosocial and spiritual components to it. Our study showed the association of pain and spiritual distress and is consistent with previous reports.[33, 43, 44, 45] The presence of pain can often limit a person's ability to have meaningful interaction with others, possibly resulting in alienation. The search for meaning at the end of life also becomes difficult for patients struggling with uncontrolled symptoms and subsequently results in spiritual distress.

Most studies have demonstrated that spiritual well-being is positively correlated with better physical and psychological well-being.[4, 46] A strong faith and belief system and the ability to find meaning and purpose positively affects spiritual well-being resulting in less psychological distress.[46] Several authors have recommended pastoral care interventions aimed at strengthening spiritual well-being in patients with psychosocial issues like depression and anxiety.[47] The inverse to this relationship which is the effect of psychological distress, such as depression, on spiritual well-being has not been fully investigated. Our study showed that depression was associated with spiritual distress. A similar study of 31 palliative care patients admitted to the hospital showed that spiritual distress was positively correlated with anxiety, depression, and fatigue.[29] Although spiritual distress may manifest as symptoms of depression, depression may also augment spiritual distress, preventing patients from adopting a more fulfilling approach to the end of life.[48]

Our study affirms the interconnectedness among the physical, psychosocial, and spiritual dimensions of personhood, with the important implication that an interdisciplinary team approach is necessary to address the complex needs of palliative care patients and their families. Specifically, the presence of a chaplain, who has acquired expertise in conducting spiritual assessments and providing spiritual interventions, is crucial. Good rapport between the patient and clinician is also essential for effective diagnosis and management of spiritual distress.[10]

This study has a number of limitations, including the small sample size, the retrospective data collection, and the use of an assessment tool for spiritual pain that has not been fully validated. Although this clinical assessment tool has content and face validity, further studies are required to examine its reliability, validity, and responsiveness to change. Importantly, spiritual pain as a construct also needs to be better defined through both qualitative and quantitative studies. Finally, we only examined spiritual pain when patients were first admitted to the APCU, which may not be representative of patients' experience. Multiple visits may be required before patients could fully engage at a very personal level and discuss their spiritual and existential concerns. Further research is required.

As patients approach death, the inward journey aimed to answer the questions of life's meaning occurs frequently. Clinicians must acknowledge the spiritual dimension of patients as an integral component of their personhood. Assessment for spiritual wellness and distress is, therefore, crucial in addressing end-of-life needs. Our findings support the interconnectedness among physical, psychological, and spiritual distress. An interprofessional approach to patient's suffering is essential in improving care at the end of life.

Table 1: Patient demographics

	No spiritual distress (%)[a], N=63	Spiritual distress present (%)[a], N=50
Mean age, in years (standard deviation)	64 (14.3)	55 (14.6)[b]
Gender		
• Female	28 (44)	17 (34)
• Male	35 (56)	33 (66)
Ethnicity		
• African American	11 (18)	10 (20)
• Hispanic	7 (11)	9 (16)
• Caucasian	40 (64)	29 (58)
• Asian	5 (8)	2 (4)

Median length of APCU stay in days (interquartile range)	8 (5–11)	7 (6–13)
Religion		
• Christian	48 (76)	44 (81)
• Jewish	3 (5)	0 (0)
• Buddhist	2 (3)	2 (4)
• Hindu	2 (3)	0 (0)
• Muslim	1 (2)	1 (2)
• Others	7 (11)	3 (6)
Median Edmonton Symptom Assessment scale (interquartile range)		
Pain	2 (1–4)	4 (1–7)[b]
Fatigue	4 (1–7)	4 (1–7)
Nausea	1 (0–1)	1 (1–1)
Depression	1 (0–2)	2 (1–4)[b]
Anxiety	1 (1–4)	3 (1–5)
Drowsiness	4 (1–6)	4 (1–6)
Dyspnea	2 (1–4)	2 (1–5)
Appetite	6 (3–8)	5 (2–8)
Sleep	3 (1–5)	4 (1–5)
Well-being	3 (1–5)	5 (1–5)

Abbreviation: APCU, acute palliative care unit.
[a]Unless otherwise specified.
[b]$P < .05$ in univariate analysis.

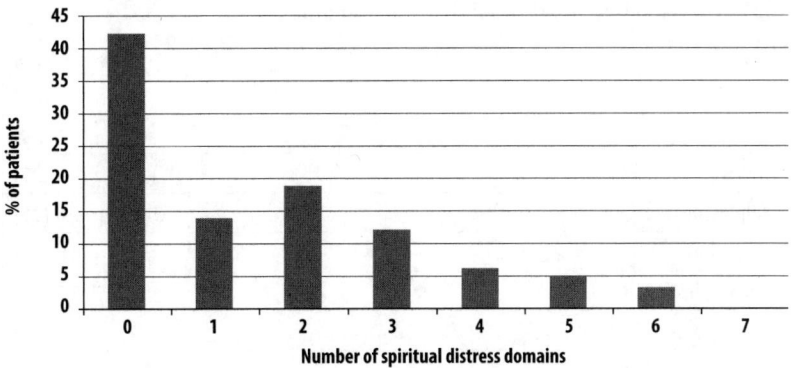

Figure 2: Number of spiritual distress domains. In this study, spiritual distress was defined as the presence of 2 or more spiritual distress domains

Table 2: Association between spiritual distress and clinical features

Characteristics and symptoms	Univariate analysis		Multivariate analysis	
	OR (95% CI)	P value	OR (95% CI)	P value
Age (per year)	0.96 (0.93–0.99)	.004	0.96 (0.93–0.99)	.012
Male gender	1.55 (0.72–3.35)	.26	–	–
Religion	1.01 (0.67–1.11)	.96	–	–
Ethnicity	1.05 (0.71–1.56)	.80	–	–
Reason for APCU admission	0.85 (0.61–1.19)	.35	–	–
Length of APCU stay (days)	1.04 (0.98–0.11)	.21	–	–
Edmonton Symptom Assessment scale				
• Pain	1.20 (1.04–1.37)	.010	–	–
• Fatigue	0.96 (0.84–1.09)	.50	–	–
• Nausea	1.10 (0.91–1.35)	.33	–	–
• Depression	1.24 (1.04–1.48)	.018	1.27 (1.04–1.56)	.02
• Anxiety	1.18 (0.997–1.40)	.05	–	–
• Drowsiness	0.97 (0.85–1.11)	.67	–	–
• Dyspnea	1.09 (0.95–1.26)	.23	–	–
• Appetite	0.97 (0.86–1.09)	.59	–	–
• Sleep	1.07 (0.93–1.24)	.34	–	–
• Well-being	1.10 (0.95–1.26)	.20	–	–

Abbreviations: APCU, acute palliative care unit; CI, confidence interval; OR, odds ratio.

Table 3: Frequency of spiritual distress domains

Domains	Number of patients (%)
Despair	36 (32)
Dread	33 (29)
Broken	31 (27)
Helplessness	28 (25)
Alienation	18 (16)
Meaningless	17 (15)
Guilt/shame	10 (8)

Table 4: Multivariate logistic regression analysis for individual spiritual domains[a]

Spiritual distress domain	OR (95% CI)	P value
Despair		
• Age	0.96 (0.92–0.99)	.006
• Male gender	3.54 (1.24–10.10)	.018
• Appetite	0.83 (0.69–0.99)	.047
• Well-being	1.28 (1.03–1.57)	.023
Dread		
• Length of APCU stay	1.09 (1.01–1.17)	.032
• Anxiety	1.35 (1.09–1.68)	.007
Brokenness		
• Age	0.97 (0.94–1.0)	.048
• Length of APCU stay	1.07 (0.99–1.14)	.075
Helplessness		
• Age	0.96 (0.93–0.99)	.016
• Sleep	1.21 (1.01–1.44)	.037
Alienation		
• Pain	1.31 (1.08–1.56)	.006
• Fatigue	0.82 (0.66–1.01)	.057
Meaningless		
• Age	0.96 (0.92–0.99)	.015
Guilt/Shame		
• Anxiety	0.61 (0.38–0.97)	.038

Abbreviations: APCU, acute palliative care unit; CI, confidence interval; OR, odds ratio.
[a]Only the significant factors were shown.

Authors' note

The authors, David Hui and Maxine de la Cruz contributed equally in this study. Findings from this study were partly presented at the 2009 Multinational Association for Supportive Care in Cancer in Rome as an oral abstract.

Declaration of conflicting interests

The author(s) declared no potential conflicts of interest with respect to the research, authorship, and/or publication of this article.

Funding

The author(s) disclosed receipt of the following financial support for the research, authorship, and/or publication of this article:

Eduardo Bruera was supported in part by National Institutes of Health (grant numbers RO1CA1RO10162-01A1, RO1CA1222292-01, and RO1CA124481-01) and David Hui was funded by the Clinician Investigator Program, Royal College of Physicians and Surgeons of Canada.

References

1. Gurevich M, Devins GM, Rodin GM. Stress response syndromes and cancer: conceptual and assessment issues. *Psychosomatics.* 2002;43(4):259–281.
2. Chao CS, Chen CH, Yen M. The essence of spirituality of terminally ill patients. *J Nurs Res.* 2002;10(4):237–245.
3. McIllmurray MB, Francis B, Harman JC, Morris SM, Soothill K, Thomas C. Psychosocial needs in cancer patients related to religious belief. *Palliat Med.* 2003;17(1):49–54.
4. McClain CS, Rosenfeld B, Breitbart W. Effect of spiritual well-being on end-of-life despair in terminally-ill cancer patients. *Lancet.* 2003;361(9369):1603–1607.
5. Harding R, Higginson IJ, Donaldson N. The relationship between patient characteristics and carer psychological status in home palliative cancer care. *Support Care Cancer.* 2003;11(10):638–643.
6. Chibnall JT, Videen SD, Duckro PN, Miller DK. Psychosocial spiritual correlates of death distress in patients with life threatening medical conditions. *Palliat Med.* 2002;16(4):331–338.
7. Puchalski C, Ferrell B, Virani R, et al. Improving the quality of spiritual care as a dimension of palliative care: the report of the Consensus Conference. *J Palliat Med.* 2009;12(10):885–904.
8. Peterman AH, Fitchett G, Brady MJ, Hernandez L, Cella D. Measuring spiritual well-being in people with cancer: the functional assessment of chronic illness therapy—spiritual well-being scale (FACIT-sp). *Ann Behav Med.* 2002;24(1):49–58.
9. Muldoon M, King N. Spirituality, health care, and bioethics. *J Relig Health.* 1995;34(4):329–349.
10. Rousseau P. Spirituality and the dying patient. *J Clin Oncol.* 2003;21(9 suppl):54s–56s.
11. Lo B, Ruston D, Kates LW, et al. Discussing religious and spiritual issues at the end of life: a practical guide for physicians. *JAMA.* 2002;287(6):749–754.
12. Nelson CJ, Rosenfeld B, Breitbart W, Galietta M. Spirituality, religion, and depression in the terminally ill. *Psychosomatics.* 2002;43(3):213–220.
13. Brady MJ, Peterman AH, Fitchett G, Mo M, Cella D. A case for including spirituality in quality of life measurement in oncology. *Psycho-Oncology.* 1999;8(5):417–428.
14. Chochinov HM, Cann BJ. Interventions to enhance the spiritual aspects of dying. *J Palliat Med.* 2005;8(suppl 1):S103–S115.
15. Keefe FJ, Affleck G, Lefebvre J, et al. Living with rheumatoid arthritis: the role of daily spirituality and daily religious and spiritual coping. *J Pain.* 2001;2(2):101–110.
16. Cassell EJ. The importance of understanding suffering for clinical ethics. *J Clin Ethics.* 1991;2(2):81–82.
17. Cassell EJ. Diagnosing suffering: a perspective. *Ann Intern Med.* 1999;131(7):531–534.

18. Rodin G, Lo C, Mikulincer M, Donner A, Gagliese L, Zimmermann C. Pathways to distress: the multiple determinants of depression, hopelessness, and the desire for hastened death in metastatic cancer patients. *Soc Sci Med.* 2009;68(3):562–569.
19. Delgado-Guay M, Parsons HA, Li Z, Palmer JL, Bruera E. Symptom distress in advanced cancer patients with anxiety and depression in the palliative care setting. *Support Care Cancer.* 2009;17(5):573–579.
20. Bruera E, Kuehn N, Miller MJ, Selmser P, Macmillan K. The Edmonton Symptom Assessment System (ESAS): a simple method for the assessment of palliative care patients. *J Palliat Care.* 1991;7(2):6–9.
21. Nash RB. Life's major spiritual issues: an emerging framework for spiritual assessment and pastoral diagnosis. *Caregiver J.* 1990;7(1):3–42.
22. Gall TL, Cornblat MW. Breast cancer survivors give voice: a qualitative analysis of spiritual factors in long-term adjustment. *Psycho-Oncology.* 2002;11(6):524–535.
23. Gall TL, Kristjansson E, Charbonneau C, Florack P. A longitudinal study on the role of spirituality in response to the diagnosis and treatment of breast cancer. *J Behav Med.* 2009;32(2): 174–186.
24. Kappeli S. Religious dimensions of suffering from and coping with cancer: a comparative study of Jewish and Christian patients. *Gynecol Oncol.* 2005;99(3 suppl 1):S135–S136.
25. True G, Phipps EJ, Braitman LE, Harralson T, Harris D, Tester W. Treatment preferences and advance care planning at end of life: the role of ethnicity and spiritual coping in cancer patients. *Ann Behav Med.* 2005;30(2):174–179.
26. Grant E, Murray SA, Kendall M, Boyd K, Tilley S, Ryan D. Spiritual issues and needs: perspectives from patients with advanced cancer and nonmalignant disease. A qualitative study. *Palliat Support Care.* 2004;2(4):371–378.
27. Breitbart W, Rosenfeld B, Pessin H, et al. Depression, hopelessness, and desire for hastened death in terminally ill patients with cancer. *JAMA.* 2000;284(22):2907–2911.
28. Kodish E, Post SG. Oncology and hope. *J Clin Oncol.* 1995;13(7):1817.
29. Hills J, Paice JA, Cameron JR, Shott S. Spirituality and distress in palliative care consultation. *J Palliat Med.* 2005;8(4):782–788.
30. Cassell EJ. The nature of suffering: physical, psychological, social, and spiritual aspects. *NLN Publ.* 1992;(15–2461):1–10.
31. Taylor B. On the experience of spirituality. *Aust J Holist Nurs.* 1999;6(3):3.
32. Balboni TA, Vanderwerker LC, Block SD, et al. Religiousness and spiritual support among advanced cancer patients and associations with end-of-life treatment preferences and quality of life. *J Clin Oncol.* 2007;25(5):555–560.
33. Mako C, Galek K, Poppito SR. Spiritual pain among patients with advanced cancer in palliative care. *J Palliat Med.* 2006;9(5):1106–1113.
34. Koenig HG. Concerns about measuring "spirituality" in research. *J Nerv Ment Dis.* 2008;196(5):349–355.
35. Jones JM, Huggins MA, Rydall AC, Rodin GM. Symptomatic distress, hopelessness, and the desire for hastened death in hospitalized cancer patients. *J Psychosom Res.* 2003;55(5):411–418.
36. Steinhauser KE, Voils CI, Clipp EC, Bosworth HB, Christakis NA, Tulsky JA. "Are you at peace?": one item to probe spiritual concerns at the end of life. *Arch Intern Med.* 2006;166(1):101–105.
37. Ellis J, Lin J, Walsh A, et al. Predictors of referral for specialized psychosocial oncology care in patients with metastatic cancer: the contributions of age, distress, and marital status. *J Clin Oncol.* 2009;27(5):699–705.
38. Hui D, Elsayem A, Li Z, De La Cruz M, Palmer JL, Bruera E. Antineoplastic therapy use in patients with advanced cancer admitted to an acute palliative care unit at a comprehensive cancer center: a simultaneous care model. *Cancer.* 2010;116(8):2036–2043.

39. Lorant V, Croux C, Weich S, Deliege D, Mackenbach J, Ansseau M. Depression and socioeconomic risk factors: 7-year longitudinal population study. *Br J Psychiatry.* 2007;190:293–298.
40. Schroevers MJ, Ranchor AV, Sanderman R. The role of social support and self-esteem in the presence and course of depressive symptoms: a comparison of cancer patients and individuals from the general population. *Soc Sci Med.* 2003;57(2):375–385.
41. Saunders C. Spiritual pain. *J Palliat Care.* 1988;4(3):29–32.
42. Clark D. "Total pain," disciplinary power and the body in the work of cicely saunders, 1958–1967. *Soc Sci Med.* 1999;49(6):727–736.
43. Wachholtz AB, Pearce MJ. Does spirituality as a coping mechanism help or hinder coping with chronic pain? *Curr Pain Headache Rep.* 2009;13(2):127–132.
44. Wachholtz AB, Pearce MJ, Koenig H. Exploring the relationship between spirituality, coping, and pain. *J Behav Med.* 2007;30(4):311–318.
45. Pargament KI, Koenig HG, Tarakeshwar N, Hahn J. Religious coping methods as predictors of psychological, physical and spiritual outcomes among medically ill elderly patients: a two-year longitudinal study. *J Health Psychol.* 2004;9(6):713–730.
46. McCoubrie RC, Davies AN. Is there a correlation between spirituality and anxiety and depression in patients with advanced cancer? *Support Care Cancer.* 2006;14(4):379–385.
47. Greenstein M, Breitbart W. Cancer and the experience of meaning: a group psychotherapy program for people with cancer. *Am J Psychother.* 2000;54(4):486–500.
48. Hungelmann J, Kenkel-Rossi E, Klassen L, Stollenwerk R. Focus on spiritual well-being: harmonious interconnectedness of mind-body-spirit—use of the JAREL spiritual well-being scale. *Geriatr Nurs.* 1996;17(6):262–266.

SECTION 3
CHAPLAINCY INTERVENTIONS AND THEIR IMPACT

Introduction

The last section in the *Reader* highlights the move between paradigms and the shift toward a focus on outcomes in chaplaincy research. Previous sections highlighted how research has identified the "what" and "for whom" of spiritual care, while this last section highlights the "why." As chaplains continue to pursue what it means to shift from a focus on presence into the realm of outcomes, research becomes even more vital for the profession. The articles selected for Section 3 employ important study designs and provide examples of important outcomes for the profession.

The first two articles in Section 3, Marin et al. (2015) and Johnson et al. (2014), examine patient and family satisfaction, one of the most common measures in chaplaincy outcome research. Concern for satisfaction is significant because, since the passage of the Patient Protection and Affordable Care Act (often referred to as Obamacare) in the US in 2010, hospitals' reimbursements are in part based on these scores.

The next four articles in Section 3, Bay et al. (2008), Berning et al. (2016), Piderman et al. (2017a), and Kestenbaum et al. (2017), focus on specific outcomes for patients associated with receiving chaplaincy care. Pay attention to the study designs and the goals of these authors. Bay et al. (2008) is one of the few chaplaincy studies that use a randomized control trial, while Berning et al. (2016), Piderman et al. (2017a), and Kestenbaum et al. (2017) describe recent efforts to develop and test chaplain interventions.

Snowden and Telfer (2017) shift our focus toward developing a measure of patient-reported outcomes of chaplaincy care. Flannelly et al. (2012) were interested in the relationship between a hospital having chaplaincy services and the rates of hospital deaths and hospice enrollments in those hospitals.

Studies like these in Section 3 seek not only to describe the work of chaplains but also to demonstrate how that work addresses the needs of patients. This is an important shift in the field of chaplaincy; it not only helps us identify best practices, but it also enables us to share important findings with members of the healthcare team, including healthcare managers.

Just as in the other sections in the *Reader*, in this section, you will see themes emerge that will allow you to bring the articles into conversation with one another. For example, consider the different ways the theme of spiritual pain is addressed by Bay et al. (2008), Berning et al. (2016), Piderman et al. (2017a), and Kestenbaum et al. (2017).

The articles in this section illustrate the types of research being done about chaplaincy outcomes. Reading them will help you develop an understanding of the different study designs and examples of important outcomes in chaplaincy care. We hope they fuel your own education and research literacy in ways that helpfully inform your work.

Article 14: Marin, D.B., Sharma, V., Sosunov, E., Egorova, N., Goldstein, R., and Handzo, G.F. (2015) Relationship Between Chaplain Visits and Patient Satisfaction

One way we can measure the impact of chaplaincy care is through patient satisfaction. This first article in Section 3 sought to explore whether there was a link between chaplaincy visits and patient satisfaction. The authors found higher ratings of patient satisfaction with their stay at the hospital among those who had been visited by a chaplain. As previously noted, this is an important finding in light of the growing emphasis in healthcare on the patient experience as well as in light of the link between quality indicators such as patient satisfaction and reimbursement.

The study comes from a team led by Deborah Marin, a psychiatrist who is the Director of the Center for Spirituality and Health and the manager for spiritual care at Mount Sinai Medical Center in New York City. This is a program that has made a major commitment to evidence-based spiritual care.

There are a number of other studies that have linked patient satisfaction with chaplaincy care; however, this study is unique in several ways. First, it uses items from two sources—the Hospital Consumer Assessment of Healthcare Providers Systems (HCAHPS) and Press Ganey—to demonstrate patient satisfaction with the hospital stay. These items are the ones used most frequently to assess patient satisfaction; the HCAHPS items are also used to determine Medicare incentive payments to hospitals. Second, the study used evidence of chaplain care from the patients' electronic medical records instead of relying on their memories of any chaplaincy care. Another impressive aspect of their design is that they used a very large sample of patients (8978) with a number of differing diagnoses. Their methods lend weight to their conclusions, shared by Donohue et al. (2017), that chaplains make important contributions to the patient experience.

In this study, the authors did not explore how patient satisfaction might be influenced by specific types of chaplain interventions. However, a second study by this team addresses this issue (Sharma et al. 2016). It was based on data that was used for the original 2015 study with several hundred additional cases. What do you think—does a specific chaplain intervention affect a patient's perception of how well spiritual needs were being met? If so, how might we investigate this?

Article 15: Johnson, J.R., Engelberg, R.A., Nielsen, E.L., Kross, E.K., Smith, N.L., Hanada, J.C., Doll O'Mahoney, S.K., and Randall Curtis, J. (2014) The Association of Spiritual Care Providers' Activities with Family Members' Satisfaction with Care after a Death in the ICU

What are the specific components of chaplains' care that impact the overall hospital experience? How important are end-of-life conversations between chaplains and families? Surveys that analyze satisfaction with hospital experience do not usually go to families who experienced a death, so we have little information about factors that shape their experience. The next article in the *Reader* demonstrates how nesting a chaplaincy study in a larger well-designed project can provide important information about the impact of chaplaincy care, in this case on families whose loved ones died in the intensive care unit (ICU) setting.

This study comes from a team, led by Dr. J. Randall Curtis, with a strong record of research focused on improving care at the end of life for ICU patients and their families. The aim of this study was to determine if spiritual care was associated with family members' satisfaction with the ICU care they and their loved ones had received.

Designed as a prospective cohort study (following a group of people over time to explore the association between exposure [chaplain care] and outcome [family satisfaction]), the research team wanted to observe both what the chaplains did as well as how families experienced their care. The team gathered data from both chaplains and family members. The prospective cohort design, where chaplain care preceded family reports of satisfaction, provides evidence that what the chaplains did impacted satisfaction. Another strength of the study is the use of well-validated surveys of family satisfaction with ICU care and satisfaction with decision-making in the ICU context.

For those with limited research experience, this article provides a guide through the basics of the research process. It clearly explains both the inclusion and exclusion criteria for study participants and is a good example of reporting descriptive statistics. These statistics in Tables 1–3 give the reader basic information about the participants and the care provided by the chaplains. The ability to read such descriptive statistics will help you evaluate some elements of the study, such as the strengths and limitations of the study sample.

The team used clustered regression models in their analysis of the data. Clustering is just as it sounds. The team needed to deal with each patient having multiple spiritual care providers (thus many surveys per patient), so they organized the information about chaplain care in a way that allowed for examining the association between chaplain activities and family satisfaction. The regression analysis included adjustment for other factors (technically, confounding factors) that might explain this association. Confounding factors are associated with both the predictors (chaplain care in this study) and the outcomes (family satisfaction in this study). When researchers find significant associations between their predictor and their outcome in regression models that have adjusted for possible confounding factors, then they can have greater confidence about their findings. Many of the studies in the *Reader* that use either logistic or multiple regression have adjusted for possible confounding factors. You may wish to review the studies that use quantitative methods and see if you can identify some of them.

Johnson et al.'s (2014) results section clearly identifies the finding for each of their study aims. When reading this section, note that the concept of statistical significance, which is important for quantitative research, simply refers to whether the results were due to chance. Statistical significance is typically identified in terms of a p-value (the result of statistical comparisons) being less than 0.05, meaning the likelihood of finding these results by chance is less than 5%. Johnson and colleagues provide a great article for becoming more comfortable reading quantitative research.

Of interest, this article also describes the frequency of 14 specific spiritual care activities the chaplains offered the patients and families in the study. The chaplain activity survey that was used to collect this information is available online (Downey et al. 2006). How do the activities identified in this study compare with those in the work by Massey et al. (2015)? End-of-life discussions, more than any other activity, appeared to have the greatest impact on family satisfaction with ICU care. Other important items included reminiscing about the patient and the total number of chaplain activities. Since the "total number of activities" impacted satisfaction, do you wonder about how the nature of the relationship with the chaplain impacted family satisfaction? Most of the chaplains providing care in this study were clinical pastoral education interns. How do you think the results would have changed if the chaplains providing care had more experience?

Article 16: Bay, P.S., Beckman, D., Trippi, J., Gunderman, R., and Terry, C. (2008) The Effect of Pastoral Care Services on Anxiety, Depression, Hope, Religious Coping, and Religious Problem Solving Styles: A Randomized Controlled Study

As the body of chaplaincy research grows, so, too, does the research that provides compelling evidence that people who are religious tend to have better health, lower mortality rates, and better coping with medical concerns. But do chaplains help facilitate these benefits, and does the impact of chaplain care differ from that of other professionals? Bay et al. (2008) examined the effects of a chaplain intervention with cardiac surgery patients on mental health variables, including anxiety, depression, and hope.

One of the most important research designs for measuring the impact of a chaplaincy intervention—or any intervention—is a randomized controlled trial (RCT). Because random assignment creates groups of participants that are equal in every way, except the intervention received by the experimental group, it provides strong evidence about whether or not the intervention had the desired effect.

Only a handful of chaplaincy studies to date have used RCTs, in large part because they are complex and expensive. An earlier, smaller RCT by Iler, Obenshain, and Camac (2001) examined the effects of chaplain care in patients with chronic obstructive pulmonary disease. Iler and colleagues (2001) did not describe the content of the chaplain visits in this study; we only know that the chaplain visited the patients daily. Bay et al.'s study (2008) is a bit of an improvement; we know that patients were visited four times, in part following a model of spiritual care in cardiac surgery described by Yim and VandeCreek (1996).

In contrast to Iler et al. (2001) and Bay et al. (2008), more information about the interventions they used is included in the studies by Berning et al. (2016), Piderman et al. (2017a), and Kestenbaum et al. (2017). These three papers are more characteristic of reports of pilot studies and the associated stages of developing and testing an intervention. In the study by Berning and colleagues (2016), the team went through stages that included identifying a need, conceptualizing an intervention that addresses the need, developing and revising the intervention based on discussion with colleagues, pilot testing the intervention for feasibility and acceptability, and gathering preliminary data on the effectiveness of the intervention. Bay's team (2008) appeared to skip several of these preliminary steps and go right to the RCT. Would these steps have improved their study in any way?

The study findings indicate that there were only minimal differences in emotional states and religious coping between the two groups at baseline, which was expected (because randomization creates groups that should be identical at the start of the study). The most significant difference between the treatment and non-treatment groups was seen in religious coping at the six-month follow-up. The experimental group's positive religious coping increased and their negative religious coping decreased. The opposite was the case for the control group. These findings support their hypothesis that chaplaincy care caused improvements in religious coping. However, there were no significant differences in depression, anxiety, hope, and the other study measures.

Readers should not conclude from Bay et al. (2008) that there is no effect of chaplaincy care on these outcomes. There are a few issues in the study design that may have prevented them from finding effects. For instance, there were low levels of anxiety and depression in the sample at baseline; it is difficult for an intervention to lower anxiety when it is low at the start. Repeating the study with a different sample, such as those with high anxiety, may yield different results.

The importance of this study is that it demonstrates that an RCT of chaplain care can be done. In addition, it showed that chaplain care appears to have a beneficial effect on religious coping among this group of patients. Doing a good RCT requires a well-designed intervention and key information that can only come from preliminary research, such as that seen in the next three articles.

Article 17: Berning, J.N., Poor, A.D., Buckley, S.M., Patel, K.R., Lederer, D.J., Goldstein, N.E., Brodie, D., and Baldwin, M.R. (2016) A Novel Picture Guide to Improve Spiritual Care and Reduce Anxiety in Mechanically Ventilated Adults in the Intensive Care Unit

The next article in Section 3 took a creative approach to working with mechanically ventilated patients. Joel Berning, the lead author of this study (2016) and a practicing chaplain at New York Presbyterian Hospital, developed picture cards to improve communication between chaplains and critically ill patients who are unable to speak. The cards were designed to help the patients identify their religious or spiritual affiliation, to express their feelings, and to request specific chaplaincy services. The team also hoped use of the cards would reduce the isolation and stress of mechanically ventilated patients. They then tested the cards using a quasi-experimental design. Quasi-experimental designs are useful tools in early stages of developing an intervention when researchers want to examine the possible causal links between an intervention and an outcome.

Berning and his team wanted to evaluate the benefits of using the communication card in spiritual care. They evaluated the benefits of the intervention with several measurements, the strongest of which was their measurement of patients' anxiety levels before and after the first chaplain visit that used picture-guided spiritual care. The patients' anxiety levels decreased, on average, 20 points on a 100-point scale. This reduction was statistically significant. But it is also interesting—visually and clinically—to see the individual changes in scores as depicted in Figure 3. Here, the scores of the 25 participants whose anxiety levels were measured pre- and post-intervention are displayed. Not everyone's anxiety levels went down; two increased and three stayed the same. Still, the vast majority of patients (20) experienced lower anxiety levels as a result of the intervention with the chaplain.

This study was conducted with one cohort of ICU patients using one chaplain. The next step in establishing the effectiveness of this intervention would be to see if use of the cards is effective in other hospitals when delivered by other chaplains. The team is in the process of planning this next step in research regarding their intervention.

Take a careful look at the spiritual care communication cards (rights for usage are available online for purchase (Vidatak 2016)). Are there patient populations in your care for whom this approach would be a feasible intervention? What, if anything, is missing from the cards to help mechanically ventilated patients express their spiritual needs and preferences for care? Are these cards appropriate for patients who are approaching the end-of-life? Given that this study was quasi-experimental, what kinds of conclusions, if any, can we draw about the relationship between the cards' usage and any decrease in stress and anxiety?

Article 18: Piderman, K.M., Radecki Breitkoptf, C., Jenkins, S.M., Lapid, M.I., Kwete, G.M., Sytsma, T.T., Lovejoy, L.A., Yoder, T.J., and Jatoi, A. (2017a) The Impact of a Spiritual Legacy Intervention in Patients with Brain Cancer and Other Neurologic Illnesses and Their Support Persons

Katherine Piderman, the first author of this study, is one of the leading chaplain-researchers in the US. Among her other work, Piderman and colleagues have reported important studies of patient expectations of chaplains (Piderman et al. 2010). This paper is one of three reports related to the Hear My Voice (HMV) project (Piderman et al. 2015, 2017b). HMV is an intervention that consists of a semi-structured interview about important features of a patient's spiritual journey (the interview can be found in Piderman et al. 2015). The interviews are recorded, transcribed, and edited in consultation with the patient. The finished product is a spiritual legacy document, which patients can share with their loved ones.

The HMV interview has some similarities with dignity therapy (Chochinov 2012) but differs in its singular focus on a patient's spiritual life. The authors of this study were looking for creative ways to engage the spiritual well-being and spiritual coping of patients with advanced brain cancer or other progressive neurodegenerative disorders, as these diseases lead to physical and mental impairments that can impact a patient's spiritual experience. The research team was also concerned with the well-being of the patients' support persons as they, too, may face spiritual or existential distress.

This paper is a pilot study to test the feasibility and acceptability of the chaplain-led spiritual life review interview and examine its effects on a variety of outcomes for both patients and their loved ones. Life review has been shown to be a potentially beneficial tool for patients and caregivers to make meaning of and increase coping with illness. Like Kestenbaum et al. (2017), this pilot study has a small sample and is not primarily designed to find significant effects on outcomes, but rather is focused on determining the acceptability and feasibility of the intervention. The team used a longitudinal exploratory approach with several measures at baseline including the FACIT-Sp-Ex and the Brief RCOPE. They examined possible intervention-related changes in the measures at one and three months after the intervention.

Completing a spiritual legacy interview and document was found to be a meaningful experience for their particular patient population. It gave the patients an effective way to reflect on their beliefs, practices and values with a trained chaplain and to have a document about their spiritual journey to share with their loved ones. Another important feature of this study is their measurement of the effects of the intervention on the patient's support persons. The 2017b paper by the team includes a very interesting report of themes in the patient interviews.

Do you think the study findings are relevant to patients with other diseases and their support persons? What additional evidence do you need, if any, before considering the implementation of this intervention? What barriers might keep you from implementing it? How could you address those barriers?

Article 19: Kestenbaum, A., Shields, M., James, J., Hocker, W., Morgan, S., Karve, S., Rabow, M.W., and Dunn, L.B. (2017) What Impact Do Chaplains Have? A Pilot Study of Spiritual AIM for Advanced Cancer Patients in Outpatient Palliative Care

Several studies have noted that while chaplains talk about our care in terms of process, chaplains' healthcare colleagues often describe their work in terms of outcomes (Cadge, Calle, and Dillinger 2011). Developing an outcome-oriented approach to our care is part of the spiritual care paradigm shift we have described. That outcome-oriented approach to care is clearly evident in the next paper.

The paper comes from a team at the University of California, San Francisco Medical Center where the Spiritual AIM (Assessment and Intervention Model) was developed (see Sheilds, Kestenbaum, and Dunn 2015). Spiritual AIM begins with assessment of one of three core spiritual needs: 1) for meaning and direction, 2) for self-worth and belonging to community, or 3) to love and be loved, often facilitated through seeking reconciliation when relationships are broken (see Table 3 in the article for examples). Unlike any other published model for spiritual assessment, Spiritual AIM also includes interventions and outcomes associated with each need. In this pilot study, the research team wanted to see if the Spiritual AIM model was feasible and tolerable in an outpatient palliative care context and if the intervention had an impact on important palliative care outcomes, such as religious and cancer-specific coping, physical outcomes, psychological outcomes, and spiritual well-being.

After a successful pilot study such as the one by this team, they could develop an RCT with a larger sample to have a more definitive test of the effects of the intervention. As you read Kestenbaum et al.'s (2017) article, consider the similarities and differences between it and Bay et al. (2008) regarding the study aims.

The results of the study point to the chaplain's care having a positive impact on several outcomes, specifically on spiritual well-being and positive religious coping. How do the three core spiritual needs in Spiritual AIM compare with the themes in the SDAT by Monod et al. (2010)? Do you think Spiritual AIM will be acceptable and effective in diverse cultural groups? Additionally, Spiritual AIM proposes that the chaplain target the primary unmet spiritual need. What if an individual exhibits more than one spiritual need?

Article 20: Snowden, A. and Telfer, I. (2017) Patient Reported Outcome Measure of Spiritual Care as Delivered by Chaplains

Who decides what chaplaincy care outcomes are the most important? Traditionally, when assessing the success of a procedure or intervention, clinical research has used biomedical markers or clinician specified outcomes (Ahmed et al. 2012). In contrast, Patient Reported Outcome Measures (PROM) are grounded in what the patient identifies as most important to him/her. This shift toward considering patients' definition of successful care and outcomes is consistent with the emphasis in healthcare on patient-centered care.

Applying that framework to chaplaincy means asking patients what they want to occur as a result of being cared for by a chaplain. Snowden and Telfer, working from Edinburgh, Scotland, describe the rigorous development of such an instrument for chaplaincy. The Scottish PROM is the first of its kind in chaplaincy research. Prior to this paper, Snowden and colleagues published three papers on the construction, operationalization, and thematic analysis of their PROM (see Snowden et al. 2013a, 2013b, and 2013c). The paper included in this *Reader* summarizes the previous reports, describes research about the validity of the PROM, and discusses the criteria that qualify it as an original PROM. Ideally, a PROM is a short instrument because patients are more likely to complete it (this one has five items), and the higher the score, the better the outcomes. Table 1 highlights the content of the PROM as well as the results of the extensive review of measures for key concepts in the PROM. The team is continuing research based on the PROM. This includes translating it and testing it in several national contexts under the auspices of the European Research Institute for Chaplains in Healthcare (ERICH 2017).

Consider the results highlighted in previous articles in the *Reader* (Raffay, Wood, and Todd 2016 and Donohue et al. 2017) and how those articles report patients' and families' views about chaplaincy care. How do their views compare to the outcomes that have been included in the PROM? What do you think about the five items selected for the PROM? Does the PROM capture the unique components of spiritual care? Can you imagine ways to use the PROM in your context? The team welcomes enquiries from those interested in using the instrument.

Article 21: Flannelly, K.J., Emanuel, L.L., Handzo, G.F., Galek, K., Silton, N.R., and Carlson, M. (2012) A National Study of Chaplaincy Services and End-of-Life Outcomes

Previous articles in this *Reader* have highlighted the importance of chaplains in end-of-life and care planning conversations (Massey et al. 2015; Johnson et al. 2014). What impact do these conversations have on the actual end-of-life care of patients? This last article of the *Reader* explores the possible association between chaplaincy services and the utilization of healthcare services at the end of life. This is important because previous research has suggested that those who are more religious frequently choose more aggressive care at the end of life (Phelps et al. 2009).

This paper is perhaps one of the only studies of chaplaincy care that uses an ecological study design. This means that, unlike the majority of the other articles in this *Reader*, this study uses data about populations or organizations and not data about individuals. Specifically, it uses data from the American Hospital Association (AHA) to identify hospitals with a chaplaincy department and data from the Dartmouth Atlas of Health Care to identify the rate of death and the rate of hospice enrollment in those hospitals.

The study comes from a team formerly at the HealthCare Chaplaincy Network led by Kevin Flannelly. Around the time when this study was conducted, this team produced a large number of important chaplaincy-related studies. In this study, Flannelly et al. (2012) focused on whether rates of hospital deaths and hospice enrollment differ between hospitals that provide chaplaincy services and hospitals that do not. Their results, that hospitals with chaplaincy departments had lower rates of in-hospital deaths and higher rates of hospice enrollment, suggest the role that chaplains may play in patient and family choices about end-of-life care. These important findings need to be further tested with research using other study designs.

The authors note that the differences in rates could be explained by another variable. What do you think? Just as with Cadge, Freese, and Christakis (2008), the AHA data does not provide any additional information about what it means for a hospital to report that they have a chaplaincy department. How do you see this challenge impacting the results? The authors identify the relatively small associations between having a chaplaincy department (their exposure or independent variable) and rates of hospital deaths and hospice enrollment (their outcome or dependent variables). Does this matter even though their results were statistically significant?

References

Ahmed, S., Berzon, R.A., Revicki, D.A., Lenderking, W.R., et al. (2012) "The use of patient-reported outcomes (PRO) within comparative effectiveness research: implications for clinical practice and health care policy." *Medical Care*, 50, 1060–1070.

Bay, P.S., Beckman, D., Trippi, J., Gunderman, R., and Terry, C. (2008) "The effect of pastoral care services on anxiety, depression, hope, religious coping, and religious problem solving styles: a randomized controlled study." *Journal of Religion & Health*, 47, 57–69.

Berning, J.N., Poor, A.D., Buckley, S.M., Patel, K.R., et al. (2016) "A novel picture guide to improve spiritual care and reduce anxiety in mechanically ventilated adults in the intensive care unit." *Annals of the American Thoracic Society*, 13, 8, 1333–1342.

Cadge, W., Calle, K., and Dillinger, J. (2011) "What do chaplains contribute to large academic hospitals? The perspectives of pediatric physicians and chaplains." *Journal of Religion & Health*, 50, 2, 300–312.

Cadge, W., Freese, J., and Christakis, N.A. (2008) "The provision of hospital chaplaincy in the United States: a national overview." *The Southern Medical Journal*, 101, 6, 626–630.

Chochinov, H.M. (2012) *Dignity Therapy: Final Words for Final Days*. New York: Oxford University Press.

Donohue, P.K., Norvell, M., Boss, R., Shepard, J., et al. (2017) "Hospital chaplains: through the eyes of parents of hospitalized children." *Journal of Palliative Medicine*, 20, 2, 1352–1358.

Downey, L., Engelberg, R.A., Shannon, S.E., and Curtis, J.R. (2006) "Measuring intensive care nurses' perspectives on family-centered end-of-life care: evaluation of three questionnaires." *American Journal of Critical Care*, 15, 6, 568–579. Accessed on 2/11/18 at depts.washington.edu/eolcare/pubs/wp-content/uploads/2011/09/spiritualcare_v3.0.pdf.

European Research Institute for Chaplains in Healthcare (ERICH) (2017) Enhancing Spiritual Care through Chaplaincy Research. Accessed on 2/11/18 at www.pastoralezorg.be/page/erich.

Flannelly, K.J., Emanuel, L.L., Handzo, G.F., Galek, K., Silton, N.R., and Carlson, M. (2012) "A national study of chaplaincy services and end-of-life outcomes." *BMC Palliative Care*, 11, 10.

Iler, W.L., Obenshain, D., and Camac, M. (2001) "The impact of daily chaplain visits from chaplains on patients with chronic obstructive pulmonary disease (COPD): a pilot study." *Chaplaincy Today*, 17, 1, 5–11.

Johnson, J.R., Engelberg, R.A., Nielsen, E.L., Kross, E.K., et al. (2014) "The association of spiritual care providers' activities with family members' satisfaction with care after a death in the ICU." *Critical Care Medicine*, 42, 9, 1991–2000.

Kestenbaum, A., Shields, M., James, J., Hocker, W., et al. (2017) "What impact do chaplains have? A pilot study of spiritual AIM for advanced cancer patients in outpatient palliative care." *Journal of Pain and Symptom Management*, 54, 5, 707–714.

Marin, D.B., Sharma, V., Sosunov, E., Egorova, N., Goldstein, R., and Handzo, G.F. (2015) "Relationship between chaplain visits and patient satisfaction." *Journal of Health Care Chaplaincy*, 21, 14–24.

Massey, K., Barnes, M.J.D., Villines, D., Goldstein, J.D., et al. (2015) "What do I do? Developing a taxonomy of chaplaincy activities and interventions for spiritual care in intensive care unit palliative care." *BMC Palliative Care*, 14, 10, 1–8.

Monod, S.M., Rochat, E., Büla, C.J., Jobin, G., Martin, E., and Spencer, B. (2010) "The spiritual distress assessment tool; an instrument to assess spiritual distress in hospitalized elderly persons." *BMC Geriatrics*, 10, 88–96.

Phelps, A.C., Maciejewski, P.K., Nilsson, M., Balboni, T.A., et al. (2009) "Religious coping and use of intensive life-prolonging care near death in patients with advanced cancer." *Journal of the American Medical Association*, 11, 1140–1147.

Piderman, K.M., Radecki Breitkopf, C., Jenkins, S.M., Lovejoy, L.A., et al. (2015) "The feasibility and educational value of *Hear My Voice*, a chaplain-led spiritual life review process for patients with brain cancers and progressive neurologic conditions." *Journal of Cancer Education*, 30, 209–212.

Piderman, K.M., Egginton, J., Ingram, C., Dose, A.M., et al. (2017b) "I'm still me: inspiration and instruction from individuals with brain cancer." *Journal of Health Care Chaplaincy*, 23, 15–33.

Piderman, K.M., Marek, D.V., Jenkins, S.M., Johnson, M.E., et al. (2010) "Predicting patients' expectations of hospital chaplains: a multisite survey." *Mayo Clinic Proceedings*, 85, 1, 1002–1010.

Piderman, K.M., Radecki Breitkopf, C., Jenkins, S.M., Lapid, M.I., et al. (2017a) "The impact of a spiritual legacy intervention in patients with brain cancer and other neurologic illnesses and their support persons." *Psycho-Oncology*, 26, 3, 346–353.

Raffay, J., Wood, E., and Todd, A. (2016) "Service user views of spiritual and pastoral (chaplaincy) in NHS mental health services: a co-produced constructivist grounded theory investigation." *BMC Psychiatry*, 16, 200.

Sharma, V., Marin, D.B, Sosunov, E., Ozbay, F., Goldstein, R., and Handzo, G.F. (2016) "The differential effects of chaplain interventions on patient satisfaction." *Journal of Health Care Chaplaincy*, 22, 3, 85–101.

Sheilds, M., Kestenbaum, A., and Dunn, LB. (2015) "Spiritual AIM and the work of the chaplain: a model for assessing spiritual needs and outcomes in relationship." *Palliative and Supportive Care*, 13, 75–89.

Snowden, A. and Telfer, I. (2017) "Patient reported outcome measure of spiritual care as delivered by chaplains." *Journal of Health Care Chaplaincy*, 23, 4, 131–155.

Snowden, A., Telfer, I., Kelly, E., Bunniss, S., and Mowat, H. (2013a) "The construction of the Lothian PROM." *The Scottish Journal of Healthcare Chaplaincy*, 16 (special ed.), 3–16.

Snowden, A., Telfer, I., Kelly, E., Bunniss, S., and Mowat, H. (2013b) "'I was able to talk about what was on my mind.' The operationalization of person centred care." *The Scottish Journal of Healthcare Chaplaincy*, 16 (special ed.), 13–26.

Snowden, A., Telfer, I., Kelly, E., Bunniss, S., and Mowat, H. (2013c) "Spiritual Care as person centered care: a thematic analysis of interventions." *The Scottish Journal of Healthcare Chaplaincy*, 16 (special ed.), 23–32.

Vidatak Innovation in Patient Communication (2016) *Vidatak Spiritual Care Communication Board*. Accessed on 29/1/18 at www.vidatak.com.

Yim, R. and VandeCreek, L. (1996) "Unbinding grief and life's losses for thriving recovery after open heart surgery: how pastoral care works in a managed care setting." *The Caregiver Journal*, 12, 2, 8–11.

ARTICLE 14

Relationship Between Chaplain Visits and Patient Satisfaction

Deborah B. Marin and Vanshdeep Sharma, *Department of Psychiatry, Icahn School of Medicine at Mount Sinai, New York, New York, USA*

Eugene Sosunov, *Office for Excellence in Patient Care, Mount Sinai Hospital, New York, New York, USA*

Natalia Egorova, *Department of Health Evidence and Policy, Icahn School of Medicine at Mount Sinai, New York, New York, USA*

Rafael Goldstein, *Department of Spiritual Care and Education, Mount Sinai Hospital, New York, New York, USA*

George F. Handzo, *HealthCare Chaplaincy, New York, New York, USA*

Address correspondence to Deborah B. Marin, MD, Department of Psychiatry, The Icahn School of Medicine at Mount Sinai, 1 Gustave Levy Place, New York, NY 10029, USA. E-mail: Deborah.marin@mssm.edu

Abstract

This prospective study investigated the relationship between chaplain visits and patient satisfaction, as measured by Hospital Consumer Assessment of Healthcare Providers and Systems (HCAHPS) and Press Ganey surveys from 8,978 patients who had been discharged from a tertiary care hospital. Controlling for patients' age, gender, race, ethnicity, language, education, faith, general health status, and medical conditions, chaplain visits increased the willingness of patients to recommend the hospital, as measured by both the HCAHPS survey (regression coefficient = 0.07, $p < .05$) and the Press Ganey survey (0.11, $p < .01$). On the Press Ganey survey, patients visited by chaplains were also more likely to endorse that staff met their spiritual needs (0.27, $p < .001$) and their emotional needs (0.10, $p < .05$). In terms of overall patient satisfaction, patients visited by a chaplain were more satisfied on both the Press Ganey survey (0.11, $p < .01$) and on the HCAHPS survey (0.17, $p < .05$). Chaplains' integration into the healthcare team improves patients' satisfaction with their hospital stay.

Marin, D.B., Sharma, V., Sosunov, E., Egorova, N., Goldstein, R., and Handzo, G.F. (2015) "Relationship between chaplain visits and patient satisfaction." *Journal of Health Care Chaplaincy*, 21, 14–24.

Key words: chaplaincy, HCAHPS, patient satisfaction, Press Ganey, spiritual care

Introduction

The majority of hospitalized patients in different clinical settings express spiritual struggle or needs (Astrow, Wexler, Texeira, He, & Sulmasy, 2007; Davison & Jhangri, 2010; Fitchett, Burton, & Sivan, 1997; Pearce, Coan, Herndon, Koenig, & Abernethy, 2012). As these patients may not be able to get the support from their religious community, it is incumbent upon the healthcare teams to provide the appropriate interventions (T.A. Balboni, Vanderwerker, & Block, 2007). The Joint Commission requires a spiritual assessment for each patient, to determine any religious affiliation and spiritual practices or beliefs which may impact patient care (Joint Commission on Accreditation of Healthcare Organizations, 2005). Between 54% and 63% of hospitals employ chaplains to fulfill these requirements (Cadge, Freese, & Christakis, 2008). Board Certified Chaplains are clinically and theologically trained professionals who provide support for patients' cultural, spiritual and religious needs, and minister independent of faith (VandeCreek & Lucas, 2001).

Studies assessing patient satisfaction

While there is evidence to suggest that meeting spiritual needs is associated with greater patient satisfaction, there are limited data to demonstrate that chaplain visits are associated with meeting the spiritual needs of patients, as well as improving patient satisfaction scores, particularly on publically reported measures of patient satisfaction (VandeCreek & Lyon, 1997). For example, in a sample of over 1.7 million patients, meeting their spiritual and emotional needs was significantly associated with patient satisfaction (Clark, Drain, & Malone, 2003). A 14-site study demonstrated that satisfaction with chaplains was significantly correlated with overall satisfaction with the hospital stay (VandeCreek, 2004). In an investigation of 3,141 patients who had been discharged from a general internal medicine service, patients were more satisfied with care provided by doctors, teamwork, and overall care if they had discussions about their religious and spiritual concerns (Williams, Meltzer, Arora, Chung, & Curlin, 2011). A study of 35 chronic obstructive pulmonary disease patients demonstrated that patients who were visited daily by a chaplain had significantly greater satisfaction with their hospital stay (Iler,

Obenshain, & Camac, 2001). A multicenter observational study, which evaluated 326 inpatients in four Midwestern hospitals, found that 94% of patients with spiritual/religious struggle found the visits of chaplains or clergy to be very helpful (Ellis, Thomlinson, Gemmill, & Harris, 2013).

Of these studies, only one used the Press Ganey survey to assess whether spiritual and emotional needs were met using a single question, and it did not present data as to whether or not patients were seen by chaplains (Clark et al., 2003). None of the studies have assessed patients' perception of care using the HCAHPS survey, the performance on which accounted for 30% of incentive payments to hospitals by the Center for Medicare and Medicaid Services' Value Based Purchasing Program in 2013 (Centers for Medicare & Medicaid Services, 2013a). We hypothesized that patients who were visited by chaplains would be more satisfied with their overall hospital experience and would endorse that their spiritual and emotional needs were met on the HCAHPS and Press Ganey surveys, respectively (Centers for Medicare & Medicaid Services, 2013c; Kaldenberg, Mylod, & Drain, 2003).

Methods

Setting

The study was performed at Mount Sinai Hospital, a 1,171-bed tertiary-care teaching hospital in New York City. The study period was between December 14, 2011 and May 1, 2013. Chaplain visits were conducted by members of the Department of Spiritual Care and Education (DSCE), which included 2 chaplains, 2 half time priests, and 7 chaplaincy interns. Reasons for visiting patients originated from rounds, when chaplains queried hospitalized patients and their families regarding any interest in speaking with a member of the DSCE, as well as referrals from nurses, patients, clergy, social workers, and other sources including volunteers, family, physicians, and other hospital staff. The priests also proactively visited patients whose religion was documented as Catholic. All encounters were recorded in an electronic database system.

Measures

Overall patient satisfaction was measured with HCAHPS and Press Ganey (Centers for Medicare & Medicaid Services, 2013c; Kaldenberg et al., 2003) surveys. Questionnaires were mailed to all eligible patients. At the time of the study, the HCAHPS survey consisted of 27 questions that assessed patients' perception of care. The two HCAHPS questions related to overall satisfaction were: 1) "What number would you use to rate this hospital during your stay?" ranging from 0 to 10, where 0 is "worst hospital possible" and 10 is "best hospital possible," and 2) "Would you recommend the hospital to your friends and family?" with a range from 1 "definitely no" to 4 "definitely yes." The two related Press Ganey questions were: 1) "Overall rating of care given at hospital," and 2) "Likelihood of your recommending this hospital to others." The two Press Ganey questions about meeting patients' spiritual and emotional needs were: 1) "Degree to which hospital staff addressed your spiritual needs," and 2) "Degree to which hospital staff addressed your emotional needs." All Press Ganey questions were rated on a 5-point scale ranging from 1 "very poor" to 5 "very good."

Patients' age, gender, race, ethnicity, as well as information about whether patients were visited by chaplains, were obtained from the hospital's databases. Patients provided their race and ethnicity and these variables were included as they have been shown to affect HCAHPS scores (Centers for Medicare & Medicaid Services, 2013b; Goldstein, Elliott, Lehrman, Hambarsoomian, & Giordano, 2010). Language spoken at home and information on education were obtained from the HCAHPS survey.

Dependent and independent variables

The dependent variables were the continuous variables representing scores of patient responses to the six questions of the HCAHPS and Press Ganey surveys. The independent variable of chaplain visits was measured in binary modality (yes/no). The choice of other independent variables followed recommendations of O'Malley et al. (O'Malley, Zaslavsky, Elliott, Zaborski, & Cleary, 2005). These independent variables were patients' faith (Christian, Jewish, Muslim, Other), age in 5-year intervals, gender, race (White, Black, Asian, Other), language spoken at home (English, Spanish, Other), education (8th Grade, Some High School, High School Graduate, Some College, College Graduate, More than 4 years College), self-reported health status (Poor, Fair, Good, Very Good, Excellent), emergency room admission (yes/no), response order quartile (1–4) and patients' diagnoses and procedures grouped into 48 clinical categories (yes/no) developed by the Agency for Healthcare Research and Quality (AHRQ) (HCUP CCS, 2012).

Statistical analyses

Chi-square and t-test statistics were used to compare patient characteristics in two groups; those visited and those not-visited by chaplains. We compared observed mean ± SE scores in the visited and not-visited groups. To adjust for confounders, we used OLS regression models. The final set of independent variables was selected using stepwise regression. Due to a variety of reasons, not all patients chose to participate in the surveys, and those who participated did not necessarily answer all questions. To reduce the non-response bias, we included the response order quartile in the list of independent variables of the models. This method has an advantage over non-response weighting through having less effect on precision (Elliott et al., 2009). When the models were fitted, estimated coefficients were used to calculate predicted values of scores for each question. These values were used to calculate the adjusted percent of positive responses for the groups of patients visited and not-visited by chaplains. All statistical analyses were performed using SAS 9.3 software package. This study was approved by Icahn School of Medicine at Mount Sinai Institutional Review Board.

Results

Within the study period, there were 67,952 hospitalizations, representing 48,734 adult patients. Patients had chaplain visits in 5,173 of these hospitalizations. Responses to the surveys were received from 8,978 patients who had been hospitalized and responded to the survey only once. Among respondents, we identified 498 (5.6%) hospitalizations during which patients were visited by chaplains. During these 498 hospitalizations, chaplains conducted 738 visits, ranging from 1 to 10 visits per hospitalization, with a median of 1 visit per hospitalization (first quartile = 1, fourth quartile = 2). The number of referrals for chaplain visits varied from 1 to 5 per hospitalization, with a median of 1 (first quartile = 1, fourth quartile = 1). Most referrals originated from chaplain rounds (74.7%), while nurses were the next most frequent source of referrals (8.7%). Self-referrals from patients were more frequent (3.4%) than referrals from social workers (1.6%) and doctors (1.1%). The remaining referrals came from other staff, clergy, family, and other sources.

Table 1: Selected characteristics of patients not-visited and visited by chaplains

Variable	Not-visited by chaplain N = 8,480	Visited by chaplain N = 498	p
Faith**			<.001
• Christian	3,944 (46.5%)	379 (76.1%)	
• Jewish	1,924 (22.7%)	46 (9.2%)	
• Muslim	157 (1.9%)	9 (1.8%)	
• Other	2,455 (29.0%)	64 (12.9%)	
Age (SD)**	55.9 (18.5)	61.3 (15.9)	<.001
Male Gender	3,382 (39.9%)	192 (38.6%)	.56
Race*			.03
• White	5,499 (64.8%)	299 (60.0%)	
• Black	937 (11.0%)	76 (15.3%)	
• Asian	438 (5.2%)	17 (3.4%)	
• Other	1,606 (18.9%)	106 (21.3%)	
Hispanic Ethnicity	2,175 (25.6%)	143 (28.7%)	.14
Education**			<.001
• 8th Grade	356 (4.2%)	27 (5.4%)	
• Some High School	484 (5.7%)	44 (8.8%)	
• High School Graduate	1,455 (17.2%)	101 (20.3%)	
• Some College	1,471 (17.3%)	105 (21.1%)	
• College Graduate	1,660 (19.6%)	90 (18.1%)	
• >4 Years in College	2,670 (31.5%)	106 (21.3%)	
Language*			.02
• English Language	6,448 (76.0%)	395 (79.3%)	
• Spanish Language	531 (6.3%)	37 (7.4%)	
• Other	601 (7.1%)	20 (4.0%)	
General Health Status**			<.001
• Poor	255 (3.0%)	31 (6.2%)	
• Fair	1,079 (12.7%)	101 (20.3%)	
• Good	2,129 (25.1%)	149 (29.9%)	
• Very Good	2,668 (31.5%)	133 (26.7%)	
• Excellent	2,077 (24.5%)	68 (13.7%)	

*$p < .05$. **$p < .001$.

Table 2: Observed scores (mean ± SE) for patients visited and not-visited by chaplains

Question	Not-visited by chaplain N = 8,480	Visited by chaplain N = 498
Overall rating of care given at hospital[a]	4.63 ± 0.01	4.72 ± 0.03**
What number would you use to rate this hospital during your stay?[b]	8.80 ± 0.02	8.97 ± 0.07*
Likelihood of your recommending this hospital to others[a]	4.59 ± 0.01	4.67 ± 0.03
Would you recommend this hospital to your friends and family?[b]	3.70 ± 0.01	3.77 ± 0.02*
Degree to which hospital staff addressed your spiritual needs[a]	4.23 ± 0.01	4.38 ± 0.04**
Degree to which hospital staff addressed your emotional needs[a]	4.38 ± 0.01	4.44 ± 0.04

[a]Press Ganey survey questions.
[b]HCAHPS survey questions.
*$p < .05$. **$p < .01$.

Characteristics of patients visited and not-visited by chaplains

Several parameters differed significantly between survey participants visited and not-visited by chaplains (Table 1). Patients visited by chaplains were more often of the Christian faith, older, black, had lower education levels, and more often spoke English and Spanish at home. The self-reported general health status was significantly worse in the group of visited patients.

Chaplain visits and patient satisfaction

Before adjustment for patient characteristics, mean scores for four questions about patient satisfaction were significantly higher for patients visited by chaplains. These were the two questions about overall rating on both HCAHPS and Press Ganey surveys, the HCAHPS question about recommending the hospital to friends and family and the question about spiritual needs (Table 2). The mean scores in responses to the question about emotional needs and the Press Ganey question about recommending the hospital did not differ significantly between visited and not-visited by chaplain groups.

After adjustment for patient characteristics, the coefficient for the variable of Chaplain Visit was significant for all questions (Table 3).

Table 3: Association between chaplain visits and patient satisfaction: regression coefficients for chaplain visits in the models for questions about patient satisfaction

Question	Coefficient	Standard Error	p
Overall rating of care given at hospital[a]	0.11**	0.04	0.001
What number would you use to rate this hospital during your stay?[b]	0.17*	0.08	0.036
Likelihood of your recommending this hospital to others[a]	0.11**	0.04	0.005
Would you recommend this hospital to your friends and family?[b]	0.07*	0.03	0.018
Degree to which hospital staff addressed your spiritual needs[a]	0.27***	0.05	<.001
Degree to which hospital staff addressed your emotional needs[a]	0.10*	0.04	0.020

[a]Press Ganey survey questions.
[b]HCAHPS survey questions.
*$p < .05$. **$p < .01$. ***$p < .001$.

Discussion

To our knowledge, this is the first study demonstrating that patients who are seen by chaplains are more satisfied with their hospital stay, as measured by HCAHPS and Press Ganey surveys. These findings were obtained when controlling for several independent variables that could affect patients' perception of care. These results are consistent with earlier findings that chaplain visits are associated with patient satisfaction (VandeCreek, 2004).

Chaplains as members of the healthcare team

Consistent with other investigations, referrals to chaplains accounted for the minority of chaplain visits (Galek, Vanderwerker, & Flannelly, 2009; Vanderwerker, Flannelly, & Galek, 2008). As noted by others, nurses are more likely than other healthcare team members to request chaplain visits (Galek et al.; Koenig, Bearon, Hover, & Travis, 1991). This may be due to the fact that nurses view spiritual care as a necessary component of overall patient care and may be more likely to request a chaplaincy intervention (Narayanasamy & Owens, 2001). The overall low referral rate by the medical team may reflect inadequate training and discomfort in inquiring about patients' spiritual or emotional needs (M. J. Balboni et al., 2013; Kuuppelomaki, 2001; Sellers & Haag, 1998). Due to the limited number of hospital chaplains and the medical teams' potential discomfort with assessing spiritual or religious needs, it has been recommended that chaplains be integrated into the healthcare team (Handzo, Cobb, Holmes, Kelly, & Sinclair, 2014; Handzo & Koenig, 2004; Lyndes et al., 2012; Puchalski et al., 2009). Chaplains' inclusion in the healthcare team helps to identify parameters for chaplaincy referral, provides an opportunity for chaplains to communicate their findings and recommendations into the treatment plan, and increases the likelihood of considering the patient as a whole (Lyndes et al.; Puchalski et al.).

Benefits of chaplain visits

It has been shown that patients who report that their spiritual needs are supported by the healthcare team are more likely to score higher on a Quality of Life scale, are less likely to have aggressive end of life care, and are more likely to enroll in hospice care (T. A. Balboni et al., 2013; T. A. Balboni, Balboni, & Paulk, 2011). Chaplain visits are helpful in several ways, including providing a reminder that God cares, prayer or scripture reading, making the hospitalization easier, giving hope, providing comfort, and helping to tap into inner strengths and resources (Piderman et al., 2010; VandeCreek, 2004). Our findings are generally consistent with those reports showing that chaplains do very well in meeting patients' spiritual/religious and emotional needs (Flannelly, Oettinger, Galek, Braun-Storck, & Kreger, 2009).

Strengths and limitations

This study has strengths in several aspects: (1) patients from different clinical services and with different diagnoses were included in the sample, (2) an outside vendor conducted the surveys, (3) there was documentation of visits by chaplains, (4) the chaplains did not know which patients would receive or return the satisfaction surveys, and (5) a minority of patients directly requested to see a chaplain. Our study has the following limitations. Drawing patients from a single medical center limits our ability to generalize the findings to other patient populations, as it has been recognized that there is geographic variation regarding how much patients are satisfied with interactions with chaplaincies (VandeCreek, 2004). Furthermore, an association between chaplain visits and patient satisfaction does not necessarily mean that there is a causative effect. This study also did not determine which chaplain interventions had an impact on patients' perception of care. HCAHPS and Press Ganey questions do not address patients' assessment about chaplaincy, as do other surveys (VandeCreek, 2004). We also did not screen for patients' spiritual or religious struggles, which may identify patients most in need of seeing a chaplain (Fitchett & Risk, 2009). Future studies should address these issues.

Conclusion

The HCAHPS and Press Ganey surveys are currently the two most commonly used surveys to assess patient satisfaction. Our study provides further support that chaplains should be an integral part of the healthcare team. Patient visits by chaplains during the course of the hospital stay leads to increased scores on patient satisfaction surveys. Historically, chaplaincy is not viewed as revenue generating. Our findings suggest that meeting patients' spiritual needs increases patient satisfaction and may also have positive fiscal consequences, given the advent of the Value Based Purchasing Program.

Acknowledgment

Electronic health record data were provided by Tatiana Arreglado MSN RN, Department of Clinical Informatics, Mount Sinai Health System, New York. Survey data were provided by Robert Fallar, PhD, Office of Excellence in Patient Care, Mount Sinai Hospital, New York. Reference preparation was provided by Barnaby Nicolas MSIS, Gustave L. and Janet W. Levy Library, Icahn School of Medicine at Mount Sinai, New York.

References

Astrow, A., Wexler, A., Texeira, K., He, M., & Sulmasy, D. (2007). Is failure to meet spiritual needs associated with cancer patients' perceptions of quality of care and their satisfaction with care? *Journal of Clinical Oncology, 25*, 5753–5757.

Balboni, M. J., Sullivan, A., Amobi, A., Phelps, A. C., Gorman, D. P., Zollfrank, A., ...Bulboni, T. A. (2013). Why is spiritual care infrequent at the end of life? Spiritual care perceptions among patients, nurses, and physicians and the role of training. *Journal of Clinical Oncology, 31*(4), 461–467. doi: 10.1200/JCO.2012.44.6443.

Balboni, T. A., Balboni, M. J., Enzinger, A. C., Gallivan, K., Paulk, M. E., Wright, A., ... Prigerson, H. G. (2013). Provision of spiritual support to patients with advanced cancer by religious communities and associations with medical care at the end of life. *JAMA Internal Medicine, 173*(12), 1109–1117. doi: 10.1001/jamainternmed.2013.903.

Balboni, T. A., Balboni, M. J., & Paulk, M. E. (2011). Support of cancer patients' spiritual needs and associations with medical care costs at the end of life. *Cancer, 117,* 5383–5391.

Balboni, T. A., Vanderwerker, L. C., & Block, S. D. (2007). Religiousness and spiritual support among advanced cancer patients and associations with end-of-life treatment preferences and quality of life. *Journal of Clinical Oncology, 25,* 555–560.

Cadge, W., Freese, J., & Christakis, N. A. (2008). The provision of hospital chaplaincy in the United States: A national overview. *Southern Medical Journal, 101*(6), 626–630. doi: 10.1097/SMJ.0b013e3181706856.

Centers for Medicare & Medicaid Services. (2013a). HCAHPS and Hospital VBP. Retrieved from www.hcahpsonline.org/HospitalVBP.aspx.

Centers for Medicare & Medicaid Services. (2013b). Mode & Patient-Mix Adjustment. Retrieved from www.hcahpsonline.org/modeadjustment.aspx.

Centers for Medicare & Medicaid Services. (2013c). Survey Instruments. Retrieved from www.hcahpsonline.org/surveyinstrument.aspx.

Clark, P. A., Drain, M., & Malone, M. P. (2003). Addressing patients' emotional and spiritual needs. *The Joint Commission Journal on Quality and Patient Safety, 29*(12), 659–670.

Davison, S. N., & Jhangri, G. S. (2010). Existential and supportive care needs among patients with chronic kidney disease. *Journal of Pain Symptom Management, 40*(6), 838–843. doi: 10.1016/j.jpainsymman.2010.03.015.

Elliott, M. N., Zaslavsky, A. M., Goldstein, E., Lehrman, W., Hambarsoomians, K., Beckett, M. K., & Giordano, L. (2009). Effects of survey mode, patient mix, and nonresponse on CAHPS® hospital survey scores: Methods. *Health Services Research, 44*(2P1), 501–518. doi: 10.1111/j.1475-6773.2008.00914.x.

Ellis, M. R., Thomlinson, P., Gemmill, C., & Harris, W. (2013). The Spiritual Needs and Resources of Hospitalized Primary Care Patients. *Journal of Religion and Health, 52*(4), 1306–1318. doi: 10.1007/s10943-012-9575-z.

Fitchett, G., Burton, L. A., & Sivan, A. B. (1997). The religious needs and resources of psychiatric inpatients. *Journal of Nervous and Mental Disease, 185*(5), 320–326.

Fitchett, G., & Risk, J. L. (2009). Screening for spiritual struggle. *Journal of Pastoral Care Counsel, 63*(1–2), 4-1-12.

Flannelly, K. J., Oettinger, M., Galek, K., Braun-Storck, A., & Kreger, R. (2009). The correlates of chaplains' effectiveness in meeting the spiritual/religious and emotional needs of patients. *Journal of Pastoral Care Counsel, 63*(1–2), 9–15.

Galek, K., Vanderwerker, L., & Flannelly, K. (2009). Topography of referrals to chaplains in the Metropolitan Chaplaincy Study. *Journal of Pastoral Care Counsel, 63*(6), 1–13.

Goldstein, E., Elliott, M. N., Lehrman, W. G., Hambarsoomian, K., & Giordano, L. A. (2010). Racial/Ethnic Differences in Patients' Perceptions of Inpatient Care Using the HCAHPS Survey. *Medical Care Research and Review, 67*(74), 74–91.

Handzo, G. F., Cobb, M., Holmes, C., Kelly, E., & Sinclair, S. (2014). Outcomes for professional health care chaplaincy: An international call to action. *Journal of Health Care Chaplaincy, 20*(2), 43–53. doi: 10.1080/08854726.2014.902713.

Handzo, G. F., & Koenig, H. G. (2004). Spiritual care: Whose job is it anyway? *Southern Medical Journal, 97*(12), 1242–1244.

HCUP CCS. (2012). Healthcare Cost and Utilization Project (HCUP). Retrieved from www.hcup-us.ahrq.gov/toolssoftware/ccs/ccs.jsp.

Iler, W., Obenshain, D., & Camac, N. (2001). The impact of daily visits from chaplains on patients with chronic obstructive pulmonary disease (COPD): A pilot study. *Chaplaincy Today, 17,* 5–11.

Joint Commission on Accreditation of Healthcare Organizations. (2005). Evaluating your spiritual assessment process. *Joint Commission, The Source, 3,* 6–7.

Kaldenberg, D. O., Mylod, D. M., & Drain, M. (2003). Patient-derived information: Satisfaction with care in acute and post-acute care environments. In N. Goldfield, M. Pine, & J. Pine (Eds.), *Measuring and managing health care quality: Procedures, techniques, and protocols* (2nd ed.), New York, NY: Aspen Publishers, pp.469–489.

Koenig, H. G., Bearon, L. B., Hover, M., & Travis, J. L., III. (1991). Religious perspectives of doctors, nurses, patients, and families. *Journal of Pastoral Care, 45*(3), 254–267.

Kuuppelomaki, M. (2001). Spiritual support for terminally ill patients: Nursing staff assessments. *Journal of Clinical Nursing, 10*(5), 660–670.

Lyndes, K. A., Fitchett, G., Berlinger, N., Cadge, W., Misasi, J., & Flanagan, E. (2012). A survey of chaplains' roles in pediatric palliative care: Integral members of the team. *Journal of Health Care Chaplaincy, 18*(1–2), 74–93. doi: 10.1080/08854726.2012.667332.

Narayanasamy, A., & Owens, J. (2001). A critical incident study of nurses' responses to the spiritual needs of their patients. *Journal of Advanced Nursing, 33*(4), 446–455.

O'Malley, A. J., Zaslavsky, A. M., Elliott, M. N., Zaborski, L., & Cleary, P. D. (2005). Case-mix adjustment of the CAHPS® Hospital survey. *Health Services Research, 40*(6 II), 2162–2181. doi: 10.1111/j.1475-6773.2005.00470.x.

Pearce, M. J., Coan, A. D., Herndon, J. E., 2nd, Koenig, H. G., & Abernethy, A. P. (2012). Unmet spiritual care needs impact emotional and spiritual well-being in advanced cancer patients. *Support Care Cancer, 20*(10), 2269–2276. doi: 10.1007/s00520-011-1335-1.

Piderman, K. M., Marek, D. V., Jenkins, S. M., Johnson, M. E., Buryska, J. F., Shanafelt, T. D., Mueller, P. S. (2010). Predicting patients' expectations of hospital chaplains: a multisite survey. *Mayo Clinic Proceedings, 85*(11), 1002–1010. doi: 10.4065/mcp.2010.0168.

Puchalski, C., Ferrell, B., Virani, R., Otis-Green, S., Baird, P., Bull, J., ...Sulmasy, D. (2009). Improving the quality of spiritual care as a dimension of palliative care: The report of the Consensus Conference. *Journal of Palliative Medicine, 12*(10), 885–904. doi: 10.1089/jpm.2009.0142.

Sellers, S. C., & Haag, B. A. (1998). Spiritual nursing interventions. *Journal of Holistic Nursing, 16*(3), 338–354.

VandeCreek, L. (2004). How satisfied are patients with the ministry of chaplains? *Journal of Pastoral Care Counsel, 58*(4), 335–342.

VandeCreek, L., & Lucas, A. M. (2001). *The discipline for pastoral care giving: Foundations for outcome oriented chaplaincy*. New York, NY: Haworth Pastoral Press.

VandeCreek, L., & Lyon, M. A. (1997). Ministry of hospital chaplains: Patient satisfaction. *Journal of Health Care Chaplaincy, 6*(2), 1–61. doi: 10.1300/J080v06n02_01.

Vanderwerker, L., Flannelly, K., & Galek, K. (2008). What do chaplains really do? III. Referrals in the New York Chaplaincy Study. *Journal of Health Care Chaplaincy, 14*, 57–73.

Williams, J. A., Meltzer, D., Arora, V., Chung, G., & Curlin, F. A. (2011). Attention to inpatients' religious and spiritual concerns: Predictors and association with patient satisfaction. *Journal of General Internal Medicine, 26*(11), 1265–1271. doi: 10.1007/s11606-011-1781-y.

ARTICLE 15

The Association of Spiritual Care Providers' Activities with Family Members' Satisfaction with Care after a Death in the ICU

Jeffrey R. Johnson, MD, MA[1], Ruth A. Engelberg, PhD[1], Elizabeth L. Nielsen, MPH[1], Erin K. Kross, MD[1], Nicholas L. Smith, PhD[2,3,4], Julie C. Hanada, MA[5], Sean K. Doll O'Mahoney, MDiv BCC[5], and J. Randall Curtis, MD, MPH[1]

1 Harborview Medical Center, Division of Pulmonary and Critical Care Medicine, Department of Medicine, University of Washington, Seattle, WA

2 Department of Epidemiology, School of Public Health, University of Washington, Seattle, WA

3 Seattle Epidemiologic Research and Information Center, Office of Research & Development, Seattle, WA

4 Group Health Research Institute, Group Health, Seattle, WA

5 Department of Spiritual Care, Harborview Medical Center, Seattle, WA

Corresponding author: J. Randall Curtis, MD, MPH, Division of Pulmonary and Critical Care Medicine, Harborview Medical Center, Box 359762, University of Washington, 325 Ninth Avenue, Seattle, Washington 98104. Phone: (206) 744-3356; Fax: (206) 744-8584, jrc@u.washington.edu.

Abstract

Objective: Spiritual distress is common in the ICU, and spiritual care providers are often called upon to provide care for patients and their families. Our goal was to evaluate the activities that spiritual care providers conduct to support patients and families, and whether those activities are associated with family satisfaction with ICU care.

Design: Prospective cohort study.

Setting: 350-bed, 65-ICU bed tertiary care teaching hospital.

Subjects: Spiritual care providers and family members of patients who died in the ICU or within 30 hours of transfer from the ICU.

Johnson, J.R., Engelberg, R.A., Nielsen, E.L., Kross, E.K., Smith, N.L., Hanada, J.C., Doll O'Mahoney, S.K., and Curtis, J.R. (2014) "The association of spiritual care providers' activities with family members' satisfaction with care after a death in the ICU." *Critical Care Medicine*, 42, 9, 1991–2000.

Measurements: Spiritual care providers completed surveys reporting their activities. Family members completed validated measures of satisfaction with care and satisfaction with spiritual care. Clustered regression was used to assess the association between activities completed by spiritual care providers and family ratings of care.

Results: Of 494 eligible patients, 275 family members completed surveys (response rate, 56%). Fifty-seven spiritual care providers received surveys relating to 268 patients, completing 285 surveys for 244 patients (response rate, 91%). Spiritual care providers commonly reported activities related to supporting religious and spiritual needs (>=90%) and providing support for family feelings (90%). Discussions about the patient's wishes for end-of-life care and a greater number of spiritual care activities performed were both associated with increased overall family satisfaction with ICU care (p<0.05). Discussions about a patient's end-of-life wishes, preparation for a family conference, and total number of activities performed were associated with improved family satisfaction with decision-making in the ICU (p<0.05).

Conclusions: Spiritual care providers engage in a variety of activities with families of ICU patients; several are associated with increased family satisfaction with ICU care in general and decision-making in the ICU specifically. These findings provide insight into spiritual care provider activities, and guidance for interventions to improve spiritual care delivered to families of critically ill patients.

Key words: intensive care, critical care, spiritual care, end-of-life care, dying, death, palliative care

Introduction

An inclusive conceptualization of spirituality is based on an individual's search for meaning and purpose in life.[1,2] For many patients facing serious illness, spirituality plays a substantial role in coping with prognosis, symptoms, and dying.[3,4,5,6] Despite this endorsement of spirituality's importance, patients report that their physicians often fail to talk with them about their spiritual needs.[7,8,9,10] Importantly, when spiritual care needs are unmet, patients rate their care more poorly[11] and medical costs are increased.[12] The Joint Commission has recognized the importance of supporting spiritual needs, including it as a component of their care standards, and attention to spiritual needs has been considered a moral obligation for healthcare institutions.[13,14]

The importance of spirituality to families has been similarly described.[15] In a survey of primary care outpatients, interest in discussions of spirituality was greatest when anticipating or experiencing the loss of a loved one, suggesting that the death of a family member is a time of substantial spiritual need for family members of critically ill patients.[9, 15] Under these circumstances, a hospital chaplain or spiritual care provider may provide welcomed care in the intensive care unit. Although a visit by a spiritual care provider has been associated with increased family satisfaction with spiritual care,[16] little is known about the specific activities spiritual care providers offer and their associations with ratings of care from the perspective of family members of patients who die in the ICU.

Our specific aims were 2-fold: Aim 1) to describe the frequency of specific activities performed by spiritual care providers for patients who eventually died in the ICU and their family members; and Aim 2) to evaluate the associations between spiritual care providers' activities and family ratings of satisfaction with care. We hypothesized that specific activities performed by spiritual care providers would be associated with higher family satisfaction with ICU care in general and spiritual care specifically. The ultimate goal of this study was to provide insights and guidance for future interventions designed to improve spiritual care for family of critically ill patients.

Materials and methods

Design and sample

Data for this study were collected as part of a "before-after" trial evaluating the effect of a multidisciplinary quality improvement intervention to improve palliative and end-of-life care in the ICU.[17] The intervention consisted of clinician education (e.g., provision of grand rounds, interactive workshops), local champions (e.g., identification and training of ICU clinician-leaders), academic detailing (e.g. meeting one-on-one with ICU directors), audit and feedback (e.g., sharing of ICU-specific family satisfaction questionnaire data with clinicians, managers and administrators), and system support (e.g., provision of order forms, communication aids). The intervention activities were extended to all members of the interdisciplinary team (e.g., physicians, nurses, spiritual care workers, social workers).

Between August 2003 and October 2005, eligible patients were identified from a 350-bed Level 1 Trauma center with 65 ICU beds in Seattle, Washington, that has had a Department of Spiritual Care since 1978. At the time of this study, there were over 50 spiritual care providers involved with

ICU patients and their families. The majority of these were interns in their first year of Clinical Pastoral Education, a nationally accredited program of education for ministry. The Clinical Pastoral Education Program is an accredited form of pastoral education for seminarians, clergy, and laity that utilizes an action/reflection model of learning under supervision. Students develop both professional pastoral identity and pastoral expertise. An accredited unit includes a minimum of 300 hours of clinical practice and 100 hours of group learning and supervision. The core methodology of the program involves individualized learning contracts, clinical practice, didactic resources, individual and group supervision, and reflection that integrate theory, practice, and personal history.

Spiritual care providers routinely screened the ICUs Monday through Friday to identify patients or families who might benefit from spiritual care and also accepted referrals from clinicians. Our current analysis includes patients who died before (n = 122) and after (n =122) the intervention and for whom we obtained spiritual care provider questionnaires.

Eligibility/Recruitment procedures

Patients: We identified consecutive eligible patients from the hospital admission, discharge, and transfer logs. Patients over the age of 18 were eligible if they died in an ICU or within 30 hours of transfer from an ICU to another hospital location. We excluded patients with ICU stays shorter than 6 hours to ensure that spiritual care providers were likely to have had an opportunity to become involved in care.

Family members: Approximately one month after a patient's death, family questionnaires were mailed to addresses obtained from the patient's medical record. Included in the packet were a cover letter, a consent form, a stamped return envelope, and a ten-dollar incentive payment. The cover letter asked that the family member or friend most involved in the patient's care complete the questionnaire. Reminders included a postcard sent at one week after the initial mailing to all potential subjects and a second packet sent to non-respondents at four to six weeks after the initial mailing.

Spiritual care providers: Within 48 hours of an eligible patient's death, a self-report questionnaire was distributed to spiritual care providers who had been identified as associated with that patient by chart review. In some cases, this included more than one spiritual care provider. The questionnaire included items related to the quantity, types, and quality of spiritual care provided to the patient and family. To enhance response rates, 2 additional reminders were provided (i.e., postcard reminder/ thank you at 1 week to all providers, additional questionnaire delivery at 3–4 weeks to non-respondents). Spiritual care providers were informed that questionnaire results were confidential and that results would not be presented in any way that allowed individuals to be identified. The Institutional Review Board at the University of Washington approved all study procedures and materials.

Spiritual care measures

The spiritual care providers' questionnaire was initially developed by the Harborview/University of Washington End-of-Life Care Research Program for completion by nurses[18, 19] and was adapted for spiritual care providers with the input of supervisors from this department. Spiritual care providers answered 14 questions about specific activities that they or other department members may have conducted to support the families with whom they were working. A composite score was created as the sum of all endorsed items for the activity types included for analysis. The survey also included demographic items to describe the characteristics of spiritual care providers (i.e., age, sex, race/ethnicity, education, years of ICU experience). The spiritual care provider activities questionnaire is available online (http://depts.washington.edu/eolcare).

Family-assessed outcome measures

Families' satisfaction with care was assessed with the Family Satisfaction in the ICU (FS-ICU) questionnaire.[20] This questionnaire has been validated using a subset of 24 out of the 34 items that families completed.[21] The validated scoring includes: 1) a total score (FS-ICU) averaged across 24 items; 2) a Satisfaction with Care (FS-Care) subscale averaged across 14 items; and 3) a Satisfaction with Decision-Making (FS-Decision-Making) score averaged across 10 items.[21] An additional question, "How well did the ICU staff meet your spiritual/religious needs," is part of the longer FS-ICU questionnaire, but is not part of the 24 items that contribute to the FS-ICU total or subscale scores. For these analyses, it was evaluated as a separate outcome. Family members' demographic information was also collected and included age, sex, race/ethnicity, education level and relationship to patient.

Analysis

For the analyses of the self-reported spiritual care providers' activities, Aim 1, we used descriptive statistics (i.e., frequencies, means, standard deviations) based on the full sample of spiritual care provider questionnaires in which we included more than one questionnaire per patient, if available.

For the analyses of associations between spiritual care providers' self-reported activities and family outcomes (Aim 2) we used robust, clustered regression models that accommodated the skewed distributions of the satisfaction scales (FS-ICU total, FS-Care, FS-Decision-Making) and accounted for the correlated data that resulted from spiritual care providers providing surveys for multiple patients; these clustered models relaxed the assumption of independence in observations and provided appropriate standard errors by which to test the proposed associations. For the single item assessing satisfaction with spiritual care services for which the assumption of equal intervals between response options was less likely to be valid, we used ordinal logistic regression.

For Aim 2 analyses, we first created a reduced sample of spiritual care provider questionnaires (n=244) in which each patient had only one spiritual care provider questionnaire. This was necessary in order to avoid cross-clustering for 32 patients who had 2 or more spiritual care provider questionnaires. The selection of surveys to retain was guided by the following principles, in the following order of priority: 1) to maximize the number of spiritual care providers represented; 2) to retain surveys with the most complete data; and 3) to balance the number of surveys included per spiritual care provider. We then excluded activities that were very frequent (>=90%) (i.e., actively addressed spiritual or religious needs, discussed spiritual or religious needs, discussed family members' feelings) or were likely to be relevant to only a subset of patients and families (i.e., addressing cultural needs, discussing intra-family disagreements) with the rationale that these activities were unlikely to provide sufficient variability to allow reliable regression analysis. This resulted in the retention of 7 activities and a summary score of the total number of activities as predictor variables.

Potential confounders included: family characteristics (i.e., age, sex, race/ethnicity, education level), patient characteristics (i.e, age, sex, marital status), and spiritual care provider characteristics (i.e., age, sex, race/ethnicity, years of ICU experience). Years of ICU experience was categorized into <1, 1–5, or >5 years of ICU experience. An individualized adjusted model was generated for each activity, outcome, and set of covariates. Covariates were included in each adjusted model if the change in the β-coefficient was greater than or equal to 20% after inclusion of the covariate, relative to the unadjusted model. We chose 20% because of the relatively large number of models examined. Intervention status was included in all adjusted models. Due to the number of tests of association, the analyses were considered hypothesis generating and we selected a p value of $<=0.05$ to signify statistical significance without adjusting for multiple comparisons.

Results
Sample
Patients: 587 eligible patients were identified during the study period. Most patients were white (77%), male (66%), and never married/partnered, widowed or divorced (57%). Mean age at time of death was 62 years, and a third of deaths were due to trauma (33%); mean length of hospital stay and ICU stay were 9.3 and 6.3 days, respectively. Patients with documented spiritual care visits had significantly longer ICU lengths of stay and lower educational achievement ($p<0.05$); they did not vary on any of the other measured variables (Table 1).

Family respondents: 494 family members were contacted to complete surveys; 275 returned a survey (56%; Figure 1). The majority of family respondents were white (82%), female (66%) and had some post-high-school education. Many (45%) were spouses of the patients. As with patients, the only statistically significant family characteristic that was associated with a documented spiritual care visit was a lower level of educational achievement (Table 2). There were 118 patients for whom a family member and a spiritual care provider completed a survey and for whom there was a spiritual care visit documented (n=64 pre-intervention; 54 post-intervention.)

Spiritual care provider respondents: Three hundred and eighteen questionnaires representing 268 patients were sent to 57 spiritual care providers (Figure 2). Two hundred and forty-four patients had at least one questionnaire returned from at least one of 49 spiritual care providers, yielding a patient-based response rate of 91% (244/268) and a spiritual care provider participation rate of 86% (49/57). The mean number of surveys distributed to these 57 providers was 5.6 (median=2, range=1–36). The mean number completed was 5.0 (median=2, range=0–34). The majority of the spiritual care providers were female (60%) and non-Hispanic white (76%). Although more than half were serving as interns in the Spiritual Care Department and had therefore had little prior experience as spiritual care providers in the ICU (<1 year, n=40%), they represented an older group of individuals (mean age, 42) with significant advanced degree training (46%).

Aim 1: Frequency of spiritual care provider activities

On average, spiritual care providers reported engaging in a large number of activities with ICU patients' family members: 102 (39%) received 10 or more of the 14 potential activities. Only 13 families (5%) were provided with none of the activities. The mean and median number of activities per patient in which spiritual care providers engaged was eight. Actively addressing (92%) and discussing (92%) spiritual or religious needs was common. Discussions related to family members' feelings (90%) and patient values (79%) were also common, as was reminiscing about the patient (80%). Discussions about (28%) and actively addressing cultural needs (27%) were less common, as were discussions regarding intra-family disagreements about plan of care (20%; Table 3).

Aim 2: Specific spiritual care provider activities and family outcomes

The specific activity, "discussed patient's wishes for end-of-life care", as well as the total number of activities were significantly associated with both higher total FS-ICU and higher FS-Decision-Making scores. Higher FS-Decision-Making scores were also significantly associated with the activity, "prepared the family for a family conference". The item, "reminisced with the family about the patient", was associated with higher families' assessment of satisfaction with having spiritual needs met in the ICU. None of the spiritual provider activities were associated with the FS-ICU-Care subscale (Table 4).

Discussion

Our study of spiritual care providers is the first study to demonstrate the number and variety of activities that they report completing while providing support for families of critically ill patients. The family-completed questionnaires suggest several of these activities are associated with higher family satisfaction with care. In our sample, we found that both families' and patients' education levels were related to provision of spiritual care, with those with less education being more likely to have had a documented spiritual care visit. Two large studies, one nationally representative and one in the South, found that individuals with less education are more likely to self-designate as religious,[22, 23] and therefore our findings may represent appropriate targeting of spiritual care for those who desire it.

We found that the total number of activities performed was associated with higher scores on the FS-ICU, a general and validated measure of satisfaction with care in the ICU. This is consistent with prior studies in which the provision of spiritual support was associated with higher quality-of-life scores near the time of death.[10, 24] One novel feature of our study is that it relates to care provided to families of patients who died in the ICU; most prior studies of spiritual care have been conducted among outpatients in oncology or palliative care clinics.[25] The finding that 70% of primary care patients would like to discuss spiritual matters with their healthcare team if their family member were to die indicates that spiritual care is needed in support of families of patients at high risk of death.[15]

In a prospective multisite study, cancer patients whose religious and spiritual care needs were poorly met by clinic staff were more likely to die in an ICU, indicating that attention to spiritual care may affect choices for intensive care at the end of life.[24] We detected a significant association between the occurrence of discussions of patients' wishes for end-of-life care and higher overall assessments of the ICU experience. It may be the case that, for family members, the opportunity to give voice to the patient's wishes and have this acknowledged by a spiritual care provider provides some support. Similarly, the association between reminiscing about the patient and satisfaction with spiritual care supports the importance of patient-focused and family-centered approaches in which the patient is seen as an important and unique person with individual values, beliefs and history. For family members, the opportunity for a spiritual care provider to learn about their loved one as an individual may be of particular value.

The FS-ICU is composed of two subscales, one representing satisfaction with the ways in which care has been delivered, and the other measuring satisfaction with the ways in which care decisions were made.[21] In contrast to the decision-making subscale and the total score, the FS-Care subscale was not significantly associated with spiritual care provider activities. This may be due, in part, to the kinds of items that are part of the FS-Care subscale; many assess the quality of care received from doctors and nurses and these may not be influenced by the activities that spiritual care providers are able to provide. However, the significant associations between spiritual care activities and higher satisfaction with ICU decision-making may suggest that one important function of spiritual care relates to comfort with and confidence in difficult decisions. This finding also supports the hypothesis that family members' experience of decision-making depends on factors beyond the provision of information, also including spiritual and emotional support.[26, 27, 28] This hypothesis is consistent with prior studies, including one in which discussions of spiritual needs during family conferences were associated with greater satisfaction with decision-making.[29] Similarly, in a study of 48 family members of patients who had died in an ICU, 23 (48%) respondents spontaneously mentioned spirituality as reassuring at the time of end-of-life decision-making.[30]

Surrogate decision-making by family members may play an important role in the psychological distress experienced by family members after a patient dies in the ICU. For example, family members who adopt passive decision-making roles exhibit greater degrees of depression and anxiety,[31] and those whose desired decision-making role is discordant from actual decision-making role bear a greater burden of future depression and PTSD.[32] The majority of patients who die in the ICU do so after a decision to withhold or withdraw life-sustaining therapy[33] and this decision-making comes with a heavy emotional and psychological cost.[34] Our findings, as well as those of others,[29, 30] suggest that good spiritual care may be one important opportunity to support family members through this decision-making process.

Our study has several limitations. First, it was conducted in a single center, and the results may not generalize to all ICU patients and families. Washington State has a less religious population than many other areas of the USA[35] and the impact of spiritual care may vary regionally. Furthermore, at the time our study was conducted, a large chaplaincy training program was in place. This resulted in, on average, less experienced spiritual care providers than may practice in other ICUs, as well as provision of spiritual care to a large proportion of families. Despite the limitation of a single-center study, our findings provide insights into the potential role of spiritual care. Second, this is an observational study, and as such causation cannot be inferred. Furthermore, spiritual care provider questionnaire items such as "actively addressed cultural needs" and "discussed intra-family disagreements" cannot be adequately addressed in an observational study, since such needs were not prospectively assessed and would only be "addressed" for cultural minorities or families with conflict. Third, we do not know how the effects of activities may have varied depending on families' spiritual needs, as we do not have indications of whether the spiritual care providers' visits were requested and by whom they were requested. Although the spiritual care provider program is designed to meet the spiritual needs of a diverse community, offering culturally sensitive emotional and spiritual support to patients, families and staff, regardless of religious, faith or spiritual tradition, families may have been reluctant to engage or accept spiritual care providers' services if they felt that their own religious traditions may not be addressed. In addition, we have no information on interactions with spiritual care practitioners who were not affiliated with the hospital, such as those representing the patients' usual church, synagogue, or mosque. Finally, due to the number of comparisons we conducted, our findings must be considered exploratory and future studies are needed to confirm them.

Our findings suggest that spiritual care providers' conversations with families about the patient as an individual, with specific reference to his or her wishes for end-of-life care, may be particularly useful for families. Spiritual care providers' activities were most strongly associated with satisfaction with families' decision-making in the ICU, which may indicate improved comfort with difficult decisions when family members feel supported by a spiritual care provider. Our results provide some direction for future studies testing interventions to improve spiritual care for family of critically ill patients; they also suggest that interventions designed to improve the delivery of spiritual care in the ICU may be associated with improvements in family members' satisfaction with decision-making.

Acknowledgments

Funding and Registration: Funded by the National Institute of Nursing Research (R01 NR005226) and the Robert Wood Johnson Foundation. Registered at ClinicalTrials.gov: NCT00685893.

Conflict of interest

The authors have no financial conflict of interest.

Copyright form disclosures

Dr. Curtis received support for article research from NIH. His institution received grant support from NIH, Robert Wood Johnson Foundation, and PCORI. Dr. Johnson received support for article research from NIH. His institution received grant support from National Institutes of Health. Dr. Engelberg received support for article research from NIH. His institution received grant support from National Institutes of Health and Patient Centered Outcomes Research Institute (PCORI). Dr. Nielsen received support for article research from NIH. Her institution received grant support from National Institutes of Health. Dr. Kross received support for article research from NIH. Her institution received grant support from National Institutes of Health K23 award. Dr. Smith received support for article research from NIH. Dr. Hanada received support for article research from NIH. Her institution received grant support from National Institutes of Health. Dr. O'Mahoney received support for article research from NIH, is employed by Harborview Medical Center, received support for development of educational presentations from University of Washington (stipend for contribution to a presentation on what chaplains need to know about mental illness in 2010), and received support for travel from the Association for Clinical Pastoral Education (ACPE Associate Supervisor). His institution received grant support from National Institutes of Health.

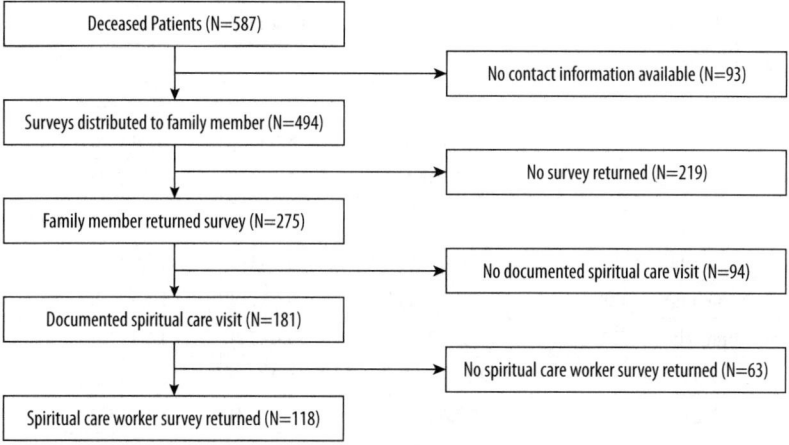

Figure 1: Flow diagram for family members

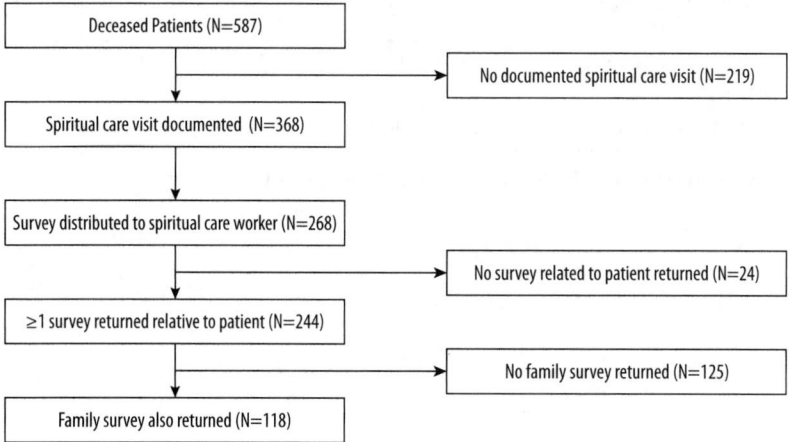

Figure 2: Flow diagram for spiritual care providers

Table 1: Patient characteristics (n=587)

Characteristic	All patients (n=587)	No spiritual care visit (n=220)	Spiritual care visit (n=367)	P*
Female, % (n)	33.9 (199)	30.5 (67)	36.0 (132)	.172
Non-Hispanic white, % (n)	77.3 (454)	79.1 (174)	76.3 (280)	.433
Marital status % (n)				.141
• Married/domestic partnership	43.1 (248)	37.3 (81)	46.6 (167)	
• Divorced/separated	22.8 (131)	25.8 (56)	20.9 (75)	
• Never partnered	18.1 (104)	18.4 (40)	17.9 (64)	
• Widowed	16.0 (92)	18.4 (40)	14.5 (52)	
Underlying cause of death, % (n)				.203
• Trauma	32.9 (193)	29.5 (65)	34.9 (128)	
• Cancer	5.1 (30)	5.5 (12)	4.9 (18)	
• Other condition	62 (364)	65.0 (143)	60.2 (221)	
Education, % (n)				.039**
• <= Eighth grade	9.0 (50)	8.7 (18)	15.5 (32)	
• Some high school	12.1 (67)	9.7 (20)	13.5 (47)	
• High school/GED	39.2 (217)	35.0 (72)	41.7 (145)	
• Some college	22.2 (123)	25.2 (52)	20.4 (71)	
• College	12.6 (70)	16.0 (33)	10.6 (37)	
• Graduate school	4.9 (27)	5.3 (11)	4.6 (16)	
Age at death, mean (SD) years	61.7 (17.6)	63.5 (17.6)	60.6 (17.5)	.054
Length of final hospital stay, mean (SD) days	9.3 (11.1)	8.3 (9.8)	9.9 (11.7)	.071
Length of final ICU stay, mean (SD) days	6.3 (8.1)	5.3 (7.5)	7.1 (8.4)	**.007**

*P-value for tests of differences between patient characteristics for those without a spiritual care visit vs. patients with a spiritual care visit.
**Less education associated with greater frequency of documented spiritual care.

Table 2: Family respondent characteristics (n=275)

Characteristic	All family respondents (n=275)	No documented spiritual care visit (n=94)	Spiritual care visit documented (n=181)	P*
Female, % (n)	65.8 (179)	67.7 (63)	64.8 (116)	.682
Non-Hispanic white, % (n)	81.9 (222)	84.8 (78)	80.4 (144)	.380
Age, mean (SD) years	56.4 (13.8)	56.5 (12.8)	56.3 (14.3)	.946
Education, median		some post-high school education	some post-high school education	.003**
Relationship to patient, % (n)				.081
• Spouse or partner	44.9 (123)	37.6 (35)	48.6 (88)	
• Child of patient	26.6 (73)	29.0 (27)	25.4 (46)	
• Parent of patient	10.6 (29)	12.9 (12)	9.4 (17)	
• Sibling	10.6 (29)	10.8 (10)	10.5 (19)	
• Other relative or close friend	5.5 (15)	7.5 (7)	4.4 (8)	
Lived with patient, % (n)	57.7 (157)	51.6 (48)	60.9 (109)	.142
Years of association with patient, mean (SD)	38.6 (15.8)	40.6 (14.9)	37.6 (16.1)	.124

*P-value for tests of differences between family characteristics of those without a documented spiritual care visit vs. those with a documented spiritual care visit.
**Less education associated with greater frequency of documented spiritual care.

Table 3: Spiritual care providers' self-reported activities*

Activity	# Valid responses	% Endorsed
Actively addressed spiritual/religious needs	285	92.3
Discussed spiritual/religious needs	284	91.5
Discussed family members' feelings	281	90.4
Reminisced about patient	282	79.8
Discussed patient's values	281	79.4
Supported family decisions regarding care	282	73.8
Encouraged talking to and touching the patient	280	61.8
Assured family that patient would be kept comfortable	276	55.1
Discussed patient's wishes for end-of-life care	282	45.4
Located private place for intra-family discussion	279	31.9
Discussed cultural needs	285	28.4
Prepared family for conference	281	27.0
Actively addressed cultural needs	281	26.7
Discussed intra-family disagreements about plan of care	281	20.3

*Activities were reported from 285 questionnaires representing 244 patients.

Table 4: Results of multivariate regression analyses,* testing associations between spiritual care provider's activities and family members' ratings of satisfaction

Linear regression used for FS-ICU, FS-Care, and FS-Decision-Making. Ordered logistic regression used for spiritual care needs met.

	FS-ICU total score					Spiritual care needs met in ICU (single item)				
Spiritual care provider's activities	N (116)	β (SE)	t	p	95% CI	N (106)	β (SE)	z	p	95% CI
Reminisced about the patient	114	5.036 (2.636)	1.91	0.065	−0.334, 10.406	105	.8216 (0.386)	2.13	**0.033**	0.065, 1.578
Discussed patient's values	114	4.585 (2.869)	1.60	0.120	−1.260, 10.429	105	0.616 (0.390)	1.58	0.114	−0.148, 1.380
Supported decisions regarding care	114	5.133 (3.068)	1.67	0.104	−1.116, 11.382	103	0.418 (0.379)	01.10	0.270	−0.325, 1.162
Encouraged talking to and touching patient	111	−2.281 (3.231)	−0.71	0.486	−8.879, 4.317	97	−0.438 (0.437)	−1.00	0.316	−1.294, 0.418
Assured family that patient would be comfortable	111	4.041 (2.689)	1.50	0.143	−1.436, 9.518	96	0.143 (0.352)	0.41	0.684	−0.546, 0.833
Discussed patient's wishes for end-of-life care	114	7.598 (2.566)	2.96	**0.006**	2.371, 12.824	100	0.844 (0.441)	1.91	0.056	−0.021, 1.709
Prepared the family for conference	112	5.165 (2.788)	1.85	0.073	−0.521, 10.850	96	0.868 (0.473)	1.84	0.066	−0.059, 1.796
Total number of activities performed	116	1.231 (.592)	2.08	**0.046**	0.024, 2.437	106	0.139 (0.073)	1.90	0.058	−0.005, 0.282

	FS-ICU: Care domain					FS-ICU: Decision-making domain				
Spiritual care provider's activities	N (117)	β (SE)	t	p	95% CI	N (116)	β (SE)	t	p	95% CI
Reminisced about the patient	115	4.381 (2.944)	1.49	0.147	−1.616, 10.378	111	3.648 (3.443)	1.06	0.298	−3.383, 10.680
Discussed patient's values	115	6.180 (3.444)	1.79	0.082	−0.834, 13.195	111	3.102 (3.665)	0.85	0.404	−4.382, 10.586
Supported decisions regarding care	111	4.586 (2.992)	1.53	0.136	−1.524, 10.696	114	6.298 (4.174)	1.51	0.141	−2.203, 14.800
Encouraged talking to and touching patient	108	−1.857 (2.718)	−0.68	0.500	−7.408, 3.694	108	−4.964 (4.002)	−1.24	0.224	−13.137, 3.210
Assured family that patient would be comfortable	108	3.157 (2.756)	1.15	0.261	−2.471, 8.785	111	4.654 (3.600)	1.29	0.205	−2.678, 11.987
Discussed patient's wishes for end-of-life care	114	4.113 (2.338)	1.76	0.088	−0.649, 8.875	114	11.723 (3.323)	3.53	**0.001**	4.955, 18.492
Prepared the family for conference	108	2.973 (2.864)	1.04	0.308	−2.885, 8.831	112	7.630 (2.282)	2.32	**0.027**	0.936, 14.323
Total number of activities performed	117	1.047 (0.573)	1.83	0.077	−0.120, 2.213	116	1.575 (0.762)	2.07	**0.047**	0.022, 3.128

*Potential covariates retained if altered β coefficient by >20%, for each specific activity, outcome, and covariate; intervention status was retained in all models

References

1. El Nawawi NM, Balboni MJ, Balboni TA. Palliative care and spiritual care: the crucial role of spiritual care in the care of patients with advanced illness. Curr Opin Support Palliat Care. 2012; 6:269–74. [PubMed: 22469668]
2. Edwards A, Pang N, Shiu V, Chan C. The understanding of spirituality and the potential role of spiritual care in end-of-life and palliative care: a meta-study of qualitative research. Palliat Med. 2010; 24:753–70. [PubMed: 20659977]
3. Puchalski CM. Spirituality in the cancer trajectory. Ann Oncol. 2012; 23 (Suppl 3):49–55. [PubMed: 22628416]
4. Grant E, Murray SA, Kendall M, Boyd K, Tilley S, Ryan D. Spiritual issues and needs: perspectives from patients with advanced cancer and nonmalignant disease. A qualitative study. Palliat Support Care. 2004; 2:371–8. [PubMed: 16594399]
5. Hampton DM, Hollis DE, Lloyd DA, Taylor J, McMillan SC. Spiritual needs of persons with advanced cancer. Am J Hosp Palliat Care. 2007; 24:42–8. [PubMed: 17347504]
6. Vallurupalli M, Lauderdale K, Balboni MJ, et al. The role of spirituality and religious coping in the quality of life of patients with advanced cancer receiving palliative radiation therapy. J Support Oncol. 2012; 10:81–7. [PubMed: 22088828]
7. Balboni TA, Vanderwerker LC, Block SD, et al. Religiousness and spiritual support among advanced cancer patients and associations with end-of-life treatment preferences and quality of life. J Clin Oncol. 2007; 25:555–60. [PubMed: 17290065]
8. Monroe MH, Bynum D, Susi B, et al. Primary care physician preferences regarding spiritual behavior in medical practice. Arch Intern Med. 2003; 163:2751–6. [PubMed: 14662629]
9. Ehman JW, Ott BB, Short TH, Ciampa RC, Hansen-Flaschen J. Do patients want physicians to inquire about their spiritual or religious beliefs if they become gravely ill? Arch Intern Med. 1999; 159:1803–6. [PubMed: 10448785]
10. Williams JA, Meltzer D, Arora V, Chung G, Curlin FA. Attention to inpatients' religious and spiritual concerns: predictors and association with patient satisfaction. J Gen Intern Med. 2011; 26:1265–71. [PubMed: 21720904]
11. Astrow AB, Wexler A, Texeira K, He MK, Sulmasy DP. Is failure to meet spiritual needs associated with cancer patients' perceptions of quality of care and their satisfaction with care? J Clin Oncol. 2007; 25:5753–7. [PubMed: 18089871]
12. Balboni T, Balboni M, Paulk ME, et al. Support of cancer patients' spiritual needs and associations with medical care costs at the end of life. Cancer. 2011; 117:5383–91. [PubMed: 21563177]
13. Sulmasy DP. Spirituality, religion, and clinical care. Chest. 2009; 135:1634–42. [PubMed: 19497898]
14. Angus DC. Charting (and publishing) the boundaries of critical illness. Am J Respir Crit Care Med. 2005; 171:938–9. [PubMed: 15849327]
15. McCord G, Gilchrist VJ, Grossman SD, et al. Discussing spirituality with patients: a rational and ethical approach. Ann Fam Med. 2004; 2:356–61. [PubMed: 15335136]
16. Wall RJ, Engelberg RA, Gries CJ, Glavan B, Curtis JR. Spiritual care of families in the intensive care unit. Crit Care Med. 2007; 35:1084–90. [PubMed: 17334245]
17. Curtis JR, Treece PD, Nielsen EL, et al. Integrating palliative and critical care: evaluation of a quality-improvement intervention. Am J Respir Crit Care Med. 2008; 178:269–75. [PubMed: 18480429]
18. Curtis JR, Patrick DL, Shannon SE, Treece PD, Engelberg RA, Rubenfeld GD. The family conference as a focus to improve communication about end-of-life care in the intensive care unit: opportunities for improvement. Crit Care Med. 2001; 29:N26–33. [PubMed: 11228570]
19. McCormick AJ, Engelberg R, Curtis JR. Social workers in palliative care: assessing activities and barriers in the intensive care unit. J Palliat Med. 2007; 10:929–37. [PubMed: 17803416]

20. Heyland DK, Tranmer JE. Group KGHIRW. Measuring family satisfaction with care in the intensive care unit: the development of a questionnaire and preliminary results. J Crit Care. 2001; 16:142–9. [PubMed: 11815899]
21. Wall RJ, Engelberg RA, Downey L, Heyland DK, Curtis JR. Refinement, scoring, and validation of the Family Satisfaction in the Intensive Care Unit (FS-ICU) survey. Crit Care Med. 2007; 35:271–9. [PubMed: 17133189]
22. Shahabi L, Powell LH, Musick MA, et al. Correlates of self-perceptions of spirituality in American adults. Ann Behav Med. 2002; 24:59–68. [PubMed: 12008795]
23. Koenig HG. Religious attitudes and practices of hospitalized medically ill older adults. Int J Geriatr Psychiatry. 1998; 13:213–24. [PubMed: 9646148]
24. Balboni TA, Paulk ME, Balboni MJ, et al. Provision of spiritual care to patients with advanced cancer: associations with medical care and quality of life near death. J Clin Oncol. 2010; 28:445–52. [PubMed: 20008625]
25. Kalish N. Evidence-based spiritual care: a literature review. Curr Opin Support Palliat Care. 2012; 6:242–6. [PubMed: 22498837]
26. Majesko A, Hong SY, Weissfeld L, White DB. Identifying family members who may struggle in the role of surrogate decision maker. Crit Care Med. 2012; 40:2281–6. [PubMed: 22809903]
27. Boyd EA, Lo B, Evans LR, et al. "It's not just what the doctor tells me:" factors that influence surrogate decision-makers' perceptions of prognosis. Crit Care Med. 2010; 38:1270–5. [PubMed: 20228686]
28. Scheunemann LP, Arnold RM, White DB. The facilitated values history: helping surrogates make authentic decisions for incapacitated patients with advanced illness. Am J Respir Crit Care Med. 2012; 186:480–6. [PubMed: 22822020]
29. Gries CJ, Curtis JR, Wall RJ, Engelberg RA. Family member satisfaction with end-of-life decision making in the ICU. Chest. 2008; 133:704–12. [PubMed: 18198256]
30. Abbott KH, Sago JG, Breen CM, Abernethy AP, Tulsky JA. Families looking back: one year after discussion of withdrawal or withholding of life-sustaining support. Crit Care Med. 2001; 29:197–201. [PubMed: 11176185]
31. Anderson WG, Arnold RM, Angus DC, Bryce CL. Passive decision-making preference is associated with anxiety and depression in relatives of patients in the intensive care unit. J Crit Care. 2009; 24:249–54. [PubMed: 19327283]
32. Gries CJ, Engelberg RA, Kross EK, et al. Predictors of symptoms of posttraumatic stress and depression in family members after patient death in the ICU. Chest. 2010; 137:280–7. [PubMed: 19762549]
33. Prendergast TJ, Claessens MT, Luce JM. A national survey of end-of-life care for critically ill patients. Am J Respir Crit Care Med. 1998; 158:1163–7. [PubMed: 9769276]
34. Azoulay E, Pochard F, Kentish-Barnes N, et al. Risk of post-traumatic stress symptoms in family members of intensive care unit patients. Am J Respir Crit Care Med. 2005; 171:987–94. [PubMed: 15665319]
35. [Accessed June 28, 2012] US Religions Landscape Survey. 2008. http://religions.pewforum.org/maps Available at: http://religions.pewforum.org/maps

ARTICLE 16

The Effect of Pastoral Care Services on Anxiety, Depression, Hope, Religious Coping, and Religious Problem Solving Styles: A Randomized Controlled Study

Paul S. Bay.* Daniel Beckman.* James Trippi.ˣ
Richard Gunderman.♦ Colin Terry†

* Chaplaincy and Pastoral Education, Clarian Health Partners, I-65 at 21st Street, P.O. Box 1367, Indianapolis, IN 46206-1367, USA e-mail: pbay@clarian.org

* CORVAS Cardiothoracic & Vascular Solutions, Clarian Health Partners, I-65 at 21st Street, P.O. Box 1367, Indianapolis, IN 46206-1367, USA

ˣ The Care Group, Clarian Health Partners, I-65 at 21st Street, P.O. Box 1367, Indianapolis, IN 46206-1367, USA

♦ Methodist Research Institute, Clarian Health Partners, I-65 at 21st Street, P.O. Box 1367, Indianapolis, IN 46206-1367, USA

† School of Medicine, Indiana University, Indianapolis, USA

Received: 11 December 2006 / Accepted: 1 May 2007 / Published online: 24 May 2007

© Blanton-Peale Institute 2007

Author Biography: Dr. Paul S. Bay received his Doctorate of Ministry degree from Christian Theological Seminary of Indianapolis, Indiana in 1997. He is Cardiovascular Care Chaplain for Clarian Health Partners which includes Indiana University Hospital, Methodist Hospital, and Riley Hospital for Children. In addition to being a Board Certified Chaplain he is also a Clinical Member of the American Association for Marriage and Family Therapy. He is the recipient of a National Institute for Healthcare Research, John Templeton Spirituality & Medicine Award and other grants of the Religion and Spiritual Integration Values of Clarian Health. Paul currently divides his time between research and patient care through the cardiovascular interdisciplinary team and heart transplant team.

Abstract

This randomized controlled study measured the effect of chaplain interventions on coronary artery bypass graft (CABG) patients over time. One hundred sixty-six CABG patients, received pre- and post-surgery testing at 1 month and 6 months with four instruments. Five chaplain visits were made to the intervention group, the control group received none. Comparison scores for anxiety, depression, hope, positive and

Bay, P.S., Beckman, D., Trippi, J., Gunderman, R., and Terry, C. (2008) "The effect of pastoral care services on anxiety, depression, hope, religious coping, and religious problem solving styles: a randomized controlled study." *Journal of Religion & Health*, 47, 57–69.

negative religious coping, and religious coping styles were analyzed. Significant difference was found between groups in positive religious coping (PRC) ($p = .023$) and negative religious coping (NRC) ($p = .046$) scores over time. PRC increased in intervention group, decreased in the control group while NRC decreased in intervention group and increased in the control group. Demographics were comparable between groups. Moderate chaplain visits (average total visits time, 44 min) may be effective in helping CABG patients increase positive religious coping and decrease negative religious coping.

Key words: CABG, chaplain, religious coping, anxiety, depression, hope

Introduction

Research studies in recent decades examine religious faith and practice to determine their associations to health, medical concerns, and mortality. Koenig, McCullough, and Larson (2001) summarize 1,200 of these studies and 400 research reviews. They describe studies regarding religion and mental health, religion and physical disorders, and the relationship of religion to the use of health services. In general, they conclude that an active religious life is associated with better health, improved coping with medical concerns, and reduced mortality rates.

Strikingly absent from this literature is an examination of whether and how the ministry of clergy (and other non-ordained persons) contributes to these associations. What contribution does parish ministry make to a healthy lifestyle? Does providing pastoral care services to the sick influence recovery? What contribution does this ministry make to the dying and their families? Certainly, research attention to the effect of pastoral care services merits attention because this ministry often takes place when patients and their families struggle with the meaning of illness and death, a struggle that for many has religious/spiritual overtones.

These questions are best explored by a clinical trial of the pastoral care ministry, a research design in which some persons receive pastoral care and others do not. A clinical trial, however, cannot be carried out in the usual congregational setting where this ministry typically occurs, because parish clergy are morally and administratively mandated to provide services to all in need. In contrast, hospital chaplains provide pastoral care in a context in which this difficulty is minimized. As employees of health care institutions, chaplains supplement the ministry of parish clergy to their hospitalized parishioners and provide care to patients who have no parish clergy available. Thus no one is denied pastoral care services, although it is important to note that the control group of such a clinical trial is contaminated by pastoral care provided by their parish clergy.

Hospital chaplains find clinical trials of their pastoral care ministry inviting for at least four reasons. First, chaplains provide ministry in scientific medical contexts that encourage all professionals to test the effectiveness of their work. Institutional administrators as well as medical and nursing authorities usually encourage and support the scientific investigation of this ministry. Second, the necessary methodological and statistical consultants are available in these health care institutions. Third, as health care faces continuing financial pressures, some authorities wonder how chaplains contribute to the clinical mission of institutions. Chaplains sense that such research efforts could begin to demonstrate how their ministry makes a distinct contribution. Finally, the results can inform the clinical practice of ministry, identifying pastoral best practices. In this study, the authors describe a clinical trial of pastoral care services carried out by a hospital chaplain to cardiac bypass surgery patients.

The cardiac and pastoral care literatures suggest that the pastoral care ministry merits testing. Studies have documented that hospitalized cardiac surgery patients and their families usually experience symptoms of anxiety and depression to which chaplains give attention (Duits et al., 1998; Koivula, Tarkka, Tarkka, Laippala, & Paunonen-Ilmonen, 2002a, b; Parent & Fortin, 2000; Saur et al., 2001). These emotions are especially important during the pre-surgical period because they limit the benefits of surgery (Perski et al., 1998).

The patients' religious faith and practice is associated with the management of these emotions. Harris et al. (1995) studying cardiac transplant patients, gathered data three times during the first year after surgery and found that patients who reported greater religiosity and more religious practices at 2 months post-surgery described better health and well-being at the 1-year anniversary date. They comment that "overall, religious beliefs and practices early in the post-transplant experience more strongly predicted respondents' perceptions of physical functioning than their Karnofsky scores at follow up." (p.24)

Another study (Sears, Rodrigue, Greene, Fauerbach, & Mills, 1997) also examined the role of religious coping in heart transplant patients and concluded, "Interventions that provide an opportunity to discuss religious ideas and concepts in a supportive context would likely prove to be beneficial." (p.350)

Family members of patients are also stressed because of the disease and the surgery, likely influencing the patient. In an examination of religious and non-religious emotional support, VandeCreek, Pargament,

Belavich, Cowell, and Friedel (1999) gathered data from family members waiting in the hospital during the cardiac bypass surgery. They found that private and communal prayers were a frequent means of religious support. Additional results suggested that the family members' religiosity contributed unique support after controlling for the benefits of non-religious support. They concluded that religious faith and practice made their own unique contribution to the management of waiting during the surgery situation and was neither overshadowed by nor duplicative of non-religious support. They suggested that religious support was particularly helpful because "religion is designed to provide a compelling presence during the most difficult times" (p.28) and they wondered if the provision of ministry would mobilize further religious coping during the stresses of surgery.

Using another part of the same data set, Pargament, VandeCreek, Belavich, Brant, and Perez (1999) examine religious and non-religious control while waiting during the surgery. These results demonstrate that both religious and non-religious coping methods make unique contributions to a sense of control. They conclude that patients and families may benefit from "a greater range of coping options, including religious as well as non-religious methods." (p.337)

Religious faith and practice is also associated with mortality rates. Oxman, Freeman, and Manheimer (1995) studied the association between cardiac bypass surgery patient characteristics and the risk of post-surgical death. After controlling for three biomedical causes of death, they found that those who reported receiving no strength or comfort from religion were three times more likely to die within 6 months after surgery than their peers whose religion provided at least some strength and comfort.

In another study that examined the relationship of religious faith and practice to mortality, Pargament, Koenig, Tarakeshwar, and Hahn (2001) examined the relationship between religious struggles and mortality among ill elderly patients. They defined religious struggle as including anger at God, feeling punished by God, and/or believing that the devil was at work in the illness. They concluded that patients with religious struggles suffered a 6–10% increased risk of dying during the 2-year study period. They comment, "Referral of these patients to clergy to help them work through these issues may ultimately improve clinical outcomes." (p.1885)

Finally, the authors are aware of one small clinical trial ($N = 49$) that examined the effect of pastoral care services provided to hospitalized chronic obstructive pulmonary disease patients although it was not reported as a clinical trial (Iler, Obenshain, and Camac, 2001). After randomly creating two groups, the authors provided daily chaplain visits to the intervention group during their hospitalization. The results demonstrated significantly lower anxiety at discharge among these patients ($p = .03$), a shorter length of stay (3.72 days vs. 9.0 days; $p = .002$), and increased patient satisfaction ($p = .05$). These reports suggest that a clinical trial is warranted.

The authors hypothesized that the provision of pastoral care services to cardiac bypass patients would cause significant changes in selected affective responses to the disease and surgery (anxiety, depressive symptoms, and hope), cause changes in religious coping processes, and influence the medical course of recovery. The Institutional Review Board of the host hospital approved the study.

Methods
The behavioral definition of pastoral care services
Pastoral care services in this study consisted of four behaviors. First, the hospital chaplain initiated pastoral conversations with the patients, meeting them in their rooms. Second, the chaplain encouraged the symbolic aspects of this ministry by identifying himself as the chaplain, a clergy person who is employed by the hospital to provide an ecumenical religious/spiritual ministry. The denominational affiliation of the chaplain was minimized. Third, the chaplain followed the usual protocol of reflective listening, developing a context for patients to verbalize their emotional/spiritual concerns (e.g., their worries, doubts, fears, anxieties, depressive thought, and concerns as well as joys and hopes). Fourth, the chaplain asked one pre-selected existential religious/spiritual question (described below) in the process of each visit. The question helped patients verbalize their needs, hopes, resources and grief work in the process of coping with the surgery and the recovery process. These pastoral visits constituted the interventions in the clinical trial.

Subjects
The sample size calculation was based on the study's goal of collecting data beginning when patients were hospitalized for the surgery until 6 months after surgery. The limited literature reported the anxiety level of these patients and the authors estimated that the intervention group would create anxiety scores 20% lower than the scores of the control group at 6 months post-surgery. The calculation established that a sample size of 85 subjects per group provided 80% power to detect this anxiety change at a significance level of .05.

Inclusion criteria required that patients be scheduled for bypass surgery that either used the bypass pump (CABG) or did not use it (OPCAB). They needed to be between 30 and 90 years of age, speak and read English, have telephone access, and have their surgeon's approval for participation. However, patients who met these criteria were excluded from the study if they were diagnosed with a psychiatric illness as defined by the Diagnostic and Statistical Manual-Version IV, were scheduled for cardiac valve surgery in addition to CABG or OPCAB, suffered from a principal diagnosis of heart failure with an ejection fraction (LVEF) <35%, or required ongoing renal dialysis. Further, patients were excluded post-surgically if they returned to surgery because they were bleeding at the surgery site, were experiencing renal failure, were reintubated, or suffered a stroke as a complication of surgery.

A trained assistant screened 485 patients for participation. Of these, 174 were excluded by the study criteria (73 due to a low ejection fraction, 30 who were on dialysis, 29 because the surgeon regarded them as being high risk, 12 because they were sedated and unable to complete the questionnaire or engage in conversation, and 30 due to miscellaneous reasons). Of the remaining 311 potential candidates, 107 declined and 204 (66%) were randomly assigned to a control or treatment group. Some patients ($N = 38$) did not complete the study. Of the 38 patients that did not complete the study, thirty-four had no follow-up data. The remaining four patients completed 1-month follow-up testing only. Of patients lost to the study, 15 dropped out for various personal reasons, nine suffered complications beyond those described above, eight died, three did not receive sufficient intervention visits from the chaplain, two did not have surgery after being enrolled, and one received unscheduled, additional pastoral care services. Data for all patients who completed any follow-up testing were included in the analysis. Therefore, the study results report on 170 subjects, 85 in each group. All testing and enrollment were performed by the research assistant to avoid bias by subject interaction with the chaplain.

Instruments

Patients completed four questionnaires, two of which were frequently used in psycho-social studies of cardiac surgery studies. Two others were chosen because they gathered data concerning the role of religiosity in coping with stress. They gathered data concerning anxiety, depression, hope, religious coping, and religious problem solving styles.

The Hospital Anxiety and Depression Scale (HADS) has proven useful in the study of cardiac patients (Duits et al., 1998; Johnston, Foulkes,

Johnston, Pollard, & Gudmundsdottir, 1999; Koivula et al., 2002a, 2002b; Lewin, Robertson, Cay, Irving, & Campbell, 1992; Mayou et al., 2002; Thompson & Meddis, 1990). Herrmann (1997) reported that this 14-item scale, first published in 1983, was available in multiple languages and used in more than 200 published studies in most types of medical settings worldwide. Factor analysis of the English and German versions confirmed an anxiety and a depression factor. He reported that Cronbach's alphas from multiple studies ranged from .80 to .93 for the anxiety and .81 to .90 for depression. Retest reliability after two weeks created correlations of .84 for anxiety and .85 for depression.

Researchers have frequently examined hope in cardiac patients by using the 12-item Herth Hope Index (Beckie, Beckstead, & Webb, 2001; Daly, Davidson, & Jackson, 1999; Evangelista, Doering, Dracup, Vassilakis, & Kobashigawa, 2003; Staples & Jeffrey, 1997). Developed from the Herth Hope Scale (Herth, 1992) as an abbreviated instrument for use in clinical settings, Herth reported an alpha coefficient of .97 and a two-week test-retest reliability of .91 for the instrument.

The 14-item Brief RCOPE was included in the instrument packet because the authors hypothesized that pastoral care interventions influenced the patients' religious coping processes and because the instrument's results have been correlated with health status. Developed as an abbreviated instrument from the longer RCOPE, its positive and negative subscales (seven items each) created alphas of .90 and .81, respectively. In the initial report (Pargament, Smith, Koigen, & Perez, 1998) the authors reported that the responses to these two subscales reflected attempts to manage stressful experiences as represented in the item contents (Table 1).

The 36-item Religious Problem Solving Scale Pargament et al. (1988), a three-factor instrument with 36 items, generated information concerning ways in which patients try to manage their problems in relation to God. The self-directing subscale of 12 items described trying to manage problems without involving God ($\alpha = .94$). Sample items included "After I've gone through a rough time, I try to make sense of it without relying on God" and "When faced with trouble, I deal with my feelings without God's help." The collaborative subscale described working with God to manage the problem ($\alpha = .94$). Its 12 items included "When it comes to deciding how to solve a problem, God and I work together as partners" and "When faced with a question, I work together with God to figure it out." The deferring approach turned the problem over to God ($\alpha = .91$) and included items such as "I do not think about different solutions to my problems because God provides them for me" and "Rather than trying to come up with the right solution to a problem myself, I let God decide how to deal with it." The one-week test-retest reliability ranged from .87 to .94. These styles gather information concerning two key dimensions "underlying the individual's relationship with God: the locus of responsibility for the problem-solving process, and the level of activity in the problem-solving process." (p.91)

Table 1: Short RCOPE: positive and negative coping items

Positive religious coping items	Negative religious coping items
Seek stronger connection with God	Wonder whether God has abandoned me
Seek God's love and care	Feel punished by God for lack of devotion
Seek God's help in letting go of anger	Question God's love for me
Try to put plans into action with God	Wonder what I did for God to punish me
Try to see how God might be trying to strengthen me in this situation	Wonder whether my church had abandoned me
Ask forgiveness for my sins	Decide the devil made this happen
Focus on my religion to stop worrying about my problems	Question the power of God

Note: Each item is scored on a scale of 0 = "not at all" to 3 = "a great deal."

The questionnaire responses were supplemented by four medical data concerning the course of recovery: the post-surgical length of stay in the hospital, the number of unscheduled physician office visits after the surgery, whether the patient was readmitted to the hospital, and the cost of the hospitalization.

Process

After obtaining informed consents, the research assistant supervised the patients' completion of the questionnaires before surgery. The first author, the hospital's chaplain for bypass surgery patients, conducted the clinical interventions consisting of four pastoral visits with each patient in the intervention group and one visit with their family members during the actual surgery—this visit with the patient's knowledge. When he was not available, a trained substitute conducted the visits. The three post-surgical visits were conducted in the hospital within the first 7 days after surgery.

The chaplain standardized each pastoral visit by listening to the patient's concerns and by asking one question focusing on a theme previously identified by the authors (Table 2). In the pre-surgical visit, the chaplain provided supportive pastoral care concerning the patients' self-acknowledged spiritual/psychological needs. The second visit was a family support visit during the patient's surgery. The third visit, usually on the second or third day after the surgery, helped patients identify and discuss their hopes. The fourth visit aided the patients in thinking about a positive personal future by using their religious and psychological resources. The fifth visit focused on feelings of grief related to the limitations imposed by the disease and previous personal loses. These five visits constituted a mean of 44 minutes with each patient/family.

Patients in the control group received no pastoral attention from the chaplain, the trained substitute, or other chaplains in the hospital, although patients in both groups may have been visited by their parish clergy. No patients in the intervention and control groups requested chaplaincy attention beyond that described. Had they or staff done so, they would have received appropriate pastoral care and been dropped from the study. Patients completed the questionnaires again at 1 month and 6 months post-surgery.

Table 2: Questions for use during the designated visit

First Visit: (Pre-Surgery): Focus on Spiritual/Psychological Needs
1. How do you make sense out of what you are going through?
2. What has your life been like lately? That is, what seems to be working and what seems to be not working?
3. What needs should be met for this surgery experience to work for you?
Second Visit: (Family Support During Surgery)
Third Visit: (Post-Surgery) Focus on Spiritual/Psychological Hope
1. What keeps you going?
2. After recovery what does your future look like?
3. What is it that makes getting up each morning matter?
4. What would make you fight for your health?
5. What is it that gives you peace or makes you feel calm?
Fourth Visit: (Post-Surgery) Focus on Spiritual/Psychological Resources
1. What have you done before when you've faced a stressful situation?
2. Who do you turn to when you need support?
3. Who counts on you?
4. What resources have you used in the past?
Fifth Visit: (Post-surgery) Focus: Spiritual/Psychological Aspects of Grief Work
1. What losses have you had in the last few years?
2. What have you done about previous losses?
3. What choices do you feel you have in this process?
4. How have relationships worked for you along the way?

Statistical analysis

Demographics were summarized using descriptive statistics and were compared between study groups using Student's t-tests, Chi-square tests, Fisher's exact tests and Mantel–Haenszel Chi-square tests where appropriate. Questionnaire scores for both groups were summarized for pre-surgery, 1 month, and 6 months post-surgery using mean and standard deviation (Table 3). For subjects with incomplete follow-up data (i.e., 1 month post-op only), 6 months follow-up data was imputed using the method of last observation carried forward. A generalized linear mixed model was used to compare the change in outcome scores between groups over time. Demographic variables that were unbalanced between groups were included as covariates in the model. Analyses were performed using software R (Version 2.3.0) and significance was set at $p \leq 05$.

Results

No significant differences between groups were found for age (mean = 64 years), gender (75% males), marital status (76% married; 24% single, widower, or divorced), race (91% Caucasian), or education level completed (16% less than 12 years; 48% high school graduates; 35% college graduates). Eighty-seven percent of the patients lived with another adult in their homes or apartments, and 98% reported that family members lived within 20 miles of the hospital. A majority (64%) received the CABG procedure and 58% reported they had received patient education concerning their medical condition. Religious preference was significantly different ($p = .04$) between the groups because the control group contained more Catholics (18% vs. 6% for the intervention group) and the intervention group contained more Protestants (82% vs. 68%).

Table 3: Scores for each testing period

	Control group, Mean (SD)	Intervention group, Mean (SD)
Pre-surgical baseline		
• Anxiety (HADS)	7.3 (3.7)	6.4 (3.9)
• Depression (HADS)	4.1 (3.1)	3.6 (3.0)
• Hope (Hearth Hope Index)	40.5 (5.0)	41.1 (4.7)
• Positive Religious Coping (RCOPE)	13.4 (6.3)	13.3 (6.2)
• Negative Religious Coping (RCOPE)	1.7 (2.6)	1.5 (2.2)

• Collaborative Religious Coping (RPSS)	39.7 (13.2)	39.9 (14.6)
• Self Directing Religious Coping (RPSS)	25.5 (11.5)	25.3 (12.0)
• Deferring Religious Coping (RPSS)	31.6 (11.7)	34.0 (12.9)
1 month post-surgery		
• Anxiety (HADS)	5.7 (4.1)	4.9 (3.5)
• Depression (HADS)	3.0 (3.1)	3.1 (3.0)
• Hope (Hearth Hope Index)	40.9 (5.2)	41.5 (4.7)
• Positive Religious Coping (RCOPE)	13.3 (5.7)	14.1 (6.1)
• Negative Religious Coping (RCOPE)	1.7 (2.9)	1.3 (2.4)
• Collaborative Religious Coping (RPSS)	40.2 (11.5)	41.3 (14.3)
• Self Directing Religious Coping (RPSS)	24.7 (11.0)	23.5 (12.0)
• Deferring Religious Coping (RPSS)	32.4 (11.4)	35.7 (13.0)
6 months post-surgery		
• Anxiety (HADS)	5.3 (3.9)	4.8 (3.4)
• Depression (HADS)	3.0 (3.1)	3.0 (2.9)
• Hope (Hearth Hope Index)	40.6 (4.9)	41.2 (5.0)
• Positive Religious Coping (RCOPE)	13.1 (6.0)	14.3 (5.9)
• Negative Religious Coping (RCOPE)	2.0 (3.0)	.9 (1.5)
• Collaborative Religious Coping (RPSS)	38.5 (12.7)	41.0 (13.5)
• Self Directing Religious Coping (RPSS)	24.5 (11.1)	23.1 (11.4)
• Deferring Religious Coping (RPSS)	31.4 (11.6)	34.9 (12.4)

Questionnaire scores by group for each testing time were calculated (Table 3). Since religious preferences differed significantly between groups, it was included as a covariate in the linear mixed model. The results of the overall test of the group–time interaction (Table 4) showed a marginally significant difference in the positive religious coping scores between groups over time ($p = .081$); however, there was a significant difference in the positive religious coping scores between groups at the 6 months time point ($p = .026$). Similarly, there was a marginally significant difference in the change in negative religious coping scores between groups over time ($p = .056$), and a significant difference in negative religious coping scores between groups at the 6 months time point ($p = .021$). Positive religious coping decreased over time in the control group and increased in the intervention group. Negative religious coping increased over time in the control group and decreased in the intervention group (Table 3).

Table 4: Statistical significance of questionnaire scores between groups over time

Variable (Scale)	p-Value
Anxiety (HADS)	.623
Depression (HADS)	.421
Hope (Hearth Hope Index)	.987
Positive Religious Coping (RCOPE)	.081
Negative Religious Coping (RCOPE)	.056
Collaborative Religious Coping (RPSS)	.218
Self Directing Religious Coping (RPSS)	.519
Deferring Religious Coping (RPSS)	.597

Note: Results based on the tests of the type III sums of squares for the group–time interaction term in the linear mixed model.

No significant differences between groups were found regarding anxiety, depression, hope, or the self-directing, deferring or collaborative subscales of the Religious Problem Solving Scale. The number of hospital readmissions, unscheduled physician office visits, post-surgery length of stay and the cost of hospitalization were not significantly different between groups.

Discussion

The literature does not sufficiently examine whether and how the provision of pastoral care services to hospitalized patients contributes to the helpful relationship of religion to health, illness, and mortality. While this is admittedly difficult to study in the parish setting, the hospital context of chaplains offers an opportunity for clinical trials. In this study, a hospital chaplain provides pastoral care services to an intervention group of cardiac bypass patients. The control group receives no pastoral care from the chaplain.

The results support the hypothesis that providing these services causes changes in religious coping. In the literature, increased positive religious coping is associated with fewer symptoms of psychological stress (Pargament et al., 1998) and better mental health (Koenig, Pargament, & Nielsen, 1998). Negative religious coping is tied to depression, poorer quality of life and psychological symptoms (Pargament et al., 1998).

This suggests that pastoral care services, as defined and delivered in this project, improve the patients' emotional/spiritual adjustment to the surgery. In contrast, those who received no pastoral care services from the chaplain demonstrate religious coping that is linked to more problematic adjustments.

The anxiety, depressive feelings, and hope scores did not significantly change over time and five possible reasons for the lack of change are described. The first possibility is that our calculation that the intervention would create anxiety and depression scores 20% lower in the intervention group than the control group was unrealistic based on the natural trajectory of decrease in anxiety and depression over time. This decrease experienced by both the control group and intervention group is supported by the literature on CABG patients' recovery. Since there were no studies measuring the effect of pastoral interventions on CABG patients at the time we started our study, an optimistic estimate of change was hypothesized.

A second possibility is that the provision of pastoral care services really does not impact anxiety, depressive feelings, or hope. While this possibility must not be dismissed, patients frequently report at the end of pastoral care visits that they feel much better emotionally and psychologically.

The third possibility pertains to the questionnaires. Concerning anxiety, the baseline scores reflect somewhat more anxiety in these patients than that reported in some other studies. Thus, while anxiety was somewhat heightened, patients seem to manage it by choosing surgeons in whom they place notable confidence. Further, the surgeons who participated in this study (and most surgeons) possess reputations that reflected surgical success. They openly display confidence in their skills and experience. Perhaps this surgeon–patient relationship was of sufficient power to mask anxiety changes due to the intervention services.

Concerning depressive feeling, the range of scores for non-clinical samples in the literature is 3.40–3.59 (Stordal et al., 2001). Depression scores at the baseline time period in this study are 4.1 (SD = 3.1) for the control group and 3.6 (SD = 3.0) for the intervention group. These standard deviations suggest that, at baseline, the patients in this study may not have experienced depressive symptoms beyond those in the general population.

Concerning hope, the baseline scores in this study are higher than those of subjects in 12 reports reviewed. In one study (Rustoen, Wahl, Hanestad, Gjengedal, & Moum, 2004), the mean score from over 1,000 subjects in a control group from the general population (37.2 ± 4.1) is within one standard deviation of patients in the control and intervention groups at baseline (40.4 ± 5.0 and 41.1 ± 4.7, respectively). This high baseline may have decreased the probability that a significant change would be demonstrated. Another limitation was the absence of studies measuring how pastoral interventions affect hope. Therefore, the effect of change as a result of our pastoral intervention hypothesized was an estimate.

A fourth explanation for the lack of changes concerns the absence of knowledge concerning the necessary "dosage" of pastoral care services to create changes and the appropriate length of time for data gathering. Perhaps the approximately 44 min of chaplain–patient contact distributed over four visits and one visit with the family is insufficient to produce significant changes beyond those demonstrated here in religious coping. Further, gathering data 1 month and 6 months after surgery may allow any additional changes to dissipate. The clinical trial described in the literature review found lower anxiety at discharge, shorter length of stay, and increased patient satisfaction in response to a more concentrated intervention comprising daily pastoral visits of 20 min during the entire length of hospitalization with post-test data gathered immediately at discharge.

A fifth possible explanation concerns the existential religious/spiritual questions (Table 2) used in the intervention. Their content and the way they were used may not have sufficiently focused on reducing anxiety and depression, and increasing hope. Perhaps they were too general or not sufficiently focused on religious/spiritual concerns and resources. The clinical trial noted above reported that "Approximately two-thirds of the patients utilized the chaplain to vent painful or stressful emotions, share grief over their illness or other losses, or to help with conflict management within the family". (p.7) In that study, the intervention appears to be completely unstructured; perhaps the questions used in this study not only structure the intervention somewhat, but also stand in the way of patients discussing their own agenda.

In conclusion, the general literature reviewed at the time we developed our hypotheses was replete with the importance of anxiety and depression in the recovery of heart patients. However, there was no empirical evidence that pastoral interventions could influence anxiety, depression or hope in the recovery process of CABG patients. In retrospect, the hypothesis that pastoral interventions would influence these factors was not well grounded. At least four limitations must be considered when evaluating these results. First, the generalization of these results to other persons should be limited because one chaplain (and a trained substitute) provided the interventions. His or her pastoral care skill and personal/professional style surely affect outcomes, because the intervention is deeply personal and its effectiveness is couched within the context of the relationship between chaplain and patient.

Second, the study engaged cardiac bypass patients in a single major Midwest medical center. Further study is needed to determine if these results also apply to other hospitalized patients and to the provision of pastoral care services to persons in the community.

Third, this study did not screen for religiosity/spirituality; it collected only religious heritage data as a demographic characteristic. This allowed for the possibility that pastoral care services provided by parish clergy significantly varied between the groups. We did not adequately plan for this as a possible confounding variable. Researchers conducting future studies should screen out patients who are likely to receive pastoral care from their parish clergy or other pastoral persons, thereby limiting pastoral care from persons outside the study design.

Fourth, all of the outcomes were analyzed independently, as originally planned. While it is possible that all of the measures may not be completely independent of each other, no adjustment was made to the significance levels.

In summary, McIntosh and Spilka (1990) opine that "the association of religion with health is apparently as old as humanity" (p.167) and previous studies demonstrate that significant, multiple associations exist. The results of this randomized controlled trial suggest that providing pastoral care services to cardiac bypass surgery patients creates religious coping changes. Additional research is necessary to confirm these findings and their meaning.

Acknowledgments

This study was funded by the generous support of the Values Fund for Religion and Spiritual Integration in Health Care of Clarian Health Partners, Inc. We are indebted to physicians and their staff who made referrals and provided private space for confidential testing. This project was made possible by the dedicated work of Kenneth Pierce M.S., Stephen Ivy, Ph.D., Dan Young, D.Min., and Stan Jones, M.Div. We thank Larry VandeCreek, D.Min. for his help with the manuscript.

References

Beckie, T. M., Beckstead, J. W., & Webb, M. S. (2001). Modeling women's quality of life after cardiac events. *Western Journal of Nursing Research, 23*(2), 179–194.

Daly, J., Davidson, P. M., & Jackson, D. (1999). The experience of hope for survivors of acute myocardial infarction (AMI): A qualitative research study. *Australian Journal of Advanced Nursing, 16*(3), 38–44.

Duits, A. A., Duivenvoorden, H. J., Boeke, S., Taams, M. A., Mochter, B., Krauss, X. H., Passchier, J., & Erdman, R. A. M. (1998). The course of anxiety and depression in patients undergoing coronary artery bypass graft surgery. *Journal of Psychosomatic Research, 45*(2), 127–138.

Evangelista, L. S., Doering, L. V., Dracup, K., Vassilakis, M. E., & Kobashigawa, J. (2003). Hope, mood states and quality of life in female heart transplant recipients. *The Journal of Heart and Lung Transplantation, 22*(6), 681–686.

Harris, R. C., Dew, M. A., Lee, A., Amaya, M., Buches, L., Reetz, D., & Coleman, G. (1995). The role of religion in heart-transplant recipients' long-term health and well-being. *Journal of Religion and Health, 34*(1), 17–32.

Herrmann, C. (1997). International experiences with the hospital anxiety and depression scale—A review of validation data and clinical results. *Journal of Psychosomatic Research, 42*(1), 17–41.

Herth, K. (1992). Abbreviated instrument to measure hope: Development and psychometric evaluation. *Journal of Advanced Nursing, 17,* 1251–1259.

Iler, W. M., Obenshain, D., & Camac, M. (2001). The impact of daily visits from chaplains on patients with chronic obstructive pulmonary disease (COPD): A pilot study. *Chaplaincy Today, 17*(1), 5–9.

Johnston, M., Foulkes, J., Johnston, D. W., Pollard, B., & Gudmundsdottir, H. (1999). Impact on patients and partners of inpatient and extended cardiac counseling and rehabilitation: A controlled trial. *Psychosomatic Medicine, 61*(2), 225–233.

Koenig, H., McCullough, M., & Larson, D. (2001). *Handbook of religion and health.* New York: Oxford University Press.

Koenig, H. G., Pargament, K. I., & Nielsen, J. (1998). Religious coping and health status in medically ill hospitalized older adults. *The Journal of Nervous and Mental Disease, 186*(9), 513–521.

Koivula, M., Tarkka, M. T, Tarkka, M., Laippala, P., & Paunonen-Ilmonen, M. (2002a). Fear and anxiety in patients at different time-points in the coronary artery bypass process. *International Journal of Nursing Studies, 39,* 811–822.

Koivula, M., Tarkka, M. -T., Tarkka, M., Laippala, P., & Paunonen-Ilmonen M. (2002b). Fear and in-hospital social support for artery bypass grafting patients on the day before surgery. *International Journal of Nursing Studies, 39,* 415–427.

Lewin, B., Robertson, I. H., Cay, E. L., Irving, J. B., & Campbell, M. (1992). Effects of self-help post- myocardial-infarction rehabilitation on psychological adjustment and use of health services. *Lancet, 339,* 1036–1040.

Mayou, R. A., Thompson, D. R., Clements, A., Davies, C. H., Goodwin, S. J., Norwington, K., Jicks, N., & Price, J. (2002). Guideline-based early rehabilitation after myocardial infarction. A pragmatic randomised controlled trial. *Journal of Psychosomatic Research, 52,* 89–95.

McIntosh, D., & Spilka, B. (1990). Religion and physical health: The role of personal faith and control beliefs. *Research in the Social Scientific Study of Religion, 2,* 167–194.

Oxman, T. E., Freeman, D. H., & Manheimer, E. D. (1995). Lack of social participation or religious strength and comfort as risk factors for death after cardiac surgery in the elderly. *Psychosomatic Medicine, 57,* 5–15.

Parent, N., & Fortin, F. (2000). A randomized, controlled trial of vicarious experience through peer support for male first-time cardiac surgery patients: Impact on anxiety, self-efficacy expectation, and self-reported activity. *Heart & Lung, 29*(6), 389–400.

Pargament, K. I., Kennel, J., Hathaway, W., Grevengoed, N., Newman, J., & Jones, W. (1988). Religion and the problem-solving process: Three styles of coping. *Journal for the Scientific Study of Religion, 27*(1), 90–104.

Pargament, K. I., Koenig, H. G., Tarakeshwar, N., & Hahn, J. (2001). Religious struggle as a predictor of mortality among medically ill elderly patients: A 2-year longitudinal study. *Archives of Internal Medicine, 161*(15), 1881–1885.

Pargament, K. I., Smith, B. W., Koenig, H. G., & Perez, L. (1998). Patterns of positive and negative religious coping with major life stressors. *Journal for the Scientific Study of Religion, 37*(4), 710–724.

Pargament, K., VandeCreek, L., Belavich, T., Brant, C., & Perez, L. (1999). The vigil: Religion and the search for control in the hospital waiting room. *Journal of Health Psychology, 4*(3), 327–341.

Perski, A., Feleke, E., Anderson, G., Samad, B., Westerlund, H., Ericsson, C. G., & Rehnqvist, N. (1998). Emotional distress before coronary bypass grafting limits the benefits of surgery. *American Heart Journal, 136*(3), 510–517.

Rustoen, T., Wahl, A. K., Hanestad, B. R., Gjengedal, E., & Moum, T. (2004). Expressions of hope in cystic fibrosis patients: A comparison with the general population. *Heart & Lung, 33*(2), 111–118.

Saur, C. D., Granger, B. B., Muhlbaier, L. H., Forman, L. M., McKenzie, R. J., Taylor, M. C., & Smith, P. K. (2001). Depressive symptoms and outcome of coronary artery bypass grafting. *American Journal of Critical Care, 10*(1), 4–10.

Sears, S., Rodrigue, J., Greene, A., Fauerbach, P., & Mills, R. (1997). Religious coping and heart transplantation: From threat to Health. *Journal of Religion and Health, 36*(4), 345–351.

Staples, P., & Jeffrey, J. (1997). Quality of life, hope, and uncertainty of cardiac patients and their spouses before coronary artery bypass surgery. *Canadian Journal of Cardiovascular Nursing, 8*(1), 7–16.

Stordal, E., Bjartveit, K. M., Dahl, N. H., Kruger, O., Mykletun, A., & Dahl, A. A. (2001). Depression in relation to age and gender in the general population: The Nord-Trondelag Health Study (HUNT). *Acta Psychiatrica Scandinavica, 104*(3), 210–16.

Thompson, D. R., & Meddis, R. (1990). A prospective evaluation of in-hospital counselling for first time myocardial infarction men. *Journal of Psychosomatic Research, 34*(3), 237–248.

VandeCreek, L., Pargament, K., Belavich, T., Cowell, B., & Friedel, L. (1999). The unique benefits of religious support during cardiac bypass surgery. *The Journal of Pastoral Care, 53*(1), 19–29.

Author Biography: Dr. Paul S. Bay received his Doctorate of Ministry degree from Christian Theological Seminary of Indianapolis, Indiana in 1997. He is Cardiovascular Care Chaplain for Clarian Health Partners which includes Indiana University Hospital, Methodist Hospital, and Riley Hospital for Children. In addition to being a Board Certified Chaplain he is also a Clinical Member of the American Association for Marriage and Family Therapy. He is the recipient of a National Institute for Healthcare Research, John Templeton Spirituality & Medicine Award and other grants of the Religion and Spiritual Integration Values of Clarian Health. Paul currently divides his time between research and patient care through the cardiovascular interdisciplinary team and heart transplant team.

ARTICLE 17

A Novel Picture Guide to Improve Spiritual Care and Reduce Anxiety in Mechanically Ventilated Adults in the Intensive Care Unit

Joel N. Berning[1], Armeen D. Poor[2], Sarah M. Buckley[2], Komal R. Patel[2], David J. Lederer[2,3], Nathan E. Goldstein[4,5], Daniel Brodie[2], and Matthew R. Baldwin[2]

1 NewYork-Presbyterian Hospital, Pastoral Care and Education Department, New York, New York;

2 Division of Pulmonary, Allergy, and Critical Care, Columbia University, College of Physicians and Surgeons, New York, New York;

3 Department of Epidemiology, Columbia University Mailman School of Public Health, New York, New York;

4 Department of Geriatrics and Palliative Medicine, Icahn School of Medicine at Mount Sinai, New York, New York;

5 Geriatrics Research Education and Clinical Center, James J. Peters VA Medical Center, New York, New York

(Received in original form December 21, 2015; accepted in final form April 19, 2016)

Supported by National Institutes of Health grants UL1 TR000040, KL2 TR000081, and K23AG045560. The views expressed in this article do not communicate an official position of National Institutes of Health.

Author Contributions: M.R.B. and A.D.P. had full access to all of the data in the study and take responsibility for the integrity of the data and accuracy of the data analysis. Study concept and design: M.R.B. and J.N.B. Acquisition, analysis, or interpretation of data: M.R.B., J.N.B., S.M.B., K.R.P., and A.D.P. Drafting of the manuscript: M.R.B. Critical revision of the manuscript for important intellectual content: M.R.B., J.N.B., D.B., N.E.G., and D.J.L. Statistical analysis: M.R.B. and A.D.P. Study supervision: M.R.B. and J.N.B.

Correspondence and requests for reprints should be addressed to Matthew R. Baldwin, M.D., M.S., Division of Pulmonary, Allergy, and Critical Care, 622 West 168th Street, PH-8E Room 101, New York, NY 10032.
E-mail: mrb45@cumc.columbia.edu

This article has an online supplement, which is accessible from this issue's table of contents at www.atsjournals.org

Ann Am Thorac Soc Vol 13, No 8, pp 1333–1342, Aug 2016

Berning, J.N., Poor, A.D., Buckley, S.M., Patel, K.R., Lederer, D.J., Goldstein, N.E., Brodie, D., and Baldwin, M.R. (2016) "A novel picture guide to improve spiritual care and reduce anxiety in mechanically ventilated adults in the intensive care unit." *Annals of the American Thoracic Society*, 13, 8, 1333–1342.

Copyright © 2016 by the American Thoracic Society
DOI: 10.1513/AnnalsATS.201512-831OC
Internet address: www.atsjournals.org

Abstract

Rationale: Hospital chaplains provide spiritual care that helps patients facing serious illness cope with their symptoms and prognosis, yet because mechanically ventilated patients cannot speak, spiritual care of these patients has been limited.

Objectives: To determine the feasibility and measure the effects of chaplain-led picture-guided spiritual care for mechanically ventilated adults in the intensive care unit (ICU).

Methods: We conducted a quasi-experimental study at a tertiary care hospital between March 2014 and July 2015. Fifty mechanically ventilated adults in medical or surgical ICUs without delirium or dementia received spiritual care by a hospital chaplain using an illustrated communication card to assess their spiritual affiliations, emotions, and needs and were followed until hospital discharge. Feasibility was assessed as the proportion of participants able to identify spiritual affiliations, emotions, and needs using the card. Among the first 25 participants, we performed semistructured interviews with 8 ICU survivors to identify how spiritual care helped them. For the subsequent 25 participants, we measured anxiety (on 100-mm visual analog scales [VAS]) immediately before and after the first chaplain visit, and we performed semistructured interviews with 18 ICU survivors with added measurements of pain and stress (on ±100-mm VAS).

Measurements and main results: The mean (SD) age was 59 (±16) years, median mechanical ventilation days was 19.5 (interquartile range, 7–29d), and 15 (30%) died in-hospital. Using the card, 50 (100%) identified a spiritual affiliation, 47 (94%) identified one or more emotions, 45 (90%) rated their spiritual pain, and 36 (72%) selected a chaplain intervention. Anxiety after the first visit decreased 31% (mean score change, −20; 95% confidence interval, −33 to −7). Among 28 ICU survivors, 26 (93%) remembered the intervention and underwent semistructured interviews, of whom 81% felt more capable of dealing with their hospitalization and 0% felt worse. The 18 ICU survivors who underwent additional VAS testing during semistructured follow-up interviews reported a 49-point reduction in stress (95% confidence interval, −72 to −24) and no significant change in physical pain that they attributed to picture-guided spiritual care.

Conclusions: Chaplain-led picture-guided spiritual care is feasible among mechanically ventilated adults and shows potential for reducing anxiety during and stress after an ICU admission.

Key words: spiritual therapies, palliative care, mechanical ventilators, critical care, anxiety

Mechanically ventilated patients in the intensive care unit (ICU) experience substantial psychoemotional distress, because endotracheal intubation or tracheostomy prevents the majority from speaking, and most observers cannot reliably lip-read.[1, 2, 3, 4, 5, 6] Attempts at having mechanically ventilated patients write or point to letters to spell out words have been often unsuccessful, because handwriting is often illegible and the process is time consuming.[7, 8] Nurse and chaplain interpretations of nods and gesticulations by mechanically ventilated patients are sometimes accurate, but there are also reports of misinterpretation causing significant miscommunication.[2, 9, 10] When critically ill patients are unable to self-report, nurses will often use cardiorespiratory signs, ventilator compliance, and facial expressions to identify symptoms that are present. However, similar changes in vital signs or behaviors may indicate a variety of different symptoms.[9, 11]

Communication cards may improve communication between mechanically ventilated patients and their providers,[12, 13] but only one rigorous study exists that evaluates communication cards as part of a comprehensive communication intervention with endotracheally intubated ICU patients and their nurses.[14] Since the adoption of minimized sedation as an ICU best practice,[15, 16] it has been estimated that half of mechanically ventilated patients may benefit from assistive communication tools.[17]

The Joint Commission and the National Quality Forum for Palliative Care guidelines include spiritual care as a component of their care standards,[18, 19] and studies in non-ICU settings have shown that many patients find religion or spirituality to be the most important factor enabling them to cope with serious illness.[20, 21, 22] Although previous studies in the ICU have shown that chaplain care is associated with increased family satisfaction,[23, 24] the focus has traditionally been on the family members of dying patients and not the patients themselves.[25] There is growing recognition of a need for a comprehensive approach to providing proactive spiritual support to ICU patients.[24, 25, 26, 27, 28]

Like other healthcare providers in the ICU, our chaplain experienced difficulty with lip-reading and interpreting behavioural signs in mechanically ventilated patients he saw in consultation. Therefore, he created an illustrated spiritual care communication card to facilitate the assessment of spiritual needs and guide spiritual care in mechanically ventilated adults in a systematic way that meets established criteria of the Association of Professional Chaplains' Standards of Practice for spiritual assessment and delivery of care in acute care settings.[29] The card contains four sections that allow mechanically ventilated patients to point to pictures and words that indicate their (1) spiritual or religious affiliation, (2) emotions, (3) spiritual pain, and (4) desired chaplain interventions.

We aimed to determine the feasibility and measure the effects of chaplain-led picture-guided spiritual care in mechanically ventilated adult ICU patients. We hypothesized that awake and alert mechanically ventilated adult ICU patients without delirium or dementia would be able to identify their spiritual preferences and needs using the illustrated communication card and that, in turn, the chaplain would provide spiritual care that would alleviate their psychoemotional distress during and after the ICU admission.

Methods
Study design and participants
We performed a single-center prospective cohort study at an urban, tertiary care medical center. Between March 2014 and July 2015, we screened adults 18 years of age or older with 6 or more hours of mechanical ventilation who had no history of dementia, no advanced chronic neurologic disease (e.g., amyotrophic lateral sclerosis, Parkinson's disease) or stroke with receptive or expressive aphasias, were known to understand English or Spanish, and who by ICU nurse report had a Richmond Agitation Sedation Score of 0 or −1 and followed simple commands.[30] Patients were considered eligible if they were alert and oriented to self, place, and time by nodding appropriately to orientation questions and were not delirious as measured by the Confusion Assessment Method ICU survey.[31] We screened Monday to Friday when the medical ICU (MICU) chaplain was working and available to see adult ICU patients, and on weekends when the chaplain and at least one of the other staff involved in screening and assessments were on call. We preferentially screened MICU patients, because our MICU chaplain developed the spiritual care communication card for use. When no MICU patients were eligible, we then screened surgical ICU (SICU) patients who met the above criteria and who were not already receiving care by another chaplain.

Given our patients' frequent inability to write, we obtained a waiver of signed consent and reviewed with eligible patients an information sheet that explained the study procedures. Only those who nodded in assent to participation were included in the study. The study was approved by the Columbia University Medical Center Institutional Review Board.

Picture-guided spiritual care

Our MICU chaplain (J.N.B.) developed the illustrated spiritual care communication card (Figure 1; see Figure E1 in the online supplement[1]) and provided all of the picture-guided spiritual care to study participants, speaking either in English or Spanish. He is a member of the Association of Professional Chaplains, has a Master's of Divinity, and completed six units of Clinical Pastoral Education accredited by the Association for Clinical Pastoral Education. He developed the illustrated spiritual care communication card with four sections that reflect the domains of a spiritual assessment that would be typically assessed by a chaplain through conversation but instead can be assessed by having the user point to pictures and words to: (1) identify spiritual or religious affiliations; (2) identify a range of feelings; (3) rate spiritual pain;[32] and (4) select a desired religious, spiritual, or non-spiritual intervention that a chaplain can offer (Figure 1). He developed the range of feelings a patient could identify based first on the four classes of feelings that he was trained to assess when caring for someone: anger, happiness, sadness, and fear.[33] He then intuitively added five more emotions to each class and worked with an illustrator to create cartoon faces associated with each of these emotions so that patients could describe their feelings by pointing to one or more of 24 emotions.

The chaplain first reviewed the participant's state of health by speaking with providers and reviewing the medical record. He then introduced himself to the participant and led him or her through each of the four sections of the communication card. This structured chaplain-led picture-guided spiritual care meets Standards of Practice by the Association of Professional Chaplains by evaluating relevant information pertinent to the care of a recipient's bio-psycho-social-spiritual/religious health and by implementing a culturally sensitive plan of care to promote the well-being of the recipient.[29] For participants who did not select any desired chaplain intervention, the chaplain offered well wishes specific to their hospitalization. The chaplain revisited participants during their hospitalization if they desired a chaplain intervention to be repeated (e.g., prayer) or if they had ongoing psychoemotional distress for which they desired follow-up spiritual care. During revisits, he used the communication card to guide spiritual care only if a participant remained mechanically ventilated.

---

1   Please see the original publication of this article for the link to the additional file.

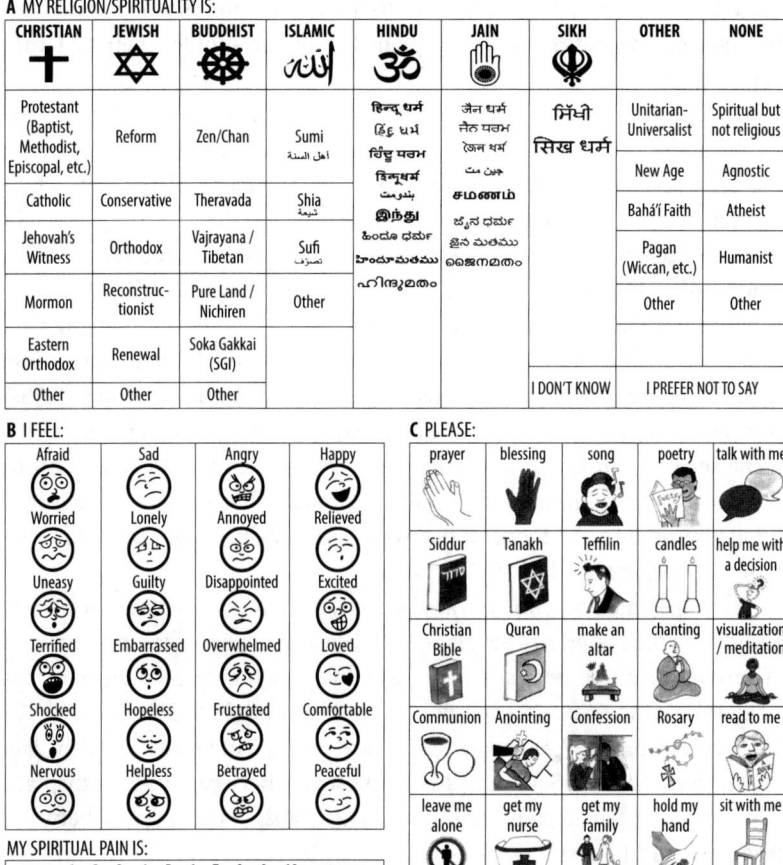

Figure 1: Spiritual care communication card (English version)

(A) Front side. Part 1: Spiritual/religious affiliation assessment. (B) Back side. Part 2: Feelings assessment; Part 3: Spiritual pain assessment; Part 4: Chaplain interventions assessment. The communication card is 11 × 17 inches and laminated. See Figure E1 in the online supplement for Spanish version.[2]

Measurements

We assessed the feasibility of using the illustrated communication card to guide spiritual care by (1) measuring the proportions of participants who were able to identify or confirm their spiritual or religious affiliation, identify at least one emotion, rate their spiritual pain on a 0 to 10 integer scale, and select at least one desired chaplain intervention when using the communication card for the first time; and by (2) measuring the time

---

2   Please see the original publication of this article for the link to the additional file.

needed to complete the four sections of the communication card and the time of the entire initial chaplain-led picture-guided spiritual care consultation.

We measured the effect of chaplain-led picture-guided spiritual care for mechanically ventilated ICU patients using a two-phase approach that is described in detail in the online supplement.[3] Briefly, because we were initially unsure how participants would react to engaging in communication about their emotions and spiritual needs, we first conducted semistructured exploratory interviews with ICU survivors from the first half of study participants (n = 25) to identify the common symptoms picture-guided spiritual care treated. On the basis of our review of these interviews, we then added 100-mm visual analog scales (VASs) to measure anxiety immediately before and after the initial chaplain visit in the second half of study participants (n = 25) and ±100-mm VAS to measure changes in stress and pain attributed to chaplain-led picture-guided spiritual care among those who survived intensive care and were awaiting hospital discharge.

Demographic and clinical variables were obtained from the electronic medical record. *A priori*, we planned subgroup analyses comparing VAS anxiety and stress scores between participants who were younger versus older, religious versus non-religious, cared for in the MICU versus SICU, and received picture-guided spiritual care in English versus Spanish. *Post hoc*, we compared VAS anxiety and stress scores between organ transplant recipients and participants without organ transplantation and between decedents and ICU survivors.

---

[3] Please see the original publication of this article for the link to the additional file.

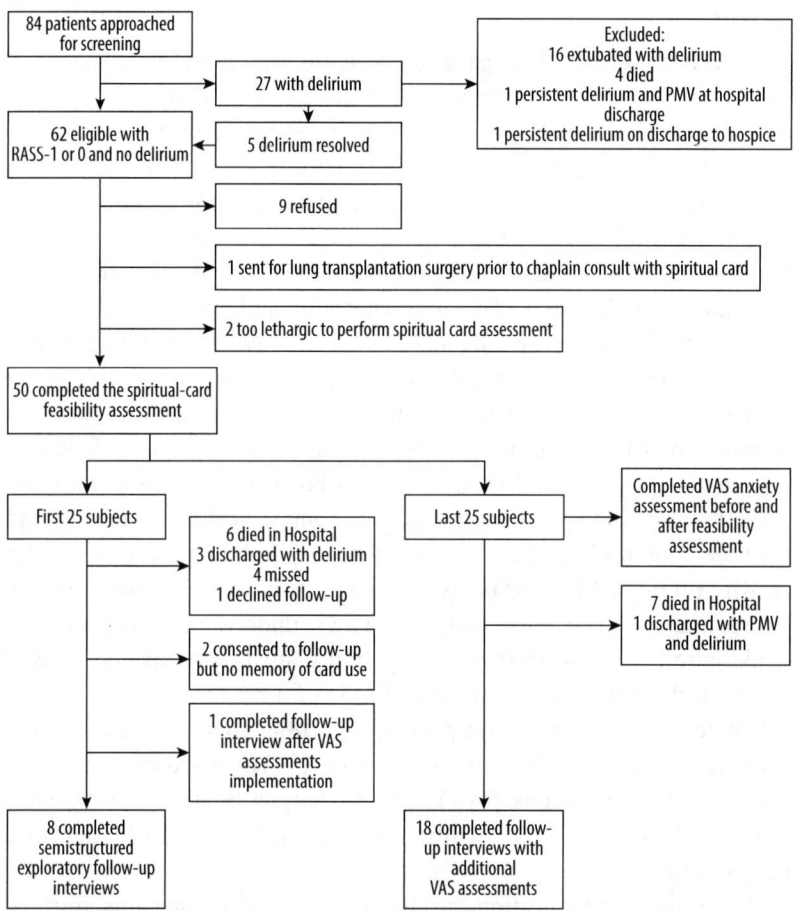

Figure 2: Study participants

PMV = prolonged mechanical ventilation; RASS = Richmond Agitation-Sedation Scale; VAS = visual analog scale.

Statistical analysis

We present categorical data using percentages and continuous data as mean (±SD) or median (interquartile range [IQR]). We compared 100-mm VAS anxiety scores immediately before and after the initial chaplain-led picture-guided spiritual care consult using the Wilcoxon signed-rank test and compared ±100-mm VAS scores measuring change in stress and pain attributed to spiritual care among ICU survivors to 0 (no change), also using Wilcoxon signed-rank test. Statistical significance was defined as a two-tailed $P < 0.05$. Analyses were performed with Stata 13.0 (Stata Corp., College Station, TX).

Results

We screened 84 adult ICU patients receiving mechanical ventilation; 27 were found to have delirium and were initially excluded, but 5 had no delirium on a subsequent day of screening and remained mechanically ventilated, resulting in 62 eligible patients. Nine (15%) declined to participate, one (1.6%) enrolled but underwent lung transplantation before receiving picture-guided spiritual care, and two (3.2%) enrolled but were too lethargic to use the card. Fifty (81%) completed a feasibility assessment on the same day after enrolling and were followed until hospital discharge. Figure 2 details participant flow through the study.

Participants had a mean (SD) age 59 (±16) years and a wide range of Acute Physiology and Chronic Health Evaluation II scores. The most common indications for mechanical ventilation were respiratory failure or distress and pneumonia. Participants were of diverse races/ethnicities, and 10 (20%) used the Spanish version of the communication card. They had multiple comorbidities (Charlson comorbidity index median [IQR], 2.5 [1–4]). Although 14 participants (28%) were solid organ or bone marrow transplantation recipients, only 6 (12%) underwent transplantation while enrolled in the study (all lung transplants). Participants received mechanical ventilation for a median (IQR) of 19.5 (7–29) days, and 23 (46%) received a tracheostomy. Forty-two (84%) met the most recent consensus definition of chronic critical illness.[34] The in-hospital mortality was 30%, 17 participants (34%) were discharged home, 17 (34%) were discharged to skilled-care facilities, and one (2%) was discharged to a hospice (Table 1).

Using the communication card for the first time, participants' spiritual affiliation was identified 100% of the time, 47 participants (94%) were able to identify one or more emotion, 45 participants (90%) rated their spiritual pain, and 36 (72%) selected a desired chaplain intervention. It took participants a median (IQR) of 8.5 minutes (5–13) to complete the four sections of the communication card, and it took the chaplain a median (IQR) of 18 (11–25) minutes to both use the card with participants and provide a desired spiritual care intervention (Table 2).

Table 1: Subject characteristics

Characteristic (n = 50)	Measure
Age (mean, SD), yr	59, 16
Male	28 (56)
Race	
• White	25 (50)

• Hispanic	12 (24)
• Black	9 (18)
• Southeast Asian	4 (8)
Card language used	
• English	40 (80)
• Spanish	10 (20)
APACHE II (mean, SD)	22, 7.0
Charlson Index (median, IQR)	2.5, 1–4
Cancer	
• Solid tumor with metastatic disease	2 (4)
• Hematologic malignancy	6 (12)
Organ transplantation	14 (28)
• Lung transplantation during hospitalization	6 (12)
• Prior lung transplantation	4 (8)
• Prior renal transplantation	3 (6)
• Prior bone marrow transplantation	1 (2)
Type of ICU	
• Medical	42 (84)
• Surgical	8 (16)
Total mechanical ventilation days (median, IQR)	19.5, 7–29
Mechanical ventilation via tracheostomy	23 (46)
Days of mechanical ventilation before picture-guided spiritual care (median, IQR)	7, 2–14
Total ICU length of stay (median, IQR)	22, 13–43
Total hospital length of stay (median, IQR)	42, 26–69
Primary ICU admission diagnosis category	
• Pulmonary	31 (62)
• Cardiac, medical	3 (6)
• Sepsis or infection	3 (6)
• Gastrointestinal	1 (2)
• Neurological	2 (4)
• Oncology	1 (2)
• Shock	3 (6)
• Surgical	5 (10)
• Vascular	1 (2)

Indication for mechanical ventilation	
• Respiratory failure or distress	6 (12)
• Pneumonia	12 (24)
• Pulmonary edema	1 (2)
• Hypoxemia	8 (16)
• ARDS	4 (8)
• Asthma	2 (4)
• Cystic fibrosis exacerbation	2 (4)
• Cardiac arrest	1 (2)
• Airway protection	6 (12)
• Postoperative	7 (14)
• Angioedema	1 (2)
Discharge disposition	
• Home	17 (34)
• Acute rehabilitation	6 (12)
• Skilled care facility	11 (22)
• Hospice	1 (2)
• Died	15 (30)

Data are presented as n (%) unless otherwise noted.
Definition of abbreviations: APACHE = Acute Physiology and Chronic Health Evaluation; ARDS = acute respiratory distress syndrome; ICU = intensive care unit; IQR = interquartile range.

Table 2: Chaplain-led picture-guided spiritual care feasibility assessment

Communication card part 1: Identify a religious or spiritual affiliation	Measure
Affiliation identified	50 (100)
Communication card used to confirm affiliation*	34 (68)
Communication card used to identify an affiliation different from what was listed in the medical record	7 (14)
Communication card used to identify an affiliation when none was listed in the medical record	9 (18)
Religion or spiritual preference	
• Catholic	28 (56)
• Jewish	5 (10)
• Nondenominational Christian	3 (6)
• Baptist	2 (4)
• Presbyterian	1 (2)
• Pentecostal	1 (2)

• Buddhist	1 (2)
• Hindu	1 (2)
• Islamic	1 (2)
• Agnostic	1 (2)
• No spiritual or religious affiliation	1 (2)
Communication card part 2: Identify emotions	
• Identified ≥1 emotion	47 (94)
• No emotions identified	3 (6)
• Types of emotions identified† (n = 47)	
− General emotion: fear	18 (38)
− General emotion: sadness	29 (62)
− General emotion: anger	23 (49)
− General emotion: happiness	23 (49)
• Groupings of emotions (n = 47)	
− Happiness only	9 (19)
− ≥1 Negative emotion only	24 (51)
− Happiness + 1 negative emotion	6 (13)
− Happiness + 2 negative emotions	3 (6)
− Happiness + 3 negative emotions	5 (11)
Communication card part 3: Rate spiritual pain	
• Able to rate spiritual pain	45 (90)
• Spiritual pain, integer scale 0–10 (mean, SD)	4.2, 3.7
• Spiritual pain score (n = 45)	
− 0	14 (31)
− 1–4	9 (20)
− 5–7	10 (22)
− 8–10	12 (27)
Communication card part 4: Identify chaplain intervention	
• Identified ≥1 desired intervention	36 (72)
• Did not identify any intervention	14 (28)
• Type of intervention identified (n = 36)	
− Religious intervention	27 (75)
» Prayer	18 (50)
» Give blessing	9 (25)
» Read Christian Bible	3 (8.3)
» Receive communion	9 (25)

cont.

» Anointing	5 (14)
» Confession	4 (11)
» Pray with rosary	8 (22)
» Make an altar	0 (0)
» Siddur	0 (0)
» Tankah	0 (0)
» Tefillin	0 (0)
» Read Quran	1 (2.8)
» Chanting music	0 (0)
− Nonreligious intervention	12 (33)
» Song	5 (14)
» Poetry	2 (5.6)
» Electronic candles	1 (2.8)
» Talk with me	2 (5.6)
» Visualization	3 (8.3)
» Read	4 (11)
» Hold hand	5 (14)
» Sit with me	3 (8.3)
» Help with a decision	1 (2.7)
− Get other help	5 (14)
» Get family	5 (14)
» Get nurse	2 (5.6)
− Leave me alone	1 (2.7)
Duration and No. of chaplain visits	
• Initial card use time, min, (median, IQR)	8.5, 5–13
• Total initial consult time, min, (median, IQR)	18, 11–25
• No. of follow-up visits with chaplain, (median, IQR)	2, 0–3
• Follow-up visit count by time, min	
− <10	64 (42)
− 11–25	42 (28)
− 26–39	23 (15)
− >40	23 (15)

Definition of abbreviation: IQR = interquartile range. Data presented as n (%) unless otherwise noted. Participants were allowed to select more than one emotion or chaplain intervention. Therefore, percentages may add to up to greater than 100%.

*The chaplain first obtained a religious affiliation from the medical record or family, and the participant nodded in acknowledgment when asked his/her preference.

†Participants pointed to cartoon faces with a descriptive word above each face (see Figure 1). There were four general emotion categories, each with specific faces: (1): fear: afraid, worried, uneasy,

terrified, shocked, nervous; (2) sadness: sad, lonely, guilty, embarrassed, hopeless, helpless; (3) anger: angry, annoyed, disappointed, overwhelmed, frustrated, betrayed; (4) happiness: happy, relieved, excited, loved, comfortable, peaceful. Numbers and percentages of specific emotions identified are listed in Table E1 in the online supplement.[4]

Table 3: Intensive care unit survivors' responses to an open-ended question about why chaplain-led picture-guided spiritual care is helpful

"It was very helpful at the time to just reset everything, to gauge where you're at and where you need to be…"
"I'm normally not the most spiritual or if you want to say religious person. The fact that there's different interventions that are universally comforting—that's really helpful because you don't know what kind of patient you have. And I think anyone would take a blessing, even if you're the most hardcore…"
"It's a relief, a guide for expression."
"It's more than just a tool; it's an outlet. You need that."
"A [chaplain visit] is soothing to the patient and family: it's ok to have all of these feelings, that I can feel serenity from sadness. It gives me permission to feel all this and that that is ok and part of the process of healing. Validation of it being ok to feel how you feel. It's ok to be upset. Patients want to impress doctors and nurses and they can't always."
"It gave me more calmness, more acceptance."
"Made me think for sure. With the numbers. How, for example, disappointed or excited I was… It made me think. Pretty helpful. Especially the feelings page. Made me think about how I felt about being afraid, disappointed. Made me think about my emotions—which was helpful. A lot of times you get overwhelmed by your feelings, especially when you're sick or in a moment of stress."
"I just felt more at peace" because "I was able to communicate."
"It may not change the physical pain, but it can help to reduce or decrease the pain by relaxing or calming the patient."
"It's helpful that it even prompts you to think about it all. When you're lying there in pain and anxiety, it's difficult to even think."
"The visit from the chaplain is extremely helpful. Talking to a chaplain or a person that has the ability to help give you interior peace and to help you with your fears and frustrations means a lot to anyone and helps you to feel better."

Excerpts of responses; all responses from all intensive care unit survivors interviewed are listed in Table E3 in the online supplement.[5]

For 34 participants (68%), identifying a spiritual affiliation consisted of the chaplain pointing to the affiliation on the card that was listed in the medical record or given by family members and observing the subject nod in acknowledgment. However, seven participants (14%) used the card to identify a spiritual affiliation that was different from what was

---

4 Please see the original publication of this article for the link to the additional file.
5 Please see the original publication of this article for the link to the additional file.

listed in the medical record. Participants had diverse spiritual or religious affiliations, with most being either Catholic (56%) or Jewish (10%), and seven (14%) identified themselves as agnostic or having no spiritual or religious affiliation (Table 2).

Participants' emotions varied widely (Table 2, Table E1[6]). Forty-eight participants (51%) felt only negative emotions (fear, sadness, and anger), and nine (19%) reported only feeling happy. Fourteen (30%) reported feeling both happy and negative emotions. On a 0 to 10 integer scale, participants' mean (SD) spiritual pain was 4.2 (±3.7) (Table 2). Among the 36 participants (72%) who selected one or more desired chaplain interventions, 75% requested religious interventions and 33% requested nonreligious interventions (Table 2). Only one subject (2.7%) indicated that he wished to be left alone after using the first three sections of the communication card. The chaplain revisited study participants during their hospitalization to provide additional spiritual care a median (IQR) of two (zero to three) times, with 70% of revisits lasting less than 25 minutes (Table 2).

Among the second half of participants (n = 25), in whom anxiety was measured by VAS immediately before and after the initial chaplain-led picture-guided spiritual care, anxiety decreased from a mean (SD) VAS score of 64 (±29) to 44 (±28) (mean absolute reduction of 20 points, 95% confidence interval [CI], –33 to –7; P = 0.002; mean relative reduction, 31%; 95% CI, –48% to –15%; P = 0.001) (Figure 3). Among 28 ICU survivors who consented to follow-up interviews, 26 (93%) remembered receiving the chaplain's picture-guided spiritual care in the ICU and completed the semistructured interviews. Eighty-one percent reported that they felt more capable of dealing with their hospitalization, 81% felt more at peace, 71% felt more connected with what is sacred, 96% would recommend chaplain-led picture-guided spiritual care to others, and 0% felt worse after receiving spiritual care (Table E2[7]). Their responses to an open-ended question about why chaplain-led picture-guided spiritual care is helpful are listed in Table 3 and Table E3[8]. Many participants report decreased anxiety and stress due to being able to communicate using the card, and several describe improved coping having recognized and acknowledged their feelings with the chaplain. On average, ICU survivors who underwent ±100-mm VAS testing at follow up (n = 18) reported mean 49-point reduction in stress (95% CI, –72 to –24; P =

---

6   Please see the original publication of this article for the link to the additional file.
7   Please see the original publication of this article for the link to the additional file.
8   Please see the original publication of this article for the link to the additional file.

0.002) and no significant change in physical pain due to chaplain-led picture-guided spiritual care (Table E2[9]).

Younger, nonreligious, English-speaking MICU participants reported slightly greater reductions in anxiety and stress than older, religious, Spanish-speaking SICU participants. Those who ultimately survived the ICU tended to report greater reductions in anxiety after the first chaplain visit than those who ultimately died or were discharged to a hospice. The four participants (8%) who underwent lung transplant during study enrollment reported a similar reduction in stress attributed to spiritual care compared with both those who underwent organ transplantation before the study period and those without organ transplantation. Given the small subsample sizes, these results should be considered preliminary and interpreted with caution (Table E4[10]).

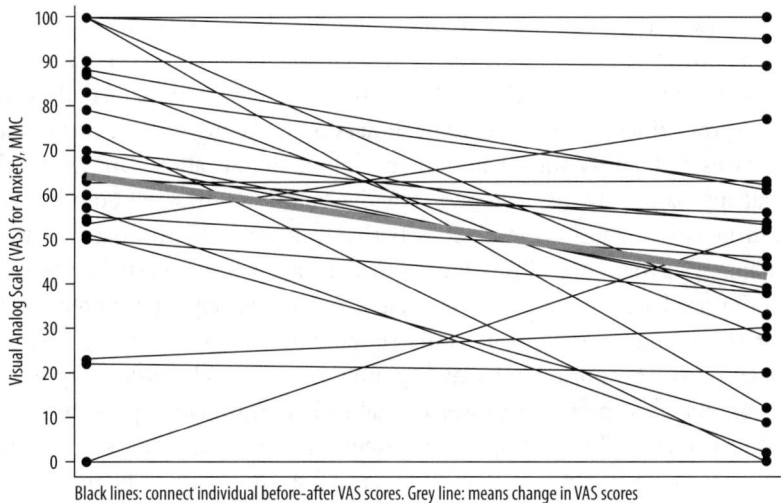

Black lines: connect individual before-after VAS scores. Grey line: means change in VAS scores

Figure 3: Visual Analog Scale (VAS) for Anxiety

Anxiety was measured with 100-mm visual analog scale (VAS) immediately before and after the first time the participant received chaplain-led picture-guided spiritual care among the second half of participants (n = 25). Anxiety decreased from a mean (SD) VAS score of 64 (29) to 44 (28) (mean absolute reduction of 20 points; 95% confidence interval, −33 to −7; P = 0.002; mean relative reduction of 31%; 95% confidence interval, −48% to −15%; P = 0.001)

---

9   Please see the original publication of this article for the link to the additional file.
10 Please see the original publication of this article for the link to the additional file.

Discussion

We have shown in a single-center cohort study that it is feasible to use a novel picture guide to assist chaplains with spiritual care for awake and alert mechanically ventilated adults in the ICU. Participants reported an immediate reduction in anxiety after receiving this care for the first time, and those who survived intensive care reported a reduction in stress that they attributed to picture-guided spiritual care. To our knowledge, this is the first clinical study to test a structured, integrative, and measurable approach to chaplain care aimed at treating anxiety and stress and improving coping in mechanically ventilated ICU patients. Using this unique spiritual assessment tool with ICU patients opens a novel area of chaplaincy and palliative care clinical research.

Picture-guided spiritual care may reduce anxiety during and stress after an ICU admission in several ways. Survivors of mechanical ventilation report feeling anxious and lonely because they cannot communicate vocally.[1, 5, 35] Using the communication board with the chaplain addresses a mechanically ventilated patient's fundamental need to express him or herself and to be understood. Having participants point to faces to identify their emotions on the communication card revealed that approximately 50% felt only negative emotions, 30% felt both happy and negative emotions, and 20% felt only happy. On the basis of the chaplain's experience of providing spiritual care to study participants, the high prevalence of happiness seemed to reflect participants' appreciation for still being alive and for family support they were receiving. Several ICU survivors reported in follow-up interviews that acknowledging their emotions with the chaplain was crucial to helping them cope with their critical illness. This finding is consistent with prior studies in non-ICU settings that have shown many patients find spiritual care to be the single most important factor enabling them to cope with a serious illness.[20, 21, 22] More than half of participants rated their spiritual pain greater than or equal to 5 on a 0 to 10 integer scale, and higher spiritual pain scores have been shown to be associated with lower spiritual quality of life and adverse physical and emotional symptoms.[32] The desired chaplain interventions that a patient selected, whether or not religious, focused on comforting the patient and improving his or her well-being in the context of both his or her spiritual pain and critical illness.

This study answers calls for more rigorous studies of spiritual and religious interventions,[36] a need to develop a comprehensive approach to assess and meet the spiritual needs of patients,[24, 26, 37, 38] and for research aimed at improving critical illness survivorship.[39] A 2012 Cochrane review found inconclusive evidence that palliative care teams with a chaplain help terminally ill patients feel emotionally supported, but note that patients' emotions and ability to cope were not well measured.[36] We specifically measured participants' emotions, showed improvement in symptoms of anxiety and stress, and elicited feedback that suggests spiritual care helps ICU survivors cope with critical illness. Prior studies have shown that chaplain-led spiritual care improves family satisfaction with end-of-life care in the ICU,[23, 24] but our study is the first to proactively and systematically engage mechanically ventilated ICU patients who are not necessarily dying. With technological advances, many critically ill patients now survive what were previously fatal illnesses,[40, 41] but survivors of mechanical ventilation are increasingly recognized to suffer from anxiety, depression, and post-traumatic stress disorder.[42, 43, 44] Our finding that chaplain-led spiritual care potentially improves stress after the ICU and helps ICU survivors' ability to cope raises the possibility that chaplain-led picture-guided spiritual care with follow up may be able to help prevent or alleviate these psychiatric sequelae of critical illness.

Our study has several limitations. A single chaplain provided all of the picture-guided spiritual care. Participants were primarily MICU patients sampled from an urban tertiary care center with several organ transplantation programs, but our subgroup analyses suggest little difference in the magnitude of anxiety and stress reduction in transplant and nontransplant patients who received mechanical ventilation. The feasibility of chaplain-led picture-guided spiritual care needs to be externally validated with other chaplains, in cardiac and pediatric ICU patients, and in other hospitals where case mix and patient care may differ. These validation studies should also evaluate the psychometrics of the spiritual care communication card and assess whether refinements to the card should be made. Although other ICU healthcare providers could potentially use parts of the card to screen for patients with spiritual care needs, we recommend at this time that only chaplains use the card, because they are formally trained in how to best engage communication on spiritual matters. We did not study how spiritual care affected end-of-life care among decedents, but prior studies have already shown a benefit.[23, 24] Future studies of chaplain-led picture-guided spiritual care should evaluate its effect on those who die in the ICU and their families' satisfaction with ICU care. We limited our measurements of symptoms to 100-mm VAS for anxiety after the first visit and stress and pain among ICU survivors at a single follow-up visit. Future studies should consider using more comprehensive and repeated assessments of symptoms,[45, 46] spiritual quality of life,[47] and coping.[48, 49, 50] to determine the optimal dose of spiritual care needed to improve well-being. Although our quasi-experimental study design shows a potential for efficacy of chaplain-led picture-guided spiritual care, there is no psychometric measurement support for asking subjects to recall stress reduction. Furthermore, only a randomized controlled trial can prove efficacy, and measurements of anxiety, depression, and post-traumatic stress disorder after hospital discharge should be considered as an outcome among ICU survivors.

In conclusion, our findings demonstrate that chaplain-led picture-guided spiritual care is feasible among awake and alert mechanically ventilated adults and suggest that it may reduce anxiety during and stress after an ICU admission. Using this novel picture guide will facilitate a paradigm shift in the role of chaplains in acute care settings. Instead of primarily being consulted just before a patient's death in the ICU, chaplains can now provide interactive spiritual support to mechanically ventilated ICU patients. This strategy represents a significant step forward in being able to integrate spiritual care with intensive care and shows promise to improve adult patients' well-being both during and after critical illness.

Author disclosures are available with the text of this article at www.atsjournals.org.

References

1. Khalaila R, Zbidat W, Anwar K, Bayya A, Linton DM, Sviri S. Communication difficulties and psychoemotional distress in patients receiving mechanical ventilation. *Am J Crit Care* 2011;20: 470–479.
2. Patak L, Gawlinski A, Fung NI, Doering L, Berg J. Patients' reports of health care practitioner interventions that are related to communication during mechanical ventilation. *Heart Lung* 2004;33:308–320.
3. Happ MB, Garrett K, Thomas DD, Tate J, George E, Houze M, Radtke J, Sereika S. Nurse-patient communication interactions in the intensive care unit. *Am J Crit Care* 2011;20:e28–e40.
4. Meltzer EC, Gallagher JJ, Suppes A, Fins JJ. Lip-reading and the ventilated patient. *Crit Care Med* 2012;40:1529–1531.
5. Tate JA, Devito Dabbs A, Hoffman LA, Milbrandt E, Happ MB. Anxiety and agitation in mechanically ventilated patients. *Qual Health Res* 2012;22:157–173.
6. Happ MB. Caring to communicate revisited. *Crit Care Med* 2012;40:1672–1673.
7. Albarran AW. A review of communication with intubated patients and those with tracheostomies within an intensive care environment. *Intensive Care Nurs* 1991;7:179–186.
8. Lawless CA. Helping patients with endotracheal and tracheostomy tubes communicate. *Am J Nurs* 1975;75:2151–2153.
9. Campbell GB, Happ MB. Symptom identification in the chronically critically ill. *AACN Adv Crit Care* 2010;21:64–79.
10. Gleason JJ. The pastoral caregiver's casebook. Valley Forge, PA: Judson Press; 2015.
11. Puntillo KA, Smith D, Arai S, Stotts N. Critical care nurses provide their perspectives of patients' symptoms in intensive care units. *Heart Lung* 2008;37:466–475.

12. Patak L, Gawlinski A, Fung NI, Doering L, Berg J, Henneman EA. Communication boards in critical care: patients' views. *Appl Nurs Res* 2006;19:182–190.
13. Stovsky B, Rudy E, Dragonette P. Comparison of two types of communication methods used after cardiac surgery with patients with endotracheal tubes. *Heart Lung* 1988;17:281–289.
14. Happ MB, Garrett KL, Tate JA, DiVirgilio D, Houze MP, Demirci JR, George E, Sereika SM. Effect of a multi-level intervention on nurse-patient communication in the intensive care unit: results of the SPEACS trial. *Heart Lung* 2014;43:89–98.
15. Barr J, Pandharipande PP. The pain, agitation, and delirium care bundle: synergistic benefits of implementing the 2013 Pain, Agitation, and Delirium Guidelines in an integrated and interdisciplinary fashion. *Crit Care Med* 2013;41:S99–S115.
16. Riker RR, Fraser GL. Altering intensive care sedation paradigms to improve patient outcomes. *Crit Care Clin* 2009;25:527–538, viii–ix.
17. Happ MB, Seaman JB, Nilsen ML, Sciulli A, Tate JA, Saul M, Barnato AE. The number of mechanically ventilated ICU patients meeting communication criteria. *Heart Lung* 2015;44:45–49.
18. Hodge DR. A template for spiritual assessment: a review of the JCAHO requirements and guidelines for implementation. *Soc Work* 2006;51:317–326.
19. Ferrell B, Connor SR, Cordes A, Dahlin CM, Fine PG, Hutton N, Leenay M, Lentz J, Person JL, Meier DE et al.; National Consensus Project for Quality Palliative Care Task Force Members. The national agenda for quality palliative care: the National Consensus Project and the National Quality Forum. *J Pain Symptom Manage* 2007;33:737–744.
20. Koenig HG, Bearon LB, Hover M, Travis JL III. Religious perspectives of doctors, nurses, patients, and families. *J Pastoral Care* 1991;45:254–267.
21. Balboni TA, Vanderwerker LC, Block SD, Paulk ME, Lathan CS, Peteet JR, Prigerson HG. Religiousness and spiritual support among advanced cancer patients and associations with end-of-life treatment preferences and quality of life. *J Clin Oncol* 2007;25:555–560.
22. Ehman JW, Ott BB, Short TH, Ciampa RC, Hansen-Flaschen J. Do patients want physicians to inquire about their spiritual or religious beliefs if they become gravely ill? *Arch Intern Med* 1999;159:1803–1806.
23. Johnson JR, Engelberg RA, Nielsen EL, Kross EK, Smith NL, Hanada JC, Doll O'Mahoney SK, Curtis JR. The association of spiritual care providers' activities with family members' satisfaction with care after a death in the ICU. *Crit Care Med* 2014;42:1991–2000.
24. Wall RJ, Engelberg RA, Gries CJ, Glavan B, Curtis JR. Spiritual care of families in the intensive care unit. *Crit Care Med* 2007;35:1084–1090.
25. Choi PJ, Curlin FA, Cox CE. "The patient is dying, please call the chaplain": the activities of chaplains in one medical center's intensive care units. *J Pain Symptom Manage* 2015;50:501–506.
26. Todres ID, Catlin EA, Thiel MM. The intensivist in a spiritual care training program adapted for clinicians. *Crit Care Med* 2005;33:2733–2736.
27. Selman L, Young T, Vermandere M, Stirling I, Leget C; Research Subgroup of European Association for Palliative Care Spiritual Care Taskforce. Research priorities in spiritual care: an international survey of palliative care researchers and clinicians. *J Pain Symptom Manage* 2014;48:518–531.
28. Sulmasy DP. Spirituality, religion, and clinical care. *Chest* 2009;135:1634–1642.
29. The Association of Professional Chaplains. Standards of practice in acute care. 2009 [accessed 2015 Jul 22]. Available from: www.professionalchaplains.org/files/professional_standards/standards_of_practice/standards_practice_professional_chaplains_acute_care.pdf.
30. Ely EW, Truman B, Shintani A, Thomason JW, Wheeler AP, Gordon S, Francis J, Speroff T, Gautam S, Margolin R, et al. Monitoring sedation status over time in ICU patients: reliability and validity of the Richmond Agitation-Sedation Scale (RASS). *JAMA* 2003;289:2983–2991.

31. Ely EW, Inouye SK, Bernard GR, Gordon S, Francis J, May L, Truman B, Speroff T, Gautum S, Margolin R, et al. Delirium in mechanically ventilated patients: validity and reliability of the confusion assessment method for the intensive care unit (CAM-ICU). *JAMA* 2001;286:2703–2710.
32. Delgado-Guay MO, Hui D, Parsons HA, Govan K, De la Cruz M, Thorney S, Bruesa E. Spirituality, religiosity, and spiritual pain in advanced cancer patients. *J Pain Symptom Manage* 2011;41:986–994.
33. Hill CE. Helping skills: facilitation exploration, insight, and action. Washington DC: American Psychological Association; 2009.
34. Kahn JM, Le T, Angus DC, Cox CE, Hough CL, White DB, Yende S, Casson SS. ProVent Study Group Investigators. The epidemiology of chronic critical illness in the United States. *Crit Care Med* 2015;43:282–287.
35. Rotondi AJ, Chelluri L, Sirio C, Mendelsohn A, Schulz R, Belle S, Im K, Donahoe M, Pinsky MR. Patients' recollections of stressful experiences while receiving prolonged mechanical ventilation in an intensive care unit. *Crit Care Med* 2002;30:746–752.
36. Candy B, Jones L, Varagunam M, Speck P, Tookman A, King M. Spiritual and religious interventions for well-being of adults in the terminal phase of disease. *Cochrane Database Syst Rev* 2012;5:CD007544.
37. Danis M, Pollack JM. The valuable contribution of spiritual care to end-of-life care in the ICU. *Crit Care Med* 2014;42:2131–2132.
38. McBride JL, Pilkington L, Arthur G. Development of brief pictorial instruments for assessing spirituality in primary care. *J Ambul Care Manage* 1998;21:53–61.
39. Iwashyna TJ. Survivorship will be the defining challenge of critical care in the 21st century. *Ann Intern Med* 2010;153:204–205.
40. Spragg RG, Bernard GR, Checkley W, Curtis JR, Gajic O, Guyatt G, Hall J, Israel E, Jain M, Needham DM, et al. Beyond mortality: future clinical research in acute lung injury. *Am J Respir Crit Care Med* 2010;181:1121–1127.
41. Lerolle N, Trinquart L, Bornstain C, Tadié JM, Imbert A, Diehl JL, Fagon JY, Guérot E. Increased intensity of treatment and decreased mortality in elderly patients in an intensive care unit over a decade. *Crit Care Med* 2010;38:59–64.
42. Mikkelsen ME, Christie JD, Lanken PN, Biester RC, Thompson BT, Bellamy SL, Localio AR, Demissie E, Hopkins RO, Angus DC. The adult respiratory distress syndrome cognitive outcomes study: long-term neuropsychological function in survivors of acute lung injury. *Am J Respir Crit Care Med* 2012;185:1307–1315.
43. Davydow DS, Gifford JM, Desai SV, Needham DM, Bienvenu OJ. Posttraumatic stress disorder in general intensive care unit survivors: a systematic review. *Gen Hosp Psychiatry* 2008;30:421–434.
44. Wunsch H, Christiansen CF, Johansen MB, Olsen M, Ali N, Angus DC, Sørensen HT. Psychiatric diagnoses and psychoactive medication use among nonsurgical critically ill patients receiving mechanical ventilation. *JAMA* 2014;311:1133–1142.
45. Chang VT, Hwang SS, Feuerman M. Validation of the Edmonton Symptom Assessment Scale. *Cancer* 2000;88:2164–2171.
46. Nelson JE, Meier DE, Oei EJ, Nierman DM, Senzed RS, Manfredi PL, Davis SM, Morrison RS. Self-reported symptom experience of critically ill cancer patients receiving intensive care. *Crit Care Med* 2001;29:277–282.
47. Peterman AH, Fitchett G, Brady MJ, Hernandez L, Cella D. Measuring spiritual well-being in people with cancer: the functional assessment of chronic illness therapy–Spiritual Well-being Scale (FACIT-Sp). *Ann Behav Med* 2002;24:49–58.
48. Carver CS, Scheier MF, Weintraub JK. Assessing coping strategies: a theoretically based approach. *J Pers Soc Psychol* 1989;56:267–283.
49. Carver CS. You want to measure coping but your protocol's too long: consider the brief COPE. *Int J Behav Med* 1997;4:92–100.
50. Pargament KI, Koenig HG, Perez LM. The many methods of religious coping: development and initial validation of the RCOPE. *J Clin Psychol* 2000;56:519–543.

ARTICLE 18

The Impact of a Spiritual Legacy Intervention in Patients with Brain Cancers and Other Neurologic Illnesses and Their Support Persons

Katherine M. Piderman[1]*, Carmen Radecki Breitkopf[2], Sarah M. Jenkins[3], Maria I. Lapid[4], Gracia M. Kwete[5], Terin T. Sytsma[6], Laura A. Lovejoy[1], Timothy J. Yoder[1] and Aminah Jatoi[7]

1 Chaplain Services, Mayo Clinic Rochester, 200 First Street SW EI 2-130, Rochester, MN, USA

2 Division of Health Care Policy and Research, Health Sciences Research, Mayo Clinic Rochester, 200 First St. SW Charlton 6-235, Rochester, MN, USA, 55905

3 Biostatistics and Informatics, Mayo Clinic Rochester, Rochester, MN, USA

4 Psychiatry and Psychology, Mayo Clinic Rochester, Rochester, MN, USA

5 Mayo Medical School, Mayo Clinic Rochester, Rochester, MN, USA

6 Internal Medicine, Mayo Clinic Rochester, Rochester, MN, USA

7 Medical Oncology, Mayo Clinic Rochester, Rochester, MN, USA

*Correspondence to: E-mail: piderman.katherine@mayo.edu Mayo Clinic, Chaplain Services, 200 First Street SW, EI 2-130 Rochester, Minnesota, MN, USA.

Received: 25 February 2015; Revised: 1 September 2015; Accepted: 16 October 2015

Copyright © 2015 John Wiley & Sons, Ltd.

Abstract

Objective: The objectives were to assess the feasibility of using a novel, comprehensive chaplain-led spiritual life review interview to develop a personal Spiritual Legacy Document (SLD) for persons with brain tumors and other neurodegenerative diseases and to describe spiritual well-being (SWB), spiritual coping, and quality of life (QOL) of patients and their support persons (SP) before and after receipt of the SLD.

Methods: Patient-SP pairs were enrolled over a 2-year period. Assessments included the Functional Assessment of Chronic Illness Therapy-Spiritual Expanded Version, Brief Religious Coping Scale, Brief COPE Inventory,

---

Piderman, K.M., Radecki Breitkopf, C., Jenkins, S.M., Lapid, M.I., Kwete, G.M., Sytsma, T.T., Lovejoy, L.A., Yoder, T.J., and Jatoi, A. (2017) "The impact of a spiritual legacy intervention in patients with brain cancer and other neurologic illnesses and their support persons." *Psycho-Oncology*, 26, 3, 346–353.

and QOL Linear Analog Scale. Baseline assessments were completed prior to an audio-recorded spiritual life review interview with a chaplain.

Results: Thirty-two patient/SP pairs were enrolled; 27 completed baseline assessments and the interview. Twenty-four reviewed their SLD and were eligible for follow-up. A total of 15 patients and 12 SPs completed the 1-month follow-up; 10 patients and 7 SPs completed the 3-month follow-up. Patients endorsed high levels of SWB and spiritual coping at baseline. Both patients and SPs evidenced improvement on several aspects of SWB, spiritual coping, and QOL at 1 month, but patients' decreased financial well-being was also observed. Patients and SPs demonstrated favorable changes in peacefulness and positive religious coping at both time points.

Conclusions: A chaplain-led spiritual life review is a feasible intervention for patients with neurodegenerative disease and results in beneficial effects on patients and SPs.

Background

Like others with life-limiting illnesses, many individuals with primary brain tumors, brain metastases, and other neurodegenerative disorders find that spiritual issues become prominent as they grow in understanding of their diagnosis and prognosis, and engage in various treatments.[1, 2, 3, 4, 5] Their experience inevitably includes physical challenges, but also, it is common for those with neurologic diseases to experience diminishment of their mental faculties including attention, memory, verbal ability, higher reasoning, emotional stability, and even the capacity for spiritual experience. These losses contribute to spiritual and existential concerns which medical staff may not be able to address.[6, 7, 8] Additionally, spiritual well-being (SWB) is related to quality of life (QOL) and coping in those with neurologic diseases,[6, 7, 8] and unfortunately, it appears to be compromised in this population.[9] These findings suggest the need for spiritual care.

The spirituality of caregivers of those with neurologic diseases is important to consider, as they also experience spiritual and existential distress and value support.[8, 10, 11, 12] In a recent study, caregivers with higher levels of spirituality had fewer depressive symptoms and less anxiety than those with lower levels of spirituality. This relationship appears to impact the health and QOL of caregivers and may also affect the care they provide for their loved ones.[13]

The literature suggests that life review, including spiritual life review, may be helpful to patients and caregivers.[14, 15, 16, 17, 18, 19] Life review is expected to provide an opportunity for patients to increase personal meaning, self-worth, and internal coherence, qualities that have been identified as contributing to coping and well-being in patients with brain tumors and may indirectly benefit caregivers.[8, 20]

This feasibility study was developed by a multidisciplinary team interested in promoting the SWB and QOL of patients with brain cancers and other neurodegenerative processes.[21] The objectives were as follows: (1) assess the feasibility of using a novel, comprehensive chaplain-led spiritual life review process to develop a personalized Spiritual Legacy Document (SLD) for patients, and (2) describe the SWB, spiritual coping, and QOL of patients and their designated SPs at enrollment, one month, and three months following receipt of the SLD.

Methods

The study was conducted at Mayo Clinic in Rochester, MN. Enrollment began after Institutional Review Board (IRB) approval, and took place from July 2012 through August 2014. The study was advertised through presentations to health care providers and research coordinators in medical oncology, palliative care, and neurology. An IRB-approved brochure describing the study was used to facilitate recruitment. Referrals came primarily from the Medical Oncology Brain Care Team, but referrals from other clinical areas and self-referrals were also accepted. Patients were approached based on the clinician's view that they may be interested in participating. Enrollment was interrupted for several months because of unexpected medically-related absences of the principal investigator (PI).

Patient participants were English-speaking adults, ≥18 years of age, with primary brain tumors, brain metastases, or other neurodegenerative diseases who were receiving medical care at the study site. No formal assessment of mental status was performed, but patients were eligible if the referring clinician or the study team considered them capable of completing baseline assessments and participating in the interview. Eligibility also involved the enrollment of one patient-designated SP (e.g., spouse/partner, sibling, or friend) who was willing to complete questionnaires. Excluded were from those otherwise eligible were psychiatric inpatients and individuals for whom there were concerns about harm to self or others.

The spiritual legacy interview and document development

The investigators constructed a semistructured interview guide based on published sources, i.e., the Spiritual Assessment Tool known as FICA,[22, 23] questions used in Dignity Therapy,[14] and questions about spiritual struggle based on the work of Pargament and colleagues.[24] Because of their academic and clinical training in spiritual matters, board certified chaplains were thought best suited to lead the interview.[25]

Questions were adapted by the chaplain interviewers to correspond with their experience of best practices in spiritual care and spiritual counseling.[16, 19] For example, the FICA question, 'What importance does your faith have in your life?'[26] was changed to: 'Do you have any regular spiritual or religious practices that have been meaningful to you over your life time? Does your spirituality guide you as you look towards the future?' The Dignity Therapy question, 'What are the most important roles you have played in life?'[14] was changed to 'What would you consider to be God's call or your purpose in life?' Additionally, questions addressing spiritual struggle, an area not explored by FICA or Dignity Therapy, were included, e.g., 'Have you had periods in your life when you have faced questions about your faith or spiritual approach to life? Have you had tensions or conflicts with God or with your religious community? Have you struggled to live up to your spiritual values and beliefs?' (More interview questions can be found in a previous publication.[21])

All interviews were conducted by certified chaplains who had received training from the PI who is also a certified chaplain. During the training, the PI presented the interview guide to the interviewers and engaged them in discussion to promote a consistent approach. The PI encouraged the interviewers to use the questions in a semistructured way to foster a respectful, compassionate pastoral encounter. The PI also discussed responding to challenges when interviewing patients with altered verbal ability because of their neurological condition. Following the training, the PI remained available to the interviewers for questions and feedback. SPs were not excluded from the interviews, but if present, they were instructed to let the voice of the patient predominate.

Each interview was digitally audio-recorded, transcribed, and verified. A draft of each patient's personal SLD was prepared from the transcription by the research team. Each SLD was written in the first person as if the patient were speaking. The content was organized under headings that fit themes expressed in the interview. For example, a patient's early spiritual experiences might be described under headings such as 'Faith Beginnings', 'Early Life', 'Spiritual Background' and dealing with diagnosis, under headings such as 'Sharing the News', 'Finding Purpose', and 'Releasing Control in the Face of God'. A preliminary draft of the SLD was given to the patient for review and requested changes were made. The resulting document was professionally printed as an 8×8 inch booklet. Each patient was able to order 25 copies of his/her document to keep or to share with others of their choosing.

Instruments

SWB was measured by the following:

1. The Functional Assessment of Chronic Illness Therapy–Spiritual Expanded Version (FACIT-Sp-Ex), a 23-item scale, which includes faith, meaning, and peace subscales. Range 0–16. Single items include, 'I am able to forgive others for any harm they have ever caused me', 'I feel forgiven for any harm I may have ever caused', 'Throughout the course of my day, I feel a sense of thankfulness for what others bring to my life', and 'I feel hopeful'. Range 0–4.[27, 28]

2. The single SWB Linear Analog Self-Assessment (SWB LASA) item, 'How would you describe your overall SWB?' (included in a series of items assessing various QOL domains). Range 0–10.[29, 30]

Spiritual coping strategies were measured by the following:

1. The 14-item Brief Religious Coping Scale (Brief RCOPE),[31, 32] which assesses positive religious coping (demonstrating spiritual connection and well-being) and negative religious coping (demonstrating spiritual struggle). Range 0–3.

2. The two items comprising the Religion subscale from the Brief COPE Inventory (COPE) 'I've been trying to find comfort in my religion or spiritual beliefs' and 'I've been praying or meditating'. Range 1–4.[33]

QOL was measured using 12 LASA items. Overall QOL, and physical, mental, emotional, and social aspects of QOL were assessed, in addition to SWB, described previously. Range 0–10.[5, 30, 34, 35, 36]

Patients and SPs completed baseline questionnaires prior to the patient's interview with the chaplain. Follow-up questionnaires, identical to baseline questionnaires, were mailed to patients and SPs, approximately one and three months following completion of the SLD. There was a repeat mailing to non-responders, unless the investigators learned that the patient was too ill to participate or had died.

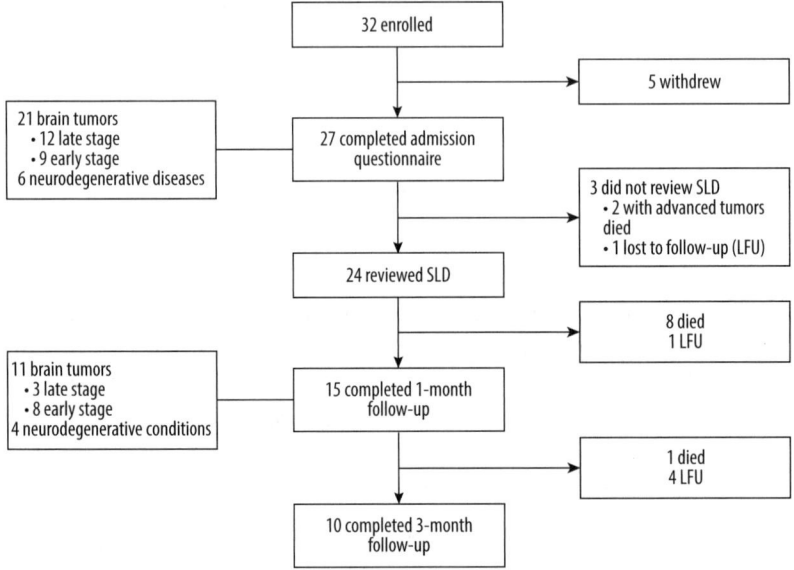

Figure 1: Patient flow diagram

Statistical methods

The responses to each instrument were summarized with means and standard deviations or frequencies and percentages (%). For most questionnaire items and scores, a higher score reflects a more positive response (exception: Negative RCOPE). The percentage of participants who improved from baseline to follow-up (any increase in score) and the percentage of participants who maintained a maximum possible score from baseline were summarized. Although the results from this exploratory study are largely descriptive in nature, we performed selected statistical comparisons to evaluate bigger differences between time points or groups. The average scores at baseline were compared between patient and SPs with linear regression models using generalized estimating equations to account for correlation within patient-SP pairs. Next, the average scores were compared between baseline and follow-up within the patient and SP groups using paired *t*-tests. Finally, the average baseline scores from the spirituality measures among the patients were compared with the estimates from the literature[29, 37] using two-sample *t*-tests. Analyses were performed using SAS. P-values less than 0.05 were considered statistically significant.

Table 1: Patient characteristics

	Died on study (n = 11)	Alive through study (n = 16)	First follow-up available (n = 15)	Total (n = 27)
Age, years				
• Mean (SD)	54.5(15.4)	50.3(14.1)	51.8(14.2)	52.0(14.5)
• Range	21.8–77.1	25.1–74.0	25.1–74.0	21.8–77.1
Gender, male	6(54.5%)	6(37.5%)	7(46.7%)	12(44.4%)
Marital status				
• Married	8(72.7%)	11(68.8%)	11(73.3%)	19(70.4%)
• Single	2(18.2%)	4(25.0%)	3(20.0%)	6(22.2%)
• Divorced or annulled	0(0.0%)	1(6.3%)	1(6.7%)	1(3.7%)
• Widowed	1(9.1%)	0(0.0%)	0(0.0%)	1(3.7%)
Education				
• High school/equivalent	3(27.3%)	0(0.0%)	0(0.0%)	3(11.1%)
• Part college/technical school	4(36.4%)	1(6.3%)	1(6.7%)	5(18.5%)
• College graduate	2(18.2%)	7(43.8%)	6(40.0%)	9(33.3%)
• Post-graduate work	2(18.2%)	8(50.0%)	8(53.3%)	10(37.0%)
Religious denomination/affiliation				
• Catholic	2(18.2%)	4(25.0%)	5(33.3%)	6(22.2%)
• Protestant	6(54.5%)	8(50.0%)	7(46.7%)	14(51.9%)
• Muslim	0(0.0%)	1(6.3%)	0(0.0%)	1(3.7%)
• No religious preference	3(27.3%)	3(18.8%)	3(20.0%)	6(22.2%)
Disease type				
• Advanced brain tumor	9(81.8%)	3(18.8%)	3(20.0%)	12(44.4%)
• Early stage brain tumor	0(0.0%)	9(56.3%)	8(53.3%)	9(33.3%)
• Other neurological disease	2(18.2%)	4(25.0%)	4(26.7%)	6(22.2%)

Results

Patient characteristics

Forty patients were approached and 32 enrolled. Those who declined participation indicated that the demands of their illness were too great or that they were not interested. Five patients were withdrawn because of illness-related complexities, leaving 27 who completed baseline questionnaires and an interview with a chaplain. Twenty-five (92.6%) patients were from the Midwestern USA. Additional patient characteristics are shown in Table 1. SPs were a spouse/partner ($n = 19$, 70.4%), parent ($n = 4$, 14.8%), sibling ($n = 3$, 11.1%), or friend ($n = 1$, 3.7%).

Among the 27 patients who were interviewed, 24 reviewed a draft of their SLD, received finalized copies, and were eligible for follow-up. Of these 24, 15 completed the 1-month follow-up questionnaire, and ten completed the 3-month follow-up questionnaire (Figure 1).

Twelve SPs completed the 1-month follow-up and seven completed the 3-month follow-up. Five SPs were present for the interview. In each case, the patient had advanced brain cancer and impaired verbal ability, but engaged in the full interview, with the SP providing detail or clarification when necessary. Four of these patients died before the first follow-up. One died before the second follow-up. (The latter dyad completed the 1-month questionnaire.)

Table 2: Baseline scores among all participants (items oriented so that higher scores are better, unless otherwise indicated), mean (standard deviation)

Item/score(range)	Patients ($n = 27$)	Support persons ($n = 27$)
FACIT-Sp-Ex(0-4/single items; 0-16/subscales)		
• Able to forgive others	3.6(0.6)	3.0(1.0) **
• Feel forgiven	3.2(0.8)	3.1(0.9)
• Thankful	3.6(0.7)	3.4(0.8)
• Hopeful	3.5(0.9)	3.1(1.0)
• Meaning subscale	14.2(2.6)	14.3(2.3)
• Peace subscale	11.3(3.3)	11.3(3.2)
• Faith subscale	13.3(3.4)	11.1(5.1) *
LASA(0-10)		
• Overall quality of life	7.6(1.9)	7.9(1.5)
• Intellectual well-being	7.4(1.7)	8.2(1.4)
• Physical well-being	6.6(2.4)	7.6(1.9)
• Emotional well-being	7.2(2.3)	7.5(2.1)
• Social activity	6.4(2.5)	6.8(2.3)
• Spiritual well-being	7.7(2.0)	7.4(2.7)

• Lack of pain frequency	6.1(3.7)	7.8(2.7)
• Lack of pain severity	6.9(2.9)	7.7(2.6)
• Lack of fatigue	5.0(2.4)	6.6(2.4) **
• Support from friends/family	8.6(2.2)	8.2(2.2)
• Financial concerns	7.3(2.6)	6.2(3.4)
• Legal concerns	8.3(2.4)	7.3(3.4)
Brief RCOPE(0–3)		
• Positive RCOPE subscale	1.8(0.9)	1.6(0.8)
• Negative RCOPE subscale[a]	0.3(0.5)	0.3(0.4)
COPE(1–4)		
• Seeking comfort in religion/spiritual beliefs	3.2(1.1)	2.9(1.2)
• Praying/meditating	3.3(1.0)	2.7(1.1) **
• Subscale: religion	3.3(1.0)	2.8(1.1) *

*$p < 0.05$. **$p < 0.01$. [a]Higher negative RCOPE score indicates more spiritual struggle.

Table 3: Comparison of data between baseline and first follow-up

Item/subscale (range)	Patients (n = 15)				Support persons (n = 12)			
	Baseline mean(SD)	Follow-up mean (SD)	Maintained maximum from baseline %	Improved from baseline %	Baseline mean(SD)	Follow-up mean (SD)	Maintained maximum from baseline %	Improved from baseline %
FACIT-Sp-Ex(0–4/single items; 0–16/subscales)								
• Able to forgive others[a]	3.7(0.6)	3.3(1.1)	46.7	13.3	3.0(1.0)	2.8(0.9)	8.3	16.7
• Feel forgiven	3.3(0.6)	3.5(0.6)	40.0	26.7	2.9(0.8)	2.7(0.8)	8.3	8.3
• Thankful	3.7(0.5)	3.7(0.5)	60.0	6.7	3.3(1.0)	3.7(0.5)	50.0	33.3
• Hopeful	3.7(0.6)	3.3(0.8)	46.7	6.7	2.9(1.1)	3.4(0.8)*	33.3	41.7
• Meaning subscale	14.3(2.6)	14.9(1.9)	40.0	33.3	14.0(2.5)	14.5(1.9)	33.3	33.3
• Peace subscale	11.4(2.8)	12.7(3.0)	6.7	60.0	11.2(4.0)	12.1(2.1)	0.0	50.0
• Faith subscale	13.7(3.0)	13.3(3.8)	33.3	20.0	10.8(5.8)	10.9(4.5)	8.3	33.3
LASA(0–10)								
• Overall quality of life	7.3(1.7)	8.0(1.1)	0.0	40.0	7.8(1.6)	8.1(1.3)	8.3	25.0
• Intellectual well-being	7.5(1.6)	7.9(1.3)	6.7	33.3	8.1(1.5)	8.6(1.2)	8.3	50.0
• Physical well-being	6.7(2.6)	7.3(1.6)	0	40.0	7.3(1.9)	8.1(1.2)	0	41.7
• Emotional well-being	7.3(2.3)	8.3(1.4)*	0.0	53.3	7.3(2.3)	7.8(1.7)	8.3	41.7
• Social activity	6.4(2.6)	7.1(2.1)	6.7	46.7	7.1(2.4)	7.3(2.4)	8.3	33.3
• Spiritual well-being	7.9(1.7)	8.7(1.3)	6.7	46.7	6.9(3.2)	7.8(2.6)**	8.3	58.3

• Lack of pain frequency	6.3(3.4)	5.5(3.2)	6.7	26.7	7.9(1.6)	7.5(2.4)	9.1	36.4
• Lack of pain severity	7.1(2.8)	6.6(2.3)	6.7	20.0	7.4(2.1)	7.6(2.7)	9.1	45.5
• Lack of fatigue	5.2(2.0)	4.9(2.6)	0	40.0	7.3(2.3)	6.2(2.2)	0	27.3
• Support from friends/family	8.7(2.1)	8.6(1.5)	20.0	40.0	8.3(2.7)	7.8(2.6)	25.0	33.3
• Financial concerns	7.4(2.5)	6.1(3.7)*	13.3	6.7	7.1(3.1)	6.8(3.2)	0.0	33.3
• Legal concerns	8.9(1.4)	7.5(3.2)	20.0	26.7	7.6(3.3)	7.6(3.0)	8.3	33.3
Brief RCOPE(0–3)								
• Positive RCOPE subscale	1.8(0.8)	2.0(0.8)**	0	80.0	1.4(0.6)	1.6(0.8)	0	54.5
• Negative RCOPE subscale[a]	0.1(0.3)	0.2(0.3)	60.0	6.7	0.2(0.4)	0.3(0.4)	54.5	18.2
COPE(1–4)								
• Seeking comfort in religion/spiritual beliefs	3.3(1.0)	3.2(1.1)	27.3	27.3	3.0(1.0)	3.2(0.9)	25.0	33.3
• Praying/meditating	3.5(0.8)	3.1(1.1)	41.7	8.3	2.9(1.0)	3.3(0.8)	33.3	41.7
• Subscale: religion	3.4(0.9)	3.1(1.0)	27.3	27.3	3.0(0.9)	3.3(0.8)	16.7	58.3

*$p < 0.05$. **$p < 0.01$ comparing average score pre versus post within patients/support persons. [a]Higher negative RCOPE score indicates more spiritual struggle.

Table 4: Summary of data among those with both follow-ups: Mean (SD)

Item/subscale(range)	Patients (n = 10)			Support persons (n = 7)		
	Baseline	Follow-up 1	Follow-up 2	Baseline	Follow-up 1	Follow-up 2
FACIT-Sp-Ex(0–4/single items; 0–16/subscales)						
• Able to forgive others	3.5(0.7)	3.6(0.5)	3.4(0.7)	2.7(1.0)	2.6(0.5)	3.0(0.9)
• Feel forgiven	3.1(0.6)	3.4(0.7)	3.4(0.7)	2.7(0.8)	2.4(0.5)	3.0(1.0)
• Thankful	3.7(0.5)	3.6(0.5)	3.8(0.4)	3.3(0.8)	3.6(0.5)	3.3(0.8)
• Hopeful	3.5(0.7)	3.1(0.9)	3.5(0.7)	3.0(1.2)	3.1(0.9)	3.1(0.9)
• Meaning subscale	14.8(1.9)	14.4(2.1)	14.2(2.8)	14.4(2.7)	14.7(1.6)	14.3(2.4)
• Peace subscale	11.0(3.4)	12.1(3.0)	13.1(2.6)	11.0(4.9)	11.9(2.5)	12.3(3.4)
• Faith subscale	12.9(3.2)	12.2(4.3)	12.1(3.7)	10.6(5.7)	11.0(3.8)	10.9(4.1)
LASA(0–10)						
• Overall quality of life	7.5(1.4)	8.2(0.8)	8.4(1.7)	8.0(1.6)	8.1(1.6)	7.9(1.3)
• Intellectual well-being	7.8(1.4)	8.2(1.2)	8.5(1.3)	8.6(1.4)	8.4(1.1)	7.6(2.1)
• Physical well-being	6.2(2.7)	7.4(1.5)	7.6(2.2)	7.1(2.4)	8.1(1.5)	7.4(1.9)
• Emotional well-being	7.4(2.1)	8.2(1.2)	8.5(1.3)	7.6(2.5)	7.9(2.0)	7.7(1.6)
• Social activity	6.7(2.6)	7.4(1.8)	7.5(2.1)	7.4(1.7)	7.0(2.8)	7.3(1.3)
• Spiritual well-being	7.6(1.9)	8.5(1.6)	8.7(1.7)	6.9(2.8)	7.7(2.3)	7.6(1.9)
• Lack of pain frequency	6.3(3.2)	5.0(2.7)	7.1(2.8)	8.0(1.4)	7.1(2.5)	7.9(2.4)
• Lack of pain severity	7.5(2.1)	6.2(2.0)	7.7(2.6)	7.1(2.2)	7.7(2.6)	6.7(3.5)

• Lack of fatigue	5.0(2.1)	5.0(2.6)	4.1(2.6)	7.9(1.2)	6.4(2.2)	5.7(2.9)
• Support from friends/family	8.8(1.5)	8.7(1.3)	9.2(0.8)	8.4(1.7)	7.4(2.8)	8.3(1.5)
• Financial concerns	8.0(1.8)	6.4(3.2)	7.8(3.1)	7.3(3.5)	8.0(2.2)	7.4(2.8)
• Legal concerns	8.9(1.6)	7.0(3.7)	8.4(2.6)	7.0(4.1)	8.1(1.7)	7.3(3.1)
Brief RCOPE(0–3)						
• Positive RCOPE subscale	1.5(0.9)	1.8(0.9)	1.8(1.0)	1.4(0.5)	1.4(0.9)	1.7(1.0)
• Negative RCOPE subscale[a]	0.0(0.1)	0.1(0.3)	0.1(0.3)	0.3(0.4)	0.3(0.3)	0.4(0.5)
COPE(1–4)						
• Seeking comfort in religion/spiritual beliefs	3.3(1.1)	2.9(1.2)	3.2(1.2)	2.9(0.9)	3.1(0.7)	3.1(1.1)
• Praying/meditating	3.4(0.8)	2.9(1.1)	3.6(1.0)	2.7(0.8)	3.0(0.8)	2.4(0.8)
• Subscale: religion	3.4(0.9)	2.9(1.1)	3.4(1.0)	2.8(0.7)	3.1(0.7)	2.8(0.7)

[a]Higher Negative RCOPE score indicates more spiritual struggle.

Baseline scores: patients and SPs (n = 27)

At baseline, patients demonstrated relatively high scores of SWB on both the FACIT-Sp-Ex and SWB LASA. The average FACIT-Sp-Ex meaning, peace, and faith subscale scores were 14.2, 11.3, and 13.3, respectively. The forgiveness, gratitude, and hope items ranged from 3.2 to 3.6. The average score for the SWB LASA was 7.7.

Patients' Brief RCOPE scores revealed moderate positive religious coping and low negative religious coping (Mean = 1.8 and 0.3, respectively), suggesting minimal spiritual distress. Patients reported high frequency of religious coping on the COPE religion subscale (Mean = 3.2 and 3.3). Finally, patient QOL ranged between 6 and 8 points, with overall average QOL = 7.6 (Table 2).

SP scores were similar to patient scores at baseline, with a few exceptions. On the FACIT-Sp-Ex, patients reported higher feelings of forgiveness for others as compared with SPs (Mean = 3.6 vs 3.0, $p < 0.01$) and had higher scores on the faith subscale (Mean = 13.3 vs 11.1, $p < 0.05$). Religious coping frequency on the COPE was significantly higher for patients (Mean = 3.3 vs 2.8, $p < 0.05$), largely because of the prayer/meditation item (Mean = 3.3 vs 2.7, $p < 0.01$). The only significant difference detected on the LASA between patients and SPs at baseline was for the fatigue item with patients reporting worse fatigue (Mean lack of fatigue = 5.0 vs 6.6, $p < 0.01$) (Table 1).

Baseline versus follow-up

FIRST FOLLOW-UP

Fifteen patients and 12 SPs completed the first follow-up assessment. Improvements in SWB were detected on the FACIT-Sp-Ex and SWB LASA in both groups. Sixty percent of patients improved on the FACIT-Sp-Ex peace subscale and over half either improved or maintained the highest score on the SWB LASA (not significant). Significant improvement was noted for SPs on the FACIT-Sp-Ex hopeful item (Mean = 2.9 to 3.4, $p < 0.05$) and the SWB LASA (Mean = 6.9 to 7.8, $p < 0.01$). Similar to patients, 50% improved on the FACIT-Sp-Ex peace subscale (not significant).

With respect to religious coping, 80% of patients improved on the positive religious coping subscale (Mean = 1.8 to 2.0, $p < 0.01$). Among SPs, 54.5% improved on the positive religious coping subscale; 58.3% improved on the COPE religion subscale (not significant).

For the QOL measures, patients' emotional well-being improved significantly (Mean = 7.3 to 8.3, $p < 0.05$); however, financial concerns grew worse (Mean = 7.4 to 6.1, $p < 0.05$). Overall QOL improved for patients from 7.3 to 8.0 (not significant). For SPs, other than the SWB LASA, no statistical improvement was noted on the LASA items (Table 3).

SECOND FOLLOW-UP

Ten patients and seven SPs completed the second follow-up. Improvements detected from baseline to 1 month on several measures of SWB, spiritual coping, and QOL improved slightly or were maintained at 3 months for both groups. The most notable was the increase on the FACIT-Sp-Ex peace subscale for both (patients: Mean = 11.0 to 12.1 to 13.1; SPs: Mean = 11.0 to 11.9 to 12.3). There were small decreases in patient and SP scores on a few items, including increased fatigue for both groups. Due to sample size limitations, no statistical testing was performed at the second follow-up (Table 4).

Conclusion

The spiritual legacy process involved in this exploratory study offered patients with brain tumors and other neurodegenerative illnesses the opportunity to reflect on and discuss important issues related to their beliefs, practices, and values with a certified chaplain. Additionally, it provided a summary document as a tangible and lasting spiritual legacy. Nearly 90% of participants were able to complete the process. This is particularly remarkable in that 9 of 24 died on study, 8 before the first follow-up. Patients' persistent, enduring commitment despite the burden of their illness demonstrates how meaningful this process was to them and suggests the feasibility and acceptability of the intervention.

Patients in this study endorsed high levels of SWB and minimal religious struggle at baseline. These scores are similar to those found in previous research.[21, 37] They suggest that disease burden did not intrude overly on the spiritual aspects of their lives, and it is even possible that it contributed to spiritual growth or strengthening.[38] Twenty-five percent of patients did not identify with a religious denomination, suggesting that religious affiliation, in itself, may not be the only contributor to SWB and spiritual coping.

At baseline, SPs scored lower than patients on measures related to faith, frequency of prayer and meditation, and forgiveness, suggesting that their experience of patient illness did not prompt the prominence of spirituality in the same way as it did for the patients. This is important information for patients' selection of support persons, i.e., if questions arise, patients could be made aware that the designated support person need not be as spiritual as they are and that they still may benefit from involvement.

This study was not powered to promote definitive statistical testing, but trends at both time points demonstrated by patients and SPs suggest that participating was helpful to them. It is particularly encouraging that the majority of patients and SPs reported more peacefulness and positive religious coping at the first follow-up and that improvement was maintained or increased for those who completed both follow-ups. Additionally, emotional well-being continued to improve for patients throughout the study.[14, 15] The reason for the decrease in patients' financial well-being is not clear. There is nothing to suggest that it is directly related to study involvement. It may or may not be related to illness, but it also is important to note that because of the small sample size, changes reported by one or two participants may have skewed the outcome.

The limitations of this study include the narrow disease focus, for it is unknown whether our observations would hold across different life-limiting conditions. Additionally, as an exploratory study, enrollment was more opportunistic than systematic, and we did not include a formal assessment of mental status to determine study eligibility. Future studies should include larger sample sizes, more diverse patient populations with regard to demographic characteristics and diagnoses, and systematic recruitment strategies to collect additional evidence on feasibility and outcomes of the intervention.

Considering the fragility and fatigue of the patients in this study and the associated stresses for those who care for them, every effort must be made to minimize respondent-burden and facilitate survey completion. Clinical applications, such as an in-depth spiritual assessment, could facilitate an abbreviated version of the SLD process and promote peacefulness at the end of life.

Acknowledgements

We are grateful for the generous financial support of a Mayo Clinic benefactor and the St. Mary's Hospital Sponsorship Board, Inc. that made this study possible. We also acknowledge with gratitude those who participated in our study in the midst of challenging illness; our co-investigators, especially Yvette Dulohery, Heidi Durland, Debra Head, James Hogg, Dean Marek, and Spence Swanson, and Mayo Clinic Media Support Services for their commitment and effort.

References

1. Beuscher L, Grando VT. Using spirituality to cope with early-stage Alzheimer's disease. *West J Nurs Res* 2009;31:583–598.
2. Delgado-Guay MO, Hui D, Parsons HA, et al. Spirituality, religiosity, and spiritual pain in advanced cancer patients. *J Pain Symptom Manage* 2011;41:986–994. DOI:10.1016/j.jpainsymman.2010.09.017.
3. Puchalski C, Ferrell BR. Making health care whole: Integrating spirituality into patient care. Templeton Press: West Conshohocken, PA, 2010.
4. Puchalski CM. A time for listening and caring: spirituality and the care of the chronically ill and dying. Oxford University Press: New York, NY, 2006.
5. Bretscher M, Rummans T, Sloan J, et al. Quality of life in hospice patients: a pilot study. *Psychosomatics* 1999;40:309–313. DOI:10.1016/S0033-3182(99)71224-7.
6. Cleary J, Ddungu H, Distelhorst SR, et al. Supportive and palliative care for metastatic breast cancer: resource allocations in low- and middle-income countries. A Breast Health Global Initiative 2013 consensus statement. *Breast* 2013;22:616–627. DOI:10.1016/j.breast.2013.07.052.
7. Nixon A, Narayanasamy A. The spiritual needs of neuro-oncology patients from patients' perspective. *J Clin Nurs* 2010;19:2259–2370. DOI:10.1111/j.1365-2702.2009.03112.x.
8. Strang S, Strang P. Spiritual thoughts, coping and 'sense of coherence' in brain tumour patients and their spouses. *Palliat Support Care* 2001;15:127–134.
9. Giovagnoli AR, Martins da Silva A, Federico A, Cornelio F. On the personal facets of quality of life in chronic neurological disorders. *Behav Neurol* 2009;21:155–163. DOI:10.3233/BEN-2009-0243.
10. Coolbrandt A, Sterckx W, Clement P, et al. Family caregivers of patients with a high-grade glioma: a qualitative study of their lived experience and needs related to professional care. *Cancer Nurs* 2014. Publish Ahead of Print. DOI:10.1097/ncc.0000000000000216.
11. Soundy A, Smith B, Butler M, Minns Lowe C, Helen D, Winward CH. A qualitative study in neurological physiotherapy and hope: beyond physical improvement. *Phys Chem Chem Phys* 2010;26:79–88. DOI:10.3109/09593980802634466.
12. Strang S, Strang P, Ternestedt BM. Existential support in brain tumour patients and their spouses. *Support Care Cancer* 2001;9:625–633.
13. Newberry AG, Choi C-WJ, Donovan HS, et al. Exploring spirituality in family caregivers of patients with primary malignant brain tumors across the disease trajectory. *Oncol Nurs Forum* 2013;40:E119–125. DOI:10.1188/13.ONF.E119-E125.
14. Chochinov HM, Kristjanson LJ, Breitbart W, et al. Effect of dignity therapy on distress and end-of-life experience in terminally ill patients: a randomised controlled trial. *Lancet Oncol* 2011;12:753–762. DOI:10.1016/ S1470-2045(11)70153-X.
15. Fitchett G, Emanuel L, Handzo G, Boyken L, Wilkie DJ. Care of the human spirit and the role of dignity therapy: a systematic review of dignity therapy research Palliative Care, Spiritual Care and Chaplaincy: The current landscape Joshua Hauser. *BMC Palliative Care* 2015;14. DOI:10.1186/s12904-015- 0007-1.
16. LeFavi RG, Wessels MH. Life review in pastoral counseling: background and efficacy for use with the terminally ill. *J of Pastoral Care & Counseling* 2003;57:281–292.
17. Piderman KM, Breitkopf CR, Jenkins SM, et al. A chaplain-led spiritual life review pilot study for patients with brain cancers and other degenerative neurologic diseases. *Rambam Maimonides Med J* 2015;6. DOI:10.5041/RMMJ.10199. eCollection 2015.
18. Piderman KM, Kung S, Jenkins SM, et al. Respecting the spiritual side of advanced cancer care: a systematic review. *Curr Oncol Rep* 2015;17:6. DOI:10.1007/s11912-014-0429-6.
19. Puchalski CM, Lunsford B, Harris MH, Miller RT. Interdisciplinary spiritual care for seriously ill and dying patients: a collaborative model. *Cancer J* 2006;12:398–416.

20. Steinhauser KE, Alexander SC, Byock IR, George LK, Olsen MK, Tulsky JA. Do preparation and life completion discussions improve functioning and quality of life in seriously ill patients? Pilot randomized control trial. *J Palliat Med* 2008;11. DOI:10.1089/jpm.2008.0078.
21. Piderman KM, Radecki Breitkopf C, Jenkins SM, et al. The feasibility and educational value of *Hear My Voice*, a chaplain-led spiritual life review process for patients with brain cancers and progressive neurologic conditions. *J Cancer Educ* 2014. DOI:10.1007/s13187-014-0686-y.
22. Anandarajah G, Hight E. Spirituality and medical practice: using the HOPE questions as a practice for spiritual assessment. *Am Fam Physician* 2001;63:81–89.
23. Puchalski C, Romer A. Taking a spiritual history allows clinicians to understand patients more fully. *J Palliat Med* 2000;3:129–137.
24. Pargament KI. Spiritually integrated psychotherapy: understanding and addressing the sacred. Guilford Press: New York, NY, 2007.
25. Piderman KM, Marek DV, Jenkins S, et al. Predicting patients' expectations of hospital chaplains: a multisite survey. *Mayo Clin Proc* 2010;85:1002–1010. DOI:10.4065/mcp.2010.0168.
26. Puchalski CM. The FICA spiritual history tool #274. *J Palliat Med* 2014;17:105–106. DOI:10.1089/jpm.2013.9458.
27. Canada AL, Murphy PE, Fitchett G, Peterman AH, Schover LR. A 3-factor model for the FACIT-Sp. *Psycho-Oncology* 2008;17:908–916. DOI: 10.1002/pon.1307.
28. Peterman AH, Fitchett G, Brady MJ, Hernandez L, Cella D. Measuring spiritual well-being in people with cancer: the functional assessment of chronic illness therapy—Spiritual Well-being Scale (FACIT- Sp). *Annals Behav Med* 2002;24:49–58.
29. Piderman KM, Johnson ME, Frost MH, et al. Spiritual quality of life in advanced cancer patients receiving radiation therapy. *Psycho-Oncology* 2014;23:216–221. DOI: 10.1002/pon.3390.
30. Rummans TA, Clark MM, Sloan JA, et al. Impacting quality of life for patients with advanced cancer with a structure multidisciplinary intervention: a randomized controlled trial. *J Clin Oncol* 2006;24:635–642.
31. Pargament KI, Koenig HG, Perez LM. The many methods of religious coping: development and initial validation of the RCOPE. *J Clin Psychol* 2000;56:519–543.
32. Pargament KI, Smith BW, Koenig HG, Perez L. Patterns of positive and negative religious coping with major life stressors. *J Sci Study Relig* 1998;37:710–724.
33. Carver CS. You want to measure coping but your protocol's too long: consider the brief COPE. *Int J Behav Med* 1997;4:92–100.
34. Grunberg SM, Groshen S, Steingass S, Zaretsky S, Meyerowitz B. Comparison of conditional quality of life terminology and visual analogue scale measurements. *Qual Life Res* 1996;5:65–72.
35. Gudex C, Dolan P, Kind P, Williams A. Health state valuations from the general public using the visual analogue scale. *Qual Life Res* 1996;5:521–531.
36. Hyland M, Sodergren S. Development of a new type of global quality of life scale, and comparison of performance and preference for 12 global scales. *Qual Life Res* 1996;5:469–480
37. Sherman AC, Simonton S, Latif U, Spohn R, Tricot G. Religious struggle and religious comfort in response to illness: health outcomes among stem cell transplant patients. *J Behav Med* 2005;28:359–367.
38. Cole BS, Hopkins CM, Tisak J, Steel JL, Carr BI. Assessing spiritual growth and spiritual decline following a diagnosis of cancer: reliability and validity of the spiritual transformation scale. *Psycho-Oncology* 2008;17:112–121.

ARTICLE 19

What Impact Do Chaplains Have? A Pilot Study of Spiritual AIM for Advanced Cancer Patients in Outpatient Palliative Care

Allison Kestenbaum, MA, MPA, BCC, ACPE Certified Educator[1]; The Rev. Michele Shields, D. Min., BCC, ACPE Certified Educator[2]; Jennifer James, MSW, MSSP[3]; The Rev. Will Hocker, M.Div., MSW, BCC[2]; Stefana Morgan, MD[4]; Shweta Karve, MD5 Michael W. Rabow, MD[6]; Laura B. Dunn, MD[5]

1 Doris A. Howell Palliative Care Service, University of California, San Diego Health; San Diego, California

2 Spiritual Care Department, University of California San Francisco Medical Center and UCSF Benioff Children's Hospital; San Francisco, California

3 Department of Social and Behavioral Sciences, School of Nursing, University of California, San Francisco; San Francisco, California

4 Department of Psychiatry, University of California, San Francisco; San Francisco, California

5 Department of Psychiatry and Behavioral Sciences, Stanford University; Stanford, California

6 Department of Medicine, University of California, San Francisco; San Francisco, California

Corresponding Author: Laura B. Dunn, MD

Professor of Psychiatry and Behavioral Sciences

Department of Psychiatry and Behavioral Sciences

Stanford University

401 Quarry Road

Stanford, CA 94305

Phone: 650-725-7709

Fax: 650-724-3144

Email: laura.dunn@stanford.edu

Kestenbaum, A., Shields, M., James, J., Hocker, W., Morgan, S., Karve, S., Rabow, MW, and Dunn, L.B. (2017) "What impact do chaplains have? A pilot study of spiritual AIM for advanced cancer patients in outpatient palliative care." *Journal of Pain and Symptom Management*, 54, 5, 707–714.

Abstract

Context: Spiritual care is integral to quality palliative care. Although chaplains are uniquely trained to provide spiritual care, studies evaluating chaplains' work in palliative care are scarce.

Objectives: The goals of this pre-post study, conducted among patients with advanced cancer receiving outpatient palliative care, were to evaluate the feasibility and acceptability of chaplain-delivered spiritual care, utilizing the Spiritual Assessment and Intervention Model ("Spiritual AIM"); and to gather pilot data on Spiritual AIM's effects on spiritual well-being, religious and cancer-specific coping, and physical and psychological symptoms.

Methods: Patients with advanced cancer (n=31) who were receiving outpatient palliative care were assigned based on chaplains' and patients' outpatient schedules, to one of three professional chaplains for three individual Spiritual AIM sessions, conducted over the course of approximately six to eight weeks. Patients completed the following measures at baseline and post-intervention: Edmonton Symptom Assessment Scale (ESAS), Steinhauser spirituality, Brief Religious Coping (Brief RCOPE), Functional Assessment of Chronic Illness Therapy—Spiritual (FACIT-Sp-12), Mini-Mental Adjustment to Cancer (Mini-MAC), Patient Dignity Inventory, Center for Epidemiological Studies—Depression (CES-D, 10-item), and Spielberger State Anxiety Inventory (STAI-S).

Results: From baseline to post-Spiritual AIM, significant increases were found on the FACIT-Sp-12 Faith subscale, the Mini-MAC Fighting Spirit subscale, and Mini-MAC Adaptive Coping factor. Two trends were observed, i.e., an increase in Positive religious coping and an increase in Fatalism (a subscale of the Mini-MAC).

Conclusion: Spiritual AIM, a brief chaplain-led intervention, holds potential to address spiritual needs, as well as religious and general coping in patients with serious illnesses.

Key words: chaplaincy, spiritual care, palliative care, cancer, spiritual distress, religious coping

Introduction

Many people turn to their spiritual resources as a means of coping;[1,2] and spiritual care is now considered an essential component of high-quality palliative care.[3, 4] Among patients with life-threatening illnesses and end-of-life (EOL) concerns, the majority want spirituality included in their care;[5] patients who reported their spiritual needs were not met reported lower quality of care and lower satisfaction with care.[6] Outcomes such as aggressiveness and costs of EOL care appear related to patients' spiritual needs. In the Coping with Cancer study, a prospective study of advanced cancer patients, patients who reported that their spiritual or religious needs were "largely or completely supported" by the clinical team ("e.g., doctors, nurses, chaplains") were more likely to receive hospice care[7] and incurred lower EOL costs of care.[8]

Notably lacking in the palliative care research literature are descriptions of *how* spiritual care is provided—by whom, using what models of assessment and intervention, and seeking what outcomes.[9, 10] Spiritual care provision in the healthcare setting too often remains shrouded in mystery.[10] In inpatient settings, although a chaplain may visit a patient (usually only once or twice), other healthcare team members often are unaware of what transpired.[10, 11, 12, 13]

Although guidelines for quality palliative care emphasize the role that any member of the interdisciplinary team may play in obtaining spiritual data,[3] and while providers of any discipline may provide space for patients to discuss existential distress,[14, 15] chaplains are uniquely trained to assess each individual's spiritual needs and develop tailored interventions.[10, 16, 17] However, without detailed descriptions or rigorous evaluations of chaplains' activities, it is difficult to characterize or evaluate professional chaplains' work.[9, 11, 17, 18]

The goals of this study, conducted in the outpatient palliative care setting, were: 1) to evaluate the feasibility and tolerability of a chaplain-delivered spiritual care intervention, which utilized a well-articulated model (Spiritual Assessment and Intervention Model; "Spiritual AIM"),[16] and 2) to evaluate the impact of Spiritual AIM on spiritual well-being, religious and cancer-specific coping, and physical and psychological symptoms.

Methods

Description of Spiritual AIM

Spiritual AIM was developed through 25 years of clinical practice and supervision, and has been taught to over a hundred diverse chaplain trainees. Spiritual AIM is one of few spiritual assessment models that articulates assessments, interventions, and outcomes, and that has been empirically studied.[19, 20] Spiritual AIM is not a questionnaire or a structured interview. Rather, the patient's spiritual need is assessed in the pastoral encounter, which focuses on the patient's primary concerns. Chaplains then choose from a set of corresponding interventions to each assessment category to inform their spiritual care to the patient. Spiritual AIM's development, theoretical underpinnings, main components, and illustrative cases are described in detail elsewhere.[16]

Spiritual AIM posits that every human being, by virtue of being human, has three fundamental or "core" spiritual needs: for meaning and direction (referred to in Spiritual AIM "shorthand" as "Meaning and Direction"); for self-worth and belonging to community ("Self-Worth"); and to love and be loved, often facilitated through seeking reconciliation when relationships are broken ("Reconciliation"). Spiritual AIM asserts that in a crisis—such as facing one's mortality—one of three core spiritual needs emerges most strongly, influencing the patient's subjective thoughts and feelings as well as affecting their observable words and behaviors. In Spiritual AIM, the chaplain's pastoral encounter requires diagnosing an individual's primary unmet spiritual need, devising and implementing a plan for addressing this need, and evaluating desired and actual outcomes of the intervention. Currently, these aspects of Spiritual AIM are conducted qualitatively by the chaplain, during meetings with the patient. The focus of Spiritual AIM is on relationships—and the idea that healing happens in relationship.

Participants

Patients with advanced cancer were recruited from an outpatient palliative care service at an academic, urban comprehensive cancer center. Inclusion criteria were an advanced cancer diagnosis (i.e., based on clinician report—the palliative care clinician expected the patient to die from their cancer within one year), receipt of concurrent oncologic and palliative care, and willingness to speak with a board-certified (or eligible) chaplain for three one-on-one visits, either in person or by telephone. Patients who had had at least one visit with their palliative care provider (an attending physician, a palliative medicine fellow, or a nurse practitioner) were offered enrollment, in order that that the palliative care provider could first address patients' presenting physical symptoms (e.g., pain, nausea) before introducing the study. If patients met inclusion criteria, providers briefly described the Spiritual AIM study, gave patients a one-page description of the study, and asked if they were willing to be contacted by the Research Coordinator.

Three chaplains (MS [n=11 patients], AK [n=10 patients], and WH [n=10 patients]) delivered the Spiritual AIM intervention. The chaplains ranged in age (32 to 57 years), faith background (United Methodist, Episcopalian, Jewish), number of years working as a chaplain (9 to 32 years), and years of experience using Spiritual AIM (3 to 22 years). Two of the chaplains were board certified, one was board certification eligible. Chaplains met weekly with researchers to promote consistency in assessment and interventions. All chaplains were trained intensively by the creator of Spiritual AIM.

Procedures

At the initial meeting with eligible participants, the Research Coordinator obtained written informed consent for the study. Participants completed baseline self-report measures on paper. This was followed by their first individual session with the chaplain. Strict randomization was not possible due to chaplains' and patients' schedules in the outpatient setting, so chaplains were assigned based on convenience of scheduling. No attempt was made to match patients to chaplains by faith, gender, or other variables, however. Two additional chaplain sessions, scheduled approximately two to three weeks apart, were held in person or by telephone, if the patient was too ill to or otherwise unable to attend a face-to-face visit. Each session lasted approximately 45 to 60 minutes, and was digitally audio recorded (for the purpose of studying Spiritual AIM) and professionally transcribed. Within two weeks after the third Spiritual AIM session, the Research Coordinator administered the same set of measures and only after patient completed these, conducted the exit interview. The chaplains were blind to patients' responses on the measures. The pre-post study was intentionally designed to gather pilot data for hypothesis generation. The scope, timeline (18 months) and budget of the project did not allow for a full randomized controlled trial of Spiritual AIM. The study design and procedures were approved prior to commencing recruitment and any study-related visits by the University of California, San Francisco Committee on Human Research.

Measures

Demographic and clinical data (cancer type) were obtained from electronic medical records with the patient's consent. The patient's religion or faith (including "none") was identified by the chaplain during visits with the patient. Patients completed the following set of self-report measures at both baseline and exit interview: Edmonton Symptom Assessment Scale (ESAS; 10 items; cancer-related symptoms);[21] Center for Epidemiological Studies-Depression (CES-D-10; 10 items; depressive symptoms);[22,23] Spielberger State Anxiety Inventory (STAI-S; 20 items; anxiety symptoms);[24] Functional Assessment of Chronic Illness Therapy-Spiritual (FACIT-Sp-12; 12 items comprising three subscales assessing spiritual well-being—i.e., Meaning, Faith, and Peace);[25,26,27,28] Steinhauser spirituality screen (one item, spiritual distress);[29] Brief RCOPE (14 items; two seven-item subscales [positive and negative religious coping]);[30] Patient Dignity Inventory (PDI; 25 items; spiritual, existential, and psychosocial distress);[31] and Mini-Mental Adjustment to Cancer scale (Mini-MAC; 29 items; cancer-related coping; five subscales [Fatalism, Fighting Spirit, Anxious Preoccupation, Helplessness/Hopelessness, Cognitive Avoidance]; also calculated as two higher-order coping constructs, i.e., Adaptive Coping [Fighting Spirit, Cognitive Avoidance, Fatalism], and Maladaptive Coping [Helplessness/Hopelessness, Anxious Preoccupation]).[32,33,34,35] The FACIT-Sp-12 and Steinhauser were chosen because they represent the widest application so far in the burgeoning field of spiritual care research of spirituality measures and because they measure spirituality, as distinct from religious coping.

Data analysis

Descriptive statistics and frequency distributions were calculated for demographic and clinical characteristics using SPSS Version 22.0. Paired t-tests were used to examine changes from baseline (pre-intervention) to post-intervention.

Results

Recruitment goals were readily achieved (n=31; original target was 30 patients) within the 18-month funded study period, nine months of which were allotted for enrollment. All patients who initiated the study completed three sessions with the chaplain, including six patients who reported no religious affiliation. None of the patients reported undue burden of these visits. All but two expressed in exit interviews that they benefited from the meetings with the chaplain.

Table 1 provides demographic and clinical characteristics of study participants. Patients had a mean age of 59.4 years (SD 9.9; range 34 to 80). A broad range of cancer types was represented. Identified core spiritual needs, as assessed by the chaplain who worked with the patient, were approximately evenly distributed across the three core spiritual needs: eleven patients were assessed as having a core spiritual need of Meaning and Direction; eleven as Self-Worth; and nine as Reconciliation.

Table 1: Demographic and clinical characteristics (n=31)

	Mean (SD)
Age (years)	59.4 (9.9) [Range: 34–80]
	n (%)
Gender	
• Female	20 (64.5%)
• Male	11 (35.5%)
Ethnicity	
• White	27 (87.1%)
• Asian	3 (9.7%)
• Hispanic	1 (3.2%)
Religious self-identification	
• Christian	18 (58.1%)
• Jewish	4 (12.9%)
• Buddhist	3 (9.7%)
• None	6 (19.4%)
Cancer type	
• Breast	6 (19%)
• Gynecologic	7 (23%)
• Gastrointestinal	5 (16%)
• Prostate	5 (16%)
• Head/neck	3 (10%)
• Other	5 (16%)

Table 2 provides baseline and post-Spiritual AIM scores on the study measures. At baseline, the sample reported low overall levels of cancer-related symptoms, "fair" to "good" overall quality of life, moderate scores on the Steinhauser spiritual well-being item, and mild to moderate levels of depressive and anxiety symptoms. There were no significant changes from baseline to post-Spiritual AIM on any of these measures.

On the FACIT-Sp-12, compared to a large sample of adult cancer survivors, our sample scored approximately one standard deviation below the mean on each subscale at baseline.[25] Post-Spiritual AIM, a significant increase was observed only on the Faith subscale of the FACIT-Sp-12.

At baseline, mean scores on the Brief RCOPE Positive and Negative religious coping subscales were lower than previously published norms.[36] Post-Spiritual AIM, there was a trend toward an increase (improvement) in Positive religious coping, while no significant change was seen in Negative religious coping.

On the Mini-MAC, we found a significant increase on the Fighting Spirit subscale and a trend toward an increase on the Fatalism subscale. When analyzed in terms of Adaptive or Maladaptive Coping, a significant increase (improvement) was observed in Adaptive Coping from baseline to post-Spiritual AIM.

Table 2: Measures of symptoms, spiritual well-being, and coping: Baseline and post-Spiritual AIM scores (n=31)

	Baseline Mean (SD)	Post-Spiritual AIM Mean (SD)	Paired samples t-test
ESAS—Total Score	25.0 (12.7)	24.4 (12.9)	t=0.465; p=0.646
Overall quality of life	3.5 (0.8)	3.5 (0.9)	t=-.215; p=0.832
Steinhauser spiritual well-being	3.1 (1.1)	3.1 (1.1)	t=-.465; p=0.646
CES-D-10	4.2 (2.2)	4.1 (2.5)	t=0.680; p=0.502
STAI-S	43.6 (12.5)	41.9 (11.3)	t=1.071; p=0.294
FACIT-Sp-12:			
Meaning	11.8 (3.9)	10.6 (4.4)	t=1.534; p=0.136
Peace	9.0 (3.6)	9.2 (4.2)	t=-0.845; p=0.405
Faith	7.1 (3.9)	8.8 (5.1)	t=-2.520; p=0.018
Patient Dignity Inventory	53.6 (14.4)	51.6 (16.5)	t=1.101; p=0.280
Brief RCOPE:			
Positive religious coping	14.0 (5.7)	15.0 (5.9)	t=-1.806; p=0.082
Negative religious coping	9.2 (2.6)	9.3 (4.1)	t=0.252; p=0.803
Mini-MAC:			
Fatalism	11.2 (2.5)	11.6 (2.4)	t=-1.794; p=0.084
Fighting spirit	10.7 (2.5)	11.8 (2.4)	t=-2.205; p=0.036
Helplessness/hopelessness	14.1 (3.9)	13.4 (5.7)	t=0.888; p=0.382
Anxious preoccupation	20.7 (5.6)	20.2 (5.0)	t=0.719; p=0.478
Cognitive avoidance	9.0 (2.1)	9.2 (2.7)	t=-0.668; p=0.510
Mini-MAC:			
Maladaptive coping	34.8 (7.7)	32.3 (12.1)	t=1.380; p=0.178
Adaptive coping	30.2 (5.4)	32.6 (5.2)	t=-2.517; p=0.018

Table 3 provides examples of qualitative material from patient-chaplain interactions, elucidating each of the main components of Spiritual AIM (assessment, intervention, and outcome) for each of the three core spiritual needs.

Table 3. Examples of assessments, interventions and outcomes for each core spiritual need in Spiritual AIM

Core spiritual need	Example of assessment marker	Patient quotation
Meaning and Direction	Patient tends to intellectualize circumstances	Something was going astray. And so the marital counseling—my wife and I thought this is the best we can do to try to analyze or objectify whatever the imbalance was.
Self-Worth and Belonging	Patient blames self, not others	When I step away from that routine, I feel like a failure… I'm a quitter, like I've always thought of myself all my life. So I'm just going back into old patterns.
Reconciliation/ To Love and Be Loved	Patient blames and mistrusts others	My husband's daughter is just this stranger who comes across as harsh, who's been hurting her father for years and years and years. She just disappears for two, three years at a time and then will call him up when she needs money or something.

Core spiritual need	Example of intervention marker	Chaplain quotation
Meaning and Direction	Chaplain asks how patient has made decisions in the past	Have there been other times in your life where you needed to reintegrate in some way? You had been taking all these classes, which sounds amazing. Is that kind of how you've done it in the past?
Self-Worth and Belonging to Community	Chaplain listens to the story of patient's illness/suffering	I'm wondering if there is more that you'd like me to know about this cancer, about the supports in your life.
Reconciliation/ To Love and Be Loved	Demonstrate ability to tolerate patient's anger	I appreciate you saying that you have a sense of what's helpful to you from a chaplain and what's not so helpful. That's good for me to hear. And it sounds like you have some concern about me as a chaplain maybe judging you or trying to push stuff on you.

cont.

Core spiritual need	Example of outcome marker	Patient quotation
Meaning and Direction	Patient identifies own primary/ prominent heart's desire (i.e., what is most important)	The chaplain helped me realize where I find spirituality… I pretty much find it in talking with people. Seems to be the place where I find the joy, the strength, the everything. And I thought that was really interesting because I have been doing that but I didn't know I was doing that.
Self-Worth and Belonging to Community	Patient's actions/ behavior suggest enhanced self-worth	The chaplain made me think a lot about where my goodness and the love that I feel as a person came from, which was settled in on my dad…
Reconciliation/ To Love and Be Loved	Patient experiences reconciliation/ forgives	I have a stepdaughter who I've had real problems with and so we talked about that. The conversations with the chaplain were good in that I will try to see my stepdaughter in as positive a light as possible, that she's not in control of her actions and her behavior and just try to kind of coexist, if for nothing else but for my husband and his relationship with his grandson.

Discussion

The unique work of chaplains deserves both careful elucidation and close examination. Empirical studies focusing specifically on chaplains' work with palliative care patients are scarce.[9] This study provides preliminary evidence for feasibility and acceptability of Spiritual AIM, a well-articulated, brief, chaplain-delivered spiritual care intervention, implemented with advanced cancer patients receiving palliative care. Conducted over a relatively short timeframe, successful recruitment and retention of advanced cancer patients from a single outpatient palliative care practice speaks to the interest of patients in incorporating spiritual care into their overall cancer care.

We observed increases from pre- to post-Spiritual AIM in several aspects of spiritual well-being: i.e., mean scores increased on both the Faith subscale of the FACIT-Sp-12 as well as the positive religious coping subscale of the Brief RCOPE. Although the Brief RCOPE's title includes the word "religious," it demonstrates utility to measure spirituality and religion. Findings should be viewed with the understanding that these represent the most widely applied and validated spiritual measures.

However, it should be noted that Spiritual AIM was developed independently of any specific assessments; therefore, it is difficult to know whether these measures are the most appropriate or sensitive to any impact of the intervention on patients. However, based on a conceptualization of the chaplain as the spiritual care specialist on the interdisciplinary care team,[37] a well-developed, chaplain-delivered spiritual care intervention should, in theory, affect spiritual and religious outcomes. If chaplains are the members of the interdisciplinary team who are most likely to explicitly discuss and/or represent the patient's relationship with God or the sacred, perhaps this relates to the trend observed in this study.

It is possible that the FACIT-Sp-12 and the Brief RCOPE, which both have some parallels to Spiritual AIM, are more sensitive to the kinds of effects that Spiritual AIM is hypothesized to exert.[26] For example, for the FACIT-Sp-12, the Faith subscale includes items about finding strength or comfort in one's faith or spiritual beliefs, feeling that one's illness has strengthened one's faith or spiritual beliefs, and feeling that "whatever happens with my illness things will be okay." It could be argued that the subscales of the FACIT-Sp-12 measure psychosocial vs. spiritual factors. Nevertheless, there is substantial evidence that the three subscales tap important constructs related to purpose, meaning, comfort, and peace that are associated with quality of life—regardless of one's specific faith or belief system.[38] In Spiritual AIM, the chaplain explores the patient's faith and spiritual beliefs and attempts to sort out which aspects may impede or facilitate peace.[16]

Spiritual AIM and RCOPE are attuned to how the patient behaves, especially their actions towards others, in the context of a serious illness. There is also a shared interest in how these actions affect relationships (with other people and God) and how they change over time.[16, 36] Each framework posits the central and critical role of "relationship"—i.e. that of the patient with the chaplain, other medical providers, family or with God. An example from the Positive religious coping subscale of the Brief RCOPE highlights this: "Tried to put my plans into action together with God." Though questions remain about explicit God language in the RCOPE and measuring the religious coping of patients for whom language about God does not resonate or who identify as non-religious. Finally, the FACIT-Sp-12 has been used successfully in other studies in patients who identify as "spiritual yet not religious."[39] Spiritual AIM and professional chaplaincy favor assessments and interventions that are feasible and effective in patients of any or no faith background.[16, 40]

The significant increases on the Fighting Spirit subscale and the Adaptive Coping factor of the Mini-MAC are intriguing. Spiritual AIM tasks chaplains with helping patients to address their own challenges, utilizing interventions tailored to each patient's core spiritual need. These findings, if replicated, might suggest that even a brief intervention like Spiritual AIM can help patients with serious or life-threatening illnesses to cope more adaptively. The trend toward an increase in Fatalism also warrants further exploration. Importantly, the "Fatalism" construct of the Mini-MAC may be conceptualized (or even better, relabeled) as gratitude or active surrender, as reflected by the items comprising the scale (e.g., "I've put myself in the hands of God;" "I count my blessings;" "I've had a good life, what's left is a bonus").[32] Further work is required to determine whether such changes can be attributed to Spiritual AIM, to some other factor(s) (e.g. religious community, supportive family, another member of the interdisciplinary team), or whether they represent a natural change over time as patients cope with illness.

While intriguing, findings of this study must be viewed cautiously. Since patients were receiving concurrent palliative care, it is possible that observed improvements were related to prior or distinct interventions by the palliative care or other providers. However, the fact that no changes were observed for physical symptoms or for several of the psychological measures argues against this possibility. However, relatively mild baseline levels on several of the symptoms scales may have limited our ability to detect changes. The study's design (pre-/post-intervention, within-subjects, single-arm study) makes it difficult to evaluate whether Spiritual AIM, rather than unobserved intervening variables, was associated with changes. Further work is needed involving larger samples of patients, randomly assigned to Spiritual AIM compared to another brief psychosocial or spiritual care intervention or to treatment-as-usual. Although Spiritual AIM is a well-articulated model, there is a need for a standardized method for teaching the intervention to providers (i.e., manualization).

These preliminary findings suggest that Spiritual AIM may hold promise as a brief, chaplain-led spiritual care intervention for patients with serious or life-limiting illnesses.

Acknowledgements

This work was funded by a grant from the John Templeton Foundation and the HealthCare Chaplaincy.

References

1. Pargament KI. *The Psychology of Religion and Coping: Theory, Research, Practice.* New York: Guilford Press; 1997.
2. Meyerson EM, Meier DE, Kestenbaum A. Honoring thy parent(s): Applying the spiritual domain in palliative care decision making. *Journal of Law and Religion* 2016;31:183–196.
3. Puchalski C, Ferrell B, Virani R, et al. Improving the quality of spiritual care as a dimension of palliative care: the report of the Consensus Conference. *J Palliat Med* 2009;12:885–904.
4. Lo B, Ruston D, Kates LW, et al. Discussing religious and spiritual issues at the end of life: a practical guide for physicians. *JAMA* 2002;287:749–754.
5. Otis-Green S, Ferrell B, Borneman T, Puchalski C, Uman G, Garcia A. Integrating spiritual care within palliative care: an overview of nine demonstration projects. *J Palliat Med* 2012;15:154–162.
6. Astrow AB, Wexler A, Texeira K, He MK, Sulmasy DP. Is failure to meet spiritual needs associated with cancer patients' perceptions of quality of care and their satisfaction with care? *J Clin Oncol* 2007;25:5753–5757.
7. Balboni TA, Paulk ME, Balboni MJ, et al. Provision of spiritual care to patients with advanced cancer: associations with medical care and quality of life near death. *J Clin Oncol* 2010;28:445–452.
8. Balboni T, Balboni M, Paulk ME, et al. Support of cancer patients' spiritual needs and associations with medical care costs at the end of life. *Cancer* 2011;117:5383–5391.
9. HealthCare Chaplaincy. *Literature Review—Testing the Efficacy of Chaplaincy Care.* New York: HealthCare Chaplaincy; 2011.
10. Cadge W. *Paging God: Religion in the Halls of Medicine.* Chicago: University of Chicago Press; 2012.
11. Massey K, Barnes MJ, Villines D, et al. What do I do? Developing a taxonomy of chaplaincy activities and interventions for spiritual care in intensive care unit palliative care. *BMC Palliat Care* 2015;14:10.
12. Fitchett G, Rasinski K, Cadge W, Curlin FA. Physicians' experience and satisfaction with chaplains: a national survey. *Archives of Internal Medicine* 2009;169:1808–1810.
13. Steinhauser KE, Olsen A, Johnson KS, et al. The feasibility and acceptability of a chaplain-led intervention for caregivers of seriously ill patients: A Caregiver Outlook pilot study. *Palliative and Supportive Care* 2016;14:456–467.
14. Lehto RH. The challenge of existential issues in acute care: nursing considerations for the patient with a new diagnosis of lung cancer. *Clin J Oncol Nurs* 2012;16:E4–E11.
15. Zollfrank AA, Trevino KM, Cadge W, et al. Teaching health care providers to provide spiritual care: a pilot study. *J Palliat Med* 2015;18:408–414.
16. Shields M, Kestenbaum A, Dunn LB. Spiritual AIM and the work of the chaplain: a model for assessing spiritual needs and outcomes in relationship. *Palliat Support Care* 2015;13:75–89.
17. Cadge W, Bandini J. The evolution of spiritual assessment tools in healthcare. *Symposium: The Religious and Secular in Medicine and Health* 2015.
18. Flannelly KJ, Weaver AJ, Handzo GF. A three-year study of chaplains' professional activities at Memorial Sloan-Kettering Cancer Center in New York City. *Psycho-Oncology* 2003;12:760–768.
19. Monod S, Martin E, Spencer B, Rochat E, Bula C. Validation of the Spiritual Distress Assessment Tool in older hospitalized patients. *BMC Geriatr* 2012;12:13.
20. Monod SM, Rochat E, Bula CJ, Jobin G, Martin E, Spencer B. The spiritual distress assessment tool: an instrument to assess spiritual distress in hospitalised elderly persons. *BMC Geriatr* 2010;10:88.
21. Chang VT, Hwang SS, Feuerman M. Validation of the Edmonton Symptom Assessment Scale. *Cancer* 2000;88:2164–2171.

22. Irwin M, Artin KH, Oxman MN. Screening for depression in the older adult: criterion validity of the 10-item Center for Epidemiological Studies Depression Scale (CES-D). *Arch Intern Med* 1999;159:1701–1704.
23. Kohout FJ, Berkman LF, Evans DA, Cornoni-Huntley J. Two shorter forms of the CES-D (Center for Epidemiological Studies Depression) depression symptoms index. *J Aging Health* 1993;5:179–193.
24. Spielberger C. *Manual for the State-Trait Anxiety Inventory (Form Y)*. Palo Alto, CA: Consulting Psychologists Press; 1983.
25. Munoz AR, Salsman JM, Stein KD, Cella D. Reference values of the Functional Assessment of Chronic Illness Therapy-Spiritual Well-Being: a report from the American Cancer Society's studies of cancer survivors. *Cancer* 2015;121:1838–1844.
26. Peterman AH, Fitchett G, Brady MJ, Hernandez L, Cella D. Measuring spiritual well-being in people with cancer: the Functional Assessment of Chronic Illness Therapy–Spiritual Well-being Scale (FACIT-Sp). *Ann Behav Med* 2002;24:49–58.
27. Johnson ME, Piderman KM, Sloan JA, et al. Measuring spiritual quality of life in patients with cancer. *J Support Oncol* 2007;5:437–442.
28. Canada AL, Murphy PE, Fitchett G, Peterman AH, Schover LR. A 3-factor model for the FACIT-Sp. *Psycho-Oncology* 2008;17:908–916.
29. Steinhauser KE, Voils CI, Clipp EC, Bosworth HB, Christakis NA, Tulsky JA. "Are you at peace?": one item to probe spiritual concerns at the end of life. *Arch Intern Med* 2006;166:101–105.
30. Pargament KI, Koenig HG, Perez LM. The many methods of religious coping: development and initial validation of the RCOPE. *J Clin Psychol* 2000;56:519–543.
31. Chochinov HM, Hassard T, McClement S, et al. The Patient Dignity Inventory: a novel way of measuring dignity-related distress in palliative care. *J Pain Symptom Manage* 2008;36:559–571.
32. Watson M, Law M, Dossantos M, Greer S, Baruch J, Bliss J. The Mini-Mac—Further Development of the Mental Adjustment to Cancer Scale. *Journal of Psychosocial Oncology* 1994;12:33–46.
33. Anagnostopoulos F, Kolokotroni P, Spanea E, Chryssochoou M. The Mini-Mental Adjustment to Cancer (Mini-MAC) scale: construct validation with a Greek sample of breast cancer patients. *Psycho-Oncology* 2006;15:79–89.
34. Czerw AI, Marek E, Deptala A. Use of the mini-MAC scale in the evaluation of mental adjustment to cancer. *Contemp Oncol (Pozn)* 2015;19:414–419.
35. Grassi L, Buda P, Cavana L, Annunziata MA, Torta R, Varetto A. Styles of coping with cancer: the Italian version of the Mini-Mental Adjustment to Cancer (Mini-MAC) scale. *Psycho-Oncology* 2005;14:115–124.
36. Pargament K, Feuille M, Burdzy D. The Brief RCOPE: Current psychometric status of a short measure of religious coping. *Religions* 2011;2:51–76.
37. Handzo G, Koenig HG. Spiritual care: whose job is it anyway? *South Med J* 2004;97:1242–1244.
38. Whitford HS, Olver IN. The multidimensionality of spiritual wellbeing: peace, meaning, and faith and their association with quality of life and coping in oncology. *Psycho-Oncology* 2012;21:602–610.
39. Bredle JM, Salsman JM, Debb SM, Arnold BJ, Cella D. Spiritual well-being as a component of health-related quality of life: The Functional Assessment of Chronic Illness Therapy—Spiritual Well-Being Scale (FACIT-Sp). *Religions* 2011;2:77–94.
40. A White Paper. Professional chaplaincy: its role and importance in healthcare. *J Pastoral Care* 2001;55:81–97.

ARTICLE 20

Patient Reported Outcome Measure of Spiritual Care as Delivered by Chaplains

Austyn Snowden, School of Health and Social Care, Edinburgh Napier University, Edinburgh, Scotland, United Kingdom

Iain Telfer, The Royal Infirmary of Edinburgh, Edinburgh, Scotland, United Kingdom

Address correspondence to Austyn Snowden, Chair in Mental Health, School of Health and Social Care, Edinburgh Napier University, 4b44, Sighthill Ct., Edinburgh EH11 4BN, Scotland, UK. E-mail: A.snowden@napier.ac.uk

Copyright © Taylor & Francis Group, LLC

Abstract

Chaplains are employed by health organizations around the world to support patients in recognizing and addressing their spiritual needs. There is currently no generalizable measure of the impact of these interventions and so the clinical and strategic worth of chaplaincy is difficult to articulate. This article introduces the Scottish PROM, an original five-item patient reported outcome measure constructed specifically to address this gap. It describes the validation process from its conceptual grounding in the spiritual care literature through face and content validity cycles. It shows that the Scottish PROM is internally consistent and unidimensional. Responses to the Scottish PROM show strong convergent validity with responses to the Warwick and Edinburgh Mental Wellbeing Scale, a generic wellbeing scale often used as a proxy for spiritual wellbeing. In summary, the Scottish PROM is fit for purpose. It measures the outcomes of spiritual care as delivered by chaplains in this study. This novel project introduces an essential and original breakthrough; the possibility of generalizable international chaplaincy research.

Key words: measurement, validity, patient reported outcome measure, chaplain, spiritual care

---

Snowden, A. and Telfer, I. (2017) "Patient reported outcome measure of spiritual care as delivered by chaplains." *Journal of Health Care Chaplaincy*, 23, 4, 131–155.

Introduction

Health services across the world employ chaplains[1] to deliver spiritual care (Cramer & Tenzek, 2012; Marin et al., 2015; Vlasblom et al., 2014). This is because people have needs over and above their physical or psychological requirements (Kelly, 2012). However, unlike physical and psychological needs it is difficult to know when someone's spiritual needs have been met, or what the outcome of meeting those needs may be. This is important for managers faced with difficult decisions as to how best to deploy limited health resources (Palfreyman, 2011). In order to make strategic decisions, planners need to understand how effective care is so they can best meet the needs of the population. They need to understand the outcome of treatment rather than just its cost (Porter & Teisberg, 2007) so they can focus resources on the most effective care. Latkovic (2013) claims that shifting to an outcomes-based payment system could save US $1 trillion. The need to be able to provide evidence of impact in terms of outcomes has never been greater.

The evidence for the impact of chaplain interventions is weak. It is known that chaplains can improve patient satisfaction with hospital stays (Marin et al., 2015), and there are many case studies of successful individual encounters (Fitchett, 2011). This is important work, but case studies and satisfaction measures are weak indicators of impact. Research hierarchies generally favor transferable, generalizable, objective data (Kirkpatrick & Kirkpatrick, 1994), certainly in decisions on funding treatment in national health services (SIGN, 2010). Chaplaincy leaders worldwide therefore recognize that outcomes of chaplaincy interventions need to be measured in order to provide a stronger evidence base (Healthcare Chaplaincy Network, 2016).

Healthcare Chaplaincy Network (2016) recently recommended that chaplains use a range of tools to measure different elements of spiritual care. The reason they had to recommend a range of tools is because there is no tool designed to specifically measure patient outcomes of chaplain interventions. The purpose of this article is to introduce the first measure designed to this end: The Scottish Patient Reported Outcome Measure (PROM).

The Scottish PROM is theoretically grounded in a Scottish interpretation of spirituality and chaplaincy. It is important to stress this cultural element early, because it is clear that chaplains deliver a range of interventions that vary according to country and context. For example, Handzo et al. (2008), in their investigation of chaplain activity in New York, found chaplains delivering religious/spiritual interventions but also more general interventions such as advocacy and counselling. Flannelly, Oettinger, Galek, Braun-Storck, and Kreger (2009) make a further distinction by incorporating emotional interventions, with different types of chaplain activity targeting different needs. It is beyond the scope of this article to attempt a synthesis of this extensive literature. The point is that chaplains worldwide deliver a wide and variable range of interventions according to need. The range of interventions is likely to change according to the local culture. In Scotland, Mowat and Swinton (2007) found the core task of Scottish chaplaincy to involve "an active process of finding people who need spiritual care, identifying the nature of the need and responding to the need through theological reflection and the sharing of spiritual practices" (p.8).

Mowat and Swinton (2007) started from the assumption that whatever chaplains did would be spiritual in nature, whether it be praying, ritual, advocacy or counselling. They then went on to deconstruct the activities of chaplains in order to clarify specialist spiritual care interventions and their impact. These activities are discussed in more detail in the following section as they underpin the development of the PROM. The impact of using this theoretical ground on the generalizability of the Scottish PROM to other cultures will be discussed later.

Methods
Patient Reported Outcome Measure and COSMIN Checklist

A patient reported outcome measure (PROM) is a measure of health, as defined by the patient, in relation to treatment they have received (Wolpert, 2014). PROMs are widely used across health services internationally, and are used to inform care planners and deliverers whether the care they provide is effective or not. The best PROMs are short, easy to understand and important to the group under study (Meadows, 2010). They are psychometrically valid and reliable, and ideally measure a unidimensional construct (Fries, Rose, & Krishnan, 2011). This article systematically details the development of the Scottish PROM to show that it meets these criteria. It follows the COSMIN criteria for reporting on the measurement properties of an original PROM (Mokkink, Terwee, Knol, et al., 2010; Mokkink, Terwee, Patrick, et al., 2010). These criteria are: theoretical underpinning, item development, face and content validity, reliability, dimensionality, and construct validity. These are discussed in turn.

Theoretical underpinning

The Scottish PROM is designed to be a single scale measure of patient outcomes of chaplaincy interventions. Higher scores on the Scottish PROM should indicate better outcomes. The first steps in the construction of the measure were to clarify patient outcomes of chaplaincy interventions. The literature was then searched for existing measures designed to quantify these outcomes.

As discussed in the introduction, because the PROM was developed in and for Scotland, it is grounded in Mowat and Swinton's (2007) seminal research, "*What Chaplains Do.*" Despite finding a broad range of activity Mowat and Swinton noted consistent recurrent elements such as chaplains listening to people and helping them to talk about what was on their mind. Key themes included honesty, control, hope, facilitating a better outlook, giving comfort, understanding, listening, and helping people achieve peace. See Snowden et al. (2012, p.7, Figure 2.1) for a complete list.

As a function of this chaplain activity people reported feeling less anxious and more at peace. They felt a greater capacity to be honest. They reported a greater sense of control and felt better understood. Therefore, while it was not their primary goal, Mowat and Swinton (2007) nevertheless generated a set of consistent consequences of chaplain activity that could be considered outcomes (Snowden, Telfer, Kelly, Bunniss, & Mowat, 2013). Outcomes of chaplain interventions included: control, peace, lessening anxiety, honesty, comfort, relief from distress, being understood, feeling hopeful, being able to cope, and having a positive outlook on life.

In order to search for existing psychometric tools designed to measure these themes the literature search string used by Mowat and Swinton (2007) was updated and expanded as follows. The following terms were combined in multiple searches in Medline, Cinahl, Psychinfo, Mendeley, Google Scholar, Cochrane library: *Chaplain* AND (patient reported outcome measure OR measure AND comfort OR hope OR intervention OR spirit* OR cope OR anxi* OR understand* OR listen* OR acknowledge* OR 'chance to talk' OR gratitude OR serenity OR peace OR control).*

Searching was an iterative process. For example, obviously the search term "measure" is incorporated within "patient reported outcome measure" and so "patient reported outcome measure" is therefore a redundant term if the purpose was to ascertain every article with the word "measure" in it. However, on some searches "measure" generated too many irrelevant results and so the longer term functioned better. In other cases, the opposite was true, when the longer measure did not generate enough relevant articles, but substituting "measure" for it revealed relevant articles on psychometric properties of spiritual care measures that would otherwise have been missed.

The end result of this theoretical phase was a set of potential outcomes of chaplaincy interventions grounded in the literature on chaplaincy and spiritual care and the identification of a number of tools designed to measure these attributes. A summary of key studies, key measures and their salience to the development of the PROM is in the Appendix.

Item development

The next phase was to turn these initial findings into items that could populate the Scottish PROM. This was achieved by inviting patient groups and chaplains to construct statements clearly connected to each theme (Snowden & Telfer, 2011). The focus at this stage was on brevity and clarity. For example, for the theme of "being listened to" the statement was: "I was listened to." Table 1 shows examples of each theme and the original statement associated with it. Comparable items from other questionnaires are also shown. While there are sometimes similarities between the items, all the Scottish PROM items are original.

The PROM items were discussed and refined over a further series of workshops with chaplains, service users, and international leaders in spiritual care throughout 2011 and 2012. The first workshop in June 2011 was attended by 40 Scottish chaplains (Snowden & Telfer, 2011). The main concern at this stage was whether the outcomes were "chaplain specific" enough. For example, hope and peace could be facilitated by any competent health professional. The spiritual element appeared missing to many, although most felt that spirituality was implicit in the items. One of the key decisions made in these workshops was that avoiding explicitly religious or mystical terms was important if the PROM was to be relevant to everybody. Scottish chaplains report that many patients, who see them and appear to benefit from their interventions, do *not* describe themselves as either spiritual or religious.

This is consistent with recent census data that shows 37% of the Scottish population declare themselves having no religion/faith, a 9% increase on the previous census.[2] Scotland is a secular nation and increasingly so. This means that adding overtly spiritual items to the PROM could exclude 37% of the Scottish population, many of whom appear to benefit from seeing a chaplain (Tennant et al., 2007). Nevertheless, this absence of religious and spiritual items continued to worry some chaplains, so a section was added to the pilot version of the PROM to ascertain spiritual traits of the participants responding. The purpose of adding the items was to see if there was any relationship between them and responses to the items in the PROM. The spiritual items were taken from Galek et al. (2005): "A need to experience love and belonging"; "A need to live an ethical and moral life"; "A need to experience beauty, music or nature;" "A need to feel hopeful"; "A need for peace and contentment"; "A need to feel thankful or grateful"; and "A need to find meaning and purpose in life" (p.64).

The pilot study showed no relationship between responses to these items and responses to the PROM, further supporting the claim that all people got equivalent benefit from seeing chaplains regardless of faith perspective (Snowden et al., 2013a). This finding that chaplains are of benefit to all people regardless of faith has helped other health professionals better understand the modern role of the healthcare chaplain. For example, in an ongoing study it has helped General Practitioners assuage fears some people have had about the religious element of chaplaincy on being referred to see them. However, this is not to say that someone's beliefs are not relevant. Chaplains need to understand a patient's faith in order to deliver individualized care. More work is needed, and in order to better understand any relationship between religiosity and chaplaincy impact, subsequent versions of the PROM have contained a shortened demographic/trait question asking people if they were spiritual/religious, both or neither.

Table 1: Themes, their origins, and associated items in the pilot PROM

Theme	Example of citation	Item in pilot PROM	Example validated scale and question
Control	Farber et al. (2010)	I am in control of my situation	Herth Hope Index (*I have a sense of direction*)
Hope	Van Gestel-Timmermans et al. (2010)	Everything is going to be ok	Herth Hope Index (*I believe in a positive outlook towards life*) BDI (*opposite: pessimism scale*)
Being listened to	Ai and McCormick (2009)	I was listened to	GESS-R (*In future I expect that I will be listened to when I speak*) Duke-UNC (*I get chances to talk to someone about problems…*)
Being understood	Gonzalez et al. (2011)	My situation was acknowledged and understood	Sources of meaning profile (*being acknowledged for personal achievements*) Ways of Coping (WAYS) (*I accepted sympathy and understanding from someone*)

Being valued	Hebert et al. (2001)	My faith and/or beliefs were valued	Spiritual Well Being Scale (*I believe that God is concerned about my problems*)
Comfort	Pargament et al. (2011)	I was able to talk about what was on my mind	Social Support Questionnaire (*Whom can you count on to console you when you were upset?*) Brief COPE (*I've been trying to find comfort in my religion or spiritual beliefs/I've been getting emotional support from others*)
Involved in decisions	Palmer and Miedany (2009)	I was involved in decisions about my care	GHQ (*I felt capable of making decisions about things*) Warwick-Edinburgh Mental Wellbeing Scale (*I've been able to make up my own mind about things*)
Honesty	Ai and McCormick (2009)	I could be honest with myself about how I was feeling	CARE (*How was the [chaplain] at being honest but not negative about your problems*)
Relief from distress	Bay et al. (2008)	My levels of anxiety had lessened	HADS (*I can sit at ease and feel relaxed*)
Relevant information	On faith: Ai and McCormick (2009) On illness: Mercer and Murphy (2008)	I found I was able to gain a better perspective on my illness	CARE (*How was the [chaplain] at: fully answering your questions, explaining clearly, giving you adequate information; not being vague*)
Cope	Bay et al. (2008)	Things seemed manageable again	[Opposite construct]: BDI screening question. (*Have you often felt helpless about the future?*)
Peace	Kannan (2008)	A sense of peace that had previously not been there	RCOPE (*Sought help from God in letting go of my anger [anger is described in this section as "an offense to peace"]*)

One of the other key purposes of the workshops was to reduce the number of items where possible. The preference is for short scales because people are more likely to complete them, and so the focus of the following workshop was to reduce the number of items down to the core and essential items (Pilkonis et al., 2011). Where one item could be considered to be subsumed within another then the subsumed item was removed. For example, "hope" is a function of "having a better outlook on life." "Distress" can be subsumed into the more general term "anxiety." The items focusing on hope and distress were therefore removed. Consensus was reached on concentrating on five key overarching outcomes: control, peace, anxiety, honesty, and having a positive outlook on life (Snowden & Telfer, 2012a). These outcomes were then turned into Likert-type items. The stem (the wording at the beginning of the PROM) included a 2-week timeframe in order to align it conceptually with comparable measures such as Warwick and Edinburgh Mental Wellbeing Scale WEMWBS. The purpose of the 2-week timeframe is to allow for reflection over a longer period of time and not just report a snapshot of experience at any given moment.

Face and content validity

The five items were then tested for face and content validity in expert panels at an international conference attended by world leaders in chaplain research (Snowden & Telfer, 2012b). At this stage, it was suggested that a free text box be added so that patients could elaborate on their outcomes should they wish to do so. The final test of face and content validity involved a pilot study of the PROM in a cohort of patients who had received spiritual care from chaplains in NHS Lothian, Scotland (Snowden et al., 2013a). The pilot study asked participants to complete and return the PROM after their episode of care had finished and also provide any comments on its relevance and understandability.

This pilot showed that the PROM was understandable and relevant to participants. The items were unambiguous. Minor amendments to the wording of the items were made as a consequence of feedback (Snowden & Telfer, 2015). For example, "I had a better outlook" was changed to "I had a positive outlook" because the latter does not infer any previous state (a worse outlook). The version tested here consisted of a stem: "In the last two weeks I have felt," and the following items: "I could be honest with myself about how I was really feeling 'Anxious';" "I had a positive outlook on my situation"; "In control of my life"; and "A sense of peace." Each item was followed by a Likert response from "none of the time" through "rarely," "some of the time," and "often" to "all of the time." This version was tested for reliability, dimensionality and convergent validity with a comparable relevant measure in a national sample of people seeing chaplains in Scotland in 2015–2016.

Reliability, dimensionality, and construct validity

The objectives of this phase of validation were to: (a) Establish the reliability of the Scottish PROM; (b) Examine the dimensionality of the Scottish PROM; and (c) Establish convergent validity of the Scottish PROM against a validated wellbeing measure. The study hypotheses were: (a) The Scottish PROM will show strong reliability; (b) The Scottish PROM will demonstrate unidimensionality; and (c) The Scottish PROM will demonstrate convergent validity with WEMWBS.

The hypotheses were tested using a non-experimental design. Project participants were all patients discharged from a community chaplaincy listening service between September 2014 and March 2016. Community chaplaincy listening (CCL) is a service delivered by chaplains in general practice healthcare centers across Scotland to people in distress. The chaplain's intervention is to listen, or more specifically "careful, agenda free listening" (Mowat, Bunniss, Snowden, & Wright, 2013, p.39). One chaplain described the listening as "Helping people unravel the events going on in their lives so that they can make meaning, find purpose and strength and a hopeful way forward" (Mowat et al., 2013, p.39).

Patients were referred to CCL by their general practitioners. Patients met with the chaplain and then had as many sessions as they needed to tell their story, consider the issues they are facing and move towards some sense of resolution or peace. Sessions routinely lasted 50 minutes and patients were free to discharge themselves from the listening service at any time, without explanation.

Ethics

Permission for the study was obtained from NHS West of Scotland research ethics committee 4 on 23rd June 2014, ref 14/WS/0083. Local R&D permissions were obtained from 11 NHS Scotland Health Boards. All people who had received CCL were included. Children under 16, people unable to consent and people who had been very recently bereaved (within 6 months) were excluded. The bereavement criterion was a stipulation of the ethics committee. Data were collected over 18-month period 2014–2016. The CCL program began in 2011.

Procedure

People who had attended CCL who had been subsequently discharged from the service were sent a questionnaire pack. The pack contained the Scottish PROM and the Warwick and Edinburgh Mental Wellbeing Scale

(WEMWBS). The WEMWBS was chosen as the comparator because it is a popular measure of general mental wellbeing (Stewart-Brown, 2013; Stewart-Brown et al., 2009) and so should demonstrate some convergence with the Scottish PROM. Furthermore, the WEMWBS has been used in a UK study where chaplains wanted to measure their impact (Kevern & Hill, 2015), and so there is the possibility of benchmarking scores on the PROM. Finally, WEMWBS has been validated in many different populations and countries and can therefore be considered to be consistently measuring wellbeing in general (Bartram, Yadegarfar, Sinclair, & Baldwin, 2011; Stewart-Brown, 2014). The questionnaires also asked basic demographic questions about age, gender and whether the person was religious, spiritual, both or neither.

Scotland has fourteen health boards responsible for health services within their geographical locality. Eleven NHS Scotland boards participated in the study. Each board area had a PROM "champion," a chaplain who coordinated research activity associated with this project in his or her own area. Following discharge from CCL the chaplain listener forwarded details of discharge to the PROM champion. The champion then forwarded a numbered (anonymized) study questionnaire to the patient. The patient then completed the questionnaire (or not) and returned it to the study administrator in the self-addressed envelope. The administrator then sent the completed anonymized database to the principal investigator. This process was designed to ensure anonymity.

Analytic plan

Each of the five items from the Scottish PROM was coded as below with the exception of the negatively worded item about anxiety, which was reverse coded: None of the Time = 0, Rarely = 1, Some of the time = 2, Most of the Time = 3, All of the time = 4. Missing data were treated as follows: where one of the five items was omitted an average of the other scores was used to replace that item. Where more than one item was omitted the whole set of responses were omitted from analysis. This scoring key gave a maximum possible score of 20. The hypotheses were tested in the following way.

Hypothesis 1: The Scottish PROM will show strong reliability

Reliability is the ability of a tool to measure a concept in a consistent way (Spiliotopoulou, 2009). Polit and Beck (2008) use the example of a scale designed to measure empathy in nursing. Such a scale should only consist of relevant items such as compassion, and not for example contain an item about diagnostic competence. Internal consistency (reliability) is a measure of how well the items measure the same trait.

Reliability is usually analyzed using Cronbach's alpha, a measure of interrelatedness between item responses (Kottner & Streiner, 2010). Results from the pilot study had demonstrated that the five PROM items showed strong internal consistency in a sample of 37 patients ($\alpha = 0.84$) (Snowden, Telfer, Kelly, Bunniss, & Mowat, 2013). Cronbach's alpha was repeated in this study using SPSS version 22. Data were imported into SPSS version 22 and a reliability analysis run.

Hypothesis 2: The Scottish PROM will represent a unidimensional construct

One of the limitations of Cronbach's alpha is that it does not test for dimensionality. Ideally the Scottish PROM should be unidimensional in that it only measures one underlying construct (Gustafsson & Aberg-Bengtsson, 2010), in this case the outcome of spiritual care. However, Cronbach's alpha could demonstrate strong internal consistency even if the scale under study was multidimensional, as long as people responded in a consistent manner. Therefore, an additional test is required to examine dimensionality (Falissard, 1999).

The most rigorous method of testing for dimensionality involves Rasch analysis (Bond & Fox, 2007; Fries et al., 2011). However, Rasch analysis requires at least five responses in each Likert category for meaningful analysis (Linacre, 2006) and in a study with a modest sample size this may not happen. The best alternative is to undertake a principal component analysis (PCA), where unidimensionality would be indicated by a one factor solution (Williams, Brown, & Onsman, 2012). Bartlett's test for sphericity was run to check correlations between the variables, and linearity and outliers were checked using scatterplot (Lund & Lund, 2015). These assumptions were met and so PCA was run in SPSS version 22.

Hypothesis 3: The Scottish PROM will demonstrate convergent validity with WEMWBS

In order to establish that the Scottish PROM was measuring a relevant concept it was compared with an existing validated measure. For example, the two tests above could show that the PROM was reliable and unidimensional but would not tell us if the tool was measuring anything relevant. In order to do this, responses to the Scottish PROM need to be compared with responses to a relevant measure. The chosen relevant measure was the Warwick and Edinburgh Mental Wellbeing Scale, because of its use in other studies measuring wellbeing in people having had spiritual care interventions (Morgan & Tan, 2015; Stewart-Brown, 2014) and its excellent validity in a range of populations (Maheswaran et al., 2012; Tennant et al., 2007). A moderate to high positive correlation between the Scottish PROM and WEMWBS would be considered good evidence of convergent validity (Mokkink, Terwee, Patrick, et al., 2010) because the Scottish PROM should be measuring an aspect of wellbeing (as measured by WEMWBS) but not be identical. That is, the correlation should not be extremely high, because if this were the case the Scottish PROM would be measuring the same construct as the WEMWBS and thus be redundant.

A principal component analysis (PCA) was run on the five-item Scottish PROM. The suitability of PCA was assessed prior to analysis. Monotonicity was checked using scatterplot and then following normality tests correlations were run to test the relationship between the Scottish PROM scores and the WEMWBS scores.

Sample size calculation

Convergent validity entails examination of the correlation between PROM total score and WEMWBS total score. An exact test on GPower version 2 examining a correlation: bivariate model was run with the following assumptions: one tailed, correlation 0.5, alpha error .05, and 95% power. Total sample required was 42.

Results and discussion

The total number of PROMs sent out was 252, and 103 PROMs were returned completed, for a response rate of 41%. Mean (SD) age was 54.1 (15.2) years with a range of 19–92 years. Of those that declared their gender, there were more females ($n = 61$) than males ($n = 25$). Of the 84 respondents who declared their religion orientation, 28 described themselves as religious, 15 spiritual, four both and 37 neither. Mean (SD) total PROM score was 13 (3.3), with range 3–19.

Hypothesis 1: The Scottish PROM will show strong reliability

Item and scale statistics are in Table 2. Cronbach's alpha for the full scale was .81 indicating very good reliability. Reliability estimates using Cronbach's alpha are known to fall as a function of the number of items in the scale (Spiliotopoulou, 2009), particularly below seven items (Swailes

& McIntyre-Bhatty, 2002). Given there are only five items in this scale the result is very encouraging.

Table 2: Item scale statistics

Item-Total Statistics				
Item	Scale mean if item deleted	Scale variance if item deleted	Corrected item-total correlation	Cronbach's alpha if item deleted
I could be honest with myself about how I was really feeling	9.94	8.156	.436	.817
I had a positive outlook on my situation	10.13	7.013	.674	.752
In control of my life	10.35	6.609	.703	.740
A sense of peace	10.54	5.910	.787	.708
Anxious	10.88	7.766	.416	.828

Hypothesis 2: The Scottish PROM will represent a unidimensional construct

Inspection of the correlation matrix showed that all variables had at least one correlation coefficient greater than 0.3. The overall Kaiser-Meyer-Olkin (KMO) measure was 0.78 with individual KMO measures all greater than 0.7, classifications of "middling" to "meritorious" according to Kaiser (1974). Bartlett's test of sphericity was statistically significant ($p < .0001$), indicating that the data was likely factorizable.

PCA revealed only one component that had eigenvalue greater than one and which explained 57% total variance. Visual inspection of the scree plot indicated that just this one component should be retained, and no rotation was therefore necessary (Lund & Lund, 2015). The interpretation of the data was consistent with the Scottish PROM measuring a unidimensional construct: in this case, outcomes of chaplain intervention. Table 3 shows the component matrix for the solution, demonstrating high loadings of all items onto the single factor.

Table 3: Component coefficients

Component matrix[a]	
Item	Component 1
I could be honest with myself about how I was really feeling	.616
I had a positive outlook on my situation	.823
In control of my life	.834
A sense of peace	.896
Anxious	−.577
Extraction Method: Principal Component Analysis[a]	

[a] 1 component extracted.

Hypothesis 3: The Scottish PROM will demonstrate convergent validity with WEMWBS

A Pearson's product-moment correlation was run to assess the relationship between total Scottish PROM scores and total WEMWBS scores. Preliminary analyses showed the relationship to be linear with both variables normally distributed, as assessed by Shapiro-Wilk test ($p > .05$). There was a high positive correlation between the scores, $r(101) = .803$, $p < .0005$, with Scottish PROM scores explaining 64% of the variation in WEMWEBS scores.

General discussion

The study is the first to report on the development and testing of an original patient reported outcome measure for spiritual care as delivered by chaplains. The introduction explained the Scottish PROM originated in the literature on "what chaplains do" (Mowat & Swinton, 2007) and the outcomes associated with these activities. It showed the iterative process of improving face and content validity in partnership with service users, chaplains and chaplain researchers, before reporting brief results of pilot testing in 2012 (Snowden et al., 2012, 2013a). This article then focused on assessing the Scottish PROM's psychometric properties. These results showed the Scottish PROM to be a valid, reliable, and unidimensional scale in this population. More research should be performed to test the measure in different populations and contexts. Psychometric examination of test–retest and inter-rater reliability would further strengthen the credibility of the Scottish PROM. Nevertheless, this article represents a significant, necessary and original step towards an international generalizable measure of the outcome of chaplain interventions.

The sample size was appropriate for the study and exceeded the power analysis estimate to test the study hypotheses. The use of an external measure to establish convergent validity is a further strength. Nevertheless, there are numerous potential biases impacting upon the results, broadly characterized as information bias (e.g., recall bias) and selection bias (Sica, 2006). They are always problematic in self-report studies such as this. For example, it can never be known how the people who chose not to participate would have responded. Those who respond to survey requests tend to be motivated to represent themselves in a positive light where possible (Furnham, 1986). As a consequence, it remains unknown how well the PROM would function as a measure of outcome in the people who did not respond. All that can be claimed in this cohort was strong internal consistency of responses and a strong correlation between responses to the PROM and responses to the WEMWBS.

The response variation (range 3–19) suggests that the Scottish PROM should be able to meaningfully detect a wide range of outcomes of spiritual care. This is important because ceiling effects are often seen in measures attempting to understand the impact of clinical encounters. For example, the Care and Relational Empathy (CARE) measure (Kersten, White, & Tennant, 2012; Mercer, Maxwell, Heaney, & Watt, 2004) is a measure of patient satisfaction within a clinical consultation. It suffers from a marked ceiling effect, possibly related to the social desirability bias discussed above; the patient wants to be seen to be highly appreciative of the doctor (Pratt, Hibberd, Cameron, & Maxwell, 2015). The consequence is that most responses to CARE are bunched around a high mean, just over 45 out of a possible total score of 50.[3] In other words, most people score above 90%. As a consequence, it is not a particularly good method of differentiating one experience from another. More data is required to calibrate the PROM and establish the meaning and clinical significance of a particular score. However, the finding that the mean was relatively low (13 out of 20) and range of responses so wide is very encouraging.[4]

In relation to generalizability, the Scottish PROM was validated in a primary care chaplaincy listening service in Scotland. It is unknown whether its performance would be equivalent in say, acute care, or a different country (however, see Note 4). It was designed to function within a particular culture, and while this project succeeded, some of the cultural assumptions needed to make the measure fit for purpose in Scotland could endanger its generalizability to other countries. For example, colleagues outside Scotland have criticized the Scottish PROM for not being "chaplain specific" enough. It is difficult to respond to this criticism as it usually involves anecdotal or personal interpretations of what a chaplain is. As discussed in the introduction it is not the aim of this article to define chaplaincy beyond grounding chaplain activity in the theoretical work of Mowat and Swinton (2007), because this was the chaplain activity under study.

Furthermore, it has been suggested, particularly in light of its strong correlation with WEMWBS, that the Scottish PROM measures mental wellbeing and not spiritual wellbeing. This argument hinges on mental and spiritual wellbeing being separate factors. Many psychologists take this stance, and attempt to identify items that are uniquely spiritual in order to construct or identify distinct spiritual factors within wellbeing measures. For example, Visser, Garssen, and Vingerhoets (2016) tested a model hypothesizing meaningfulness and trust as uniquely spiritual factors in a wellbeing measure, with peace and pleasure among others as general wellbeing factors. The idea is that by drawing such distinctions people's spiritual wellbeing can be distinguished from people's general wellbeing. As a result, the unique added value of the chaplain can be identified. Unfortunately, they found trust did not fit the model and so concluded that it should be considered a general factor of wellbeing. Findings such as these are quite common, and even when found in a single study, factor structures often fail to replicate in subsequent studies (Snowden, Watson, Stenhouse, & Hale, 2015). Visser et al. (2016) conclude their article by suggesting that a sense of meaning and purpose in life, acceptance, caring for others, connectedness with nature, transcendent experiences, and spiritual activities should be considered uniquely spiritual activities. Certainly, spiritual activities should be considered spiritual activities, but this clearly begs the question of what those could be. We would argue that the rest are not necessarily uniquely spiritual.

The Scottish PROM took a different conceptual journey. Its purpose was to measure the outcomes of spiritual care as delivered by chaplains. This means it started from the assumption that chaplains deliver spiritual activities, whatever they may be. This is what they do (Mowat & Swinton, 2007). Outcomes of this care hopefully *include* mental wellbeing. The Scottish PROM therefore incorporates an element of mental wellbeing. However, if the PROM was *solely* measuring mental wellbeing, then the correlation between the PROM and the WEMWBS would be higher, because they would be measuring exactly the same thing. Results showed they were not. Rather, a strong correlation accounting for 64% variance, as found here, suggests the scales are conceptually similar up to a point, but divergent after that point. Our interpretation is that the Scottish PROM and WEMWBS represent different types of wellbeing. Because it is measuring what chaplains do, our interpretation is that the Scottish PROM measures the outcomes of spiritual care as delivered by chaplains. The measure includes mental wellbeing. It is difficult to see why it shouldn't.

There is considerable international appetite for robust, transferable measures of the impact of chaplaincy. Despite such interest no such measure has previously been developed and so chaplains and their planners have had to justify measuring aspects of spiritual care such as mood or anxiety and then describe why these particular measures may be relevant (Healthcare Chaplaincy Network, 2016). By contrast the Scottish PROM has been specifically designed and tested to provide evidence of the outcomes of chaplaincy interventions. It is the first such measure and as such there is considerable interest in its use. In the past year, the research team have been contacted by colleagues in Australia, Tasmania, England, Wales, and Canada for permission to use the tool within various spiritual care services and populations. The Scottish PROM is being translated into Dutch and Flemish. Results of these studies/projects will be published in the next few years, and will provide important information on the practical utility of the Scottish PROM in a range of settings.

The main implication for practicing chaplains is that they now have a valid, dedicated, short measure to better understand the impact of their interventions. The importance of this is clear. For example, it could be used to monitor progress. It could be used as a method of referral to chaplains from fellow health professionals. Anecdotally, it has been used as a focal point for conversation during encounters by encouraging patients to reflect on their answers. It has also been used as a means of reflection for chaplains in supervision sessions. It is not a panacea, and not meant as a replacement for any other research, but it does offer a path towards generalizable evidence of impact for chaplains that is currently missing. This type of evidence is very important as it offers policymakers a better opportunity to understand the role and function of chaplains within health teams and to see their unique impact. For example, it would be interesting to see how well fellow health professionals fared by comparison when evaluated using this measure.

In order to build on this work further research is required to examine the function of the Scottish PROM in a wider range of settings and populations. More data is needed to ascertain population norms and meaningful thresholds across a range of clinical settings. The clinical utility of the Scottish PROM in practice also needs more research. The next planned phases of research include this. They are: (a) To test the utility of the Scottish PROM as a before and after measure of chaplain intervention in CCL. This study will also test convergent validity with EQ5D and explore the cost effectiveness of chaplain interventions; (b)

Cross-cultural validity testing in Belgian and Dutch populations; (c) Analysis of the scaling properties of the PROM using Rasch Analysis; and (d) PhD project critically examining the utility of the PROM in Europe. These projects are under development and more are under consideration.

Conclusion

The Scottish PROM is a reliable, valid measure of the outcomes of chaplain interventions in Scotland. It is the first measure designed specifically for the purpose of measuring the impact of chaplain interventions. As such it gives chaplains, managers, and budget holders a new and powerful tool to evaluate the impact of chaplaincy in a generalizable and transferable manner. This is a significant step for chaplaincy, which up to now has been reliant on case studies or non-specific measures to support their case. While case studies are essential for reflection and the professional development of chaplaincy, they do not synthesize easily, and so are of limited use to budget holders tasked with allocating ever decreasing healthcare resources to an ever increasing population. Recognizing this problem, a new approach has emerged, with scholars attempting to identify uniquely spiritual elements of healthcare so that the singular contribution of the chaplain can be articulated with a much higher degree of generalizability. Thus far, however, this project has proved intractable for two reasons: (a) there is no consensus on what a spiritual factor would consist of, and (b) most candidates that emerge can also usually be described as pertaining to emotional or mental wellbeing, and as such are not uniquely spiritual.

The Scottish PROM escapes these criticisms because firstly it is grounded in a coherent theory of "what chaplains do." Secondly, instead of taking a separatist approach to defining spirituality it was instead constructed to understand "what it is like" to receive spiritual care. The outcome of receiving spiritual care includes improvement in mental, emotional, and general wellbeing. These distinctions are unlikely to be important for people in receipt of chaplain interventions. The Scottish PROM measures the outcomes of what chaplains do.

Funding

Funding was received from NHS Education for Scotland.

Notes

1. Most countries use the term chaplain but not all. In Australia, chaplains are referred to as "pastoral carers" for example. The term chaplain is used here throughout to refer to all employees of health services around the world whose role is to primarily look after the religious and spiritual needs of their population.
2. Scottish religious group demographics www.gov.scot/Topics/People/Equality/Equalities/ DataGrid/Religion/RelPopMig.
3. www.measuringimpact.org/s4-care-measure.
4. An Australian study with a return of over 500 Scottish PROMs showed equivalent mean and standard deviation.

References

Ai, A. L. & McCormick, T. R. (2009). Increasing diversity of Americans' faiths alongside Baby Boomers' aging: implications for chaplain intervention in health settings. *Journal of Health Care Chaplaincy, 16*(1–2), pp. 24–41. www.ncbi.nlm.nih.gov/pubmed/2018311.

Bartram, D. J., Yadegarfar, G., Sinclair, J. M. A., & Baldwin, D. S. (2011). Validation of the Warwick-Edinburgh Mental Wellbeing Scale (WEMWBS) as an overall indicator of population mental health and wellbeing in the UK veterinary profession. *Veterinary Journal, 187*(3), 397–398. doi:10.1016/j.tvjl.2010.02.010

Bay, P. S., Beckman, D., Trippi, J., Gunderman, R., & Terry, C. (2008). The effect of pastoral care services on anxiety, depression, hope, religious coping, and religious problem solving styles: A randomized controlled study. *Journal of Religion and Health, 47*(1), 57–69. doi:10.1007/s10943-007-9131-4

Bond, T. G., & Fox, C. M. (2007). *Applying the Rasch model: Fundamental measurement in the human sciences* (2nd ed.). New York, NY: Routledge.

Cramer, E. M., & Tenzek, K. E. (2012). The Chaplain profession from the employer perspective: An analysis of hospice chaplain job advertisements. *Journal of Health Care Chaplaincy, 18*(3–4), 133–150. doi:10.1080/08854726.2012.720548

Falissard, B. (1999). The unidimensionality of a psychiatric scale: A statistical point of view. *International Journal of Methods in Psychiatric Research, 8*(3), 162–167. doi:10.1002/mpr.66

Farber, E. W., Bhaju, J., Campos, P. E., Hodari, K. E., Motley, V. J., Dennary, B. E., ... Sharma, S. M. (2010). Psychological wellbeing in persons receiving HIV-related mental health services: The role of personal meaning in a stress and coping model. *General Hospital Psychiatry, 32*(1), 73–9. http://doi.org/10.1016/j.genhosppsych.2009.09.011

Fitchett, G. (2011). Making our case(s). *Journal of Health Care Chaplaincy, 17*(1–2), 3–18. doi:10.1080/08854726.2011.559829

Flannelly, K. J., Oettinger, M., Galek, K., Braun-Storck, A., & Kreger, R. (2009). The correlates of chaplains' effectiveness in meeting the spiritual/religious and emotional needs of patients. *The Journal of Pastoral Care & Counseling, 63*, 1–16. doi:10.1177/154230500906300109

Fries, J., Rose, M., & Krishnan, E. (2011). The PROMIS of better outcome assessment: Responsiveness, floor and ceiling effects, and Internet administration. *The Journal of Rheumatology, 38*(8), 1759–1764. doi:10.3899/jrheum.110402

Furnham, A. (1986). Response bias, social desirability and dissimulation. *Personality and Individual Differences, 7*(3), 385–400. doi:10.1016/0191-8869(86)90014-0

Galek, K., Flannelly, K. J., Vane, A., & Galek, R. M. (2005). Assessing a patient's spiritual needs. *Holistic Nursing Practice*, *19*(2), 62–69. Retrieved from www.shi.or.th/images/misc/200608011805260.pdf.

Gonzalez, M. T., Hartig, T., Patil, G. G., Martinsen, E. W., & Kirkevold, M. (2011). A prospective study of existential issues in therapeutic horticulture for clinical depression. *Issues in Mental Health Nursing*, *32*(1), 73–81. http://doi.org/10.3109/01612840.2010.528168

Gustafsson, J.-E., & Aberg-Bengtsson, L. (2010). Unidimensionality and Interpretability of Psychological Instruments. In S. Embretson (Ed.), *Measuring psychological constructs: Advances in model-based approaches* (pp.97–121). Washington, DC: American Psychological Association.

Handzo, G. F., Flannelly, K. J., Kudler, T., Fogg, S. L., Harding, S. R., Hasan, Y. H., ... Taylor, B. E. (2008). What do chaplains really do? II. Interventions in the New York chaplaincy study. *Journal of Health Care Chaplaincy*, *14*(1), 39–56. doi:10.1080/08854720802053853

Healthcare Chaplaincy Network. (2016). *What is quality spiritual care in healthcare and how can we measure it?* Retrieved from www.healthcarechaplaincy.org/docs/research/quality_indicators_document_2_17_16.pdf.

Hebert, R. S., Jenckes, M. W., Ford, D. E., O'Connor, D. R., & Cooper, L. A. (2001). Patient perspectives on spirituality and the patient-physician relationship. *Journal of General Internal Medicine*, *16*(10), 685–92. Retrieved from www.pubmedcentral.nih.gov/articlerender.fcgi?artid=1495274&tool=pmcentrez&rendertype=abstract.

Kaiser, H. F. (1974). An index of factor simplicity. *Psychometrika*, *39*, 31–36.

Kannan, L. M. (2008). *Spirituality and symptom self management of osteoarthritis*. University of San Diego.

Kelly, E. (2012). The development of healthcare chaplaincy. *The Expository Times*, *123*(10), 469–478. doi:10.1177/0014524612444531

Kersten, P., White, P. J., & Tennant, A. (2012). The consultation and relational empathy measure: An investigation of its scaling structure. *Disability and Rehabilitation*, *34*(6), 503–509. doi:10.3109/09638288.2011.610493

Kevern, P., & Hill, L. (2015). "Chaplains for wellbeing" in primary care: Analysis of the results of a retrospective study. *Primary Health Care Research & Development*, *16*(1), 87–99. doi:10.1017/S1463423613000492

Kirkpatrick, D. L., & Kirkpatrick, J. D. (1994). *Evaluating training programs*. San Francisco, CA: Berrett-Koehler.

Kottner, J., & Streiner, D. L. (2010). Internal consistency and Cronbach's alpha: A comment on Beeckman et al. (2010). *International Journal of Nursing Studies*, *47*(7), 926–928. doi:10.1016/j.ijnurstu.2009.12.018

Latkovic, T. (2013). *The Trillion Dollar Prize. Using outcomes-based payment to address the US healthcare financing crisis*. Retrieved from http://healthcare.mckinsey.com/sites/default/files/the-trillion-dollar-prize.pdf.

Linacre, J. M. (2006). *WINSTEPS Rasch measurement computer program*. Chicago, IL: Winsteps.com.

Lund, M., & Lund, A. (2015). *Principal components analysis in SPSS statistics*. Retrieved from https://statistics.laerd.com/premium/pca/pca-in-spss-5.php.

Maheswaran, H., Weich, S., Powell, J., & Stewart-Brown, S. (2012). Evaluating the responsiveness of the Warwick Edinburgh Mental Wellbeing Scale (WEMWBS): Group and individual level analysis. *Health and Quality of Life Outcomes*, *10*(1), 156. doi:10.1186/1477-7525-10-156

Marin, D. B., Sharma, V., Sosunov, E., Egorova, N., Goldstein, R., & Handzo, G. F. (2015). Relationship between chaplain visits and patient satisfaction. *Journal of Health Care Chaplaincy*, *21*(1), 14–24. doi:10.1080/08854726.2014.981417

Meadows, K. A. (2010). Patient-reported outcome measures: An overview. *British Journal of Community Nursing*, *16*(3), 146–151.

Mercer, S. W., Maxwell, M., Heaney, D., & Watt, G. C. (2004). The consultation and relational empathy (CARE) measure: Development and preliminary validation and reliability of an empathy-based consultation process measure. *Family Practice*, *21*(6), 699–705. doi:10.1093/fampra/cmh621

Mercer, S. W., & Murphy, D. J. (2008). Validity and reliability of the CARE Measure in secondary care. *Clinical Governance: An International Journal*, *13*(4), 269–283. doi:10.1108/14777270810912969

Mokkink, L. B., Terwee, C. B., Knol, D. L., Stratford, P. W., Alonso, J., Patrick, D. L., ... De Vet, H. C. (2010). The COSMIN checklist for evaluating the methodological quality of studies on measurement properties: A clarification of its content. *BMC Medical Research Methodology*, *10*(1), 22. doi:10.1186/1471-2288-10-22

Mokkink, L. B., Terwee, C. B., Patrick, D. L., Alonso, J., Stratford, P. W., Knol, D. L., ... De Vet, H. C. W. (2010). The COSMIN checklist for assessing the methodological quality of studies on measurement properties of health status measurement instruments: An international Delphi study. *Quality of Life Research*, *19*(4), 539–549. doi:10.1007/s11136-010-9606-8

Morgan, M., & Tan, H. (2015). *Review of literature*. Abbotsford, VIC: Spiritual Health Victoria. Retrieved from www.spiritualhealthvictoria.org.au/LiteratureRetrieve.aspx?ID = 202460.

Mowat, H., Bunniss, S., Snowden, A., & Wright, L. (2013). Listening as health care. *The Scottish Journal of Healthcare Chaplaincy*, *16*, 39–46.

Mowat, H., & Swinton, J. (2007). *What do Chaplains do? The role of the Chaplain in meeting the spiritual needs of patients*. Aberdeen, UK: Mowat Research.

Palfreyman, S. (2011). Patient-reported outcome measures and how they are used. *Nursing Older People*, *23*(1), 31–36.

Palmer, D., & Miedany, Y. (2009). Patient-reported outcome measures in rheumatology. *Nursing and Residential Care*, *11*(4), 190–194.

Pargament, K., Feuille, M., & Burdzy, D. (2011). The brief RCOPE: Current psychometric status of a short measure of religious coping. *Religions*, *2*(4), 51–76. http://doi.org/10.3390/rel2010051

Pilkonis, P. A., Choi, S., Reise, S. P., & Stover, A. M. (2011). Item banks for measuring emotional distress from the patient reported outcomes measurement information system (PROMIS): Depression, anxiety and anger. *Assessment*, *18*(3), 263–283. doi:10.1177/1073191111411667

Polit, D. F., & Beck, T. B. (2008). *Nursing research*. Philadelphia, PA: Lippincott Williams & Wilkins.

Porter, M. E., & Teisberg, E. O. (2007). How physicians can change the future of health care. *The Journal of the American Medical Association*, *297*(10), 1103–1111. doi:10.1001/jama.297.10.1103

Pratt, R., Hibberd, C., Cameron, I., & Maxwell, M. (2015). The patient centered assessment method (PCAM): Integrating the social dimensions of health into primary care. *Journal of Comorbidity*, *5*(1), 110–119. doi:10.15256/joc.2015.5.35

Sica, G. T. (2006). Bias in research studies. *Radiology*, *238*(3), 780–789. doi:10.1148/radiol.2383041109

Snowden, A., & Telfer, I. (2011). *The NHS Lothian PROM*. Edinburgh, Scotland: Spiritual Care and Bereavement Management.

Snowden, A., & Telfer, I. (2012a). *Spiritual care patient reported outcome measure – Why and what potential impact on practice?* In Chaplaincy and Enhancing Person-Centred Care. Perth, Scotland.

Snowden, A., & Telfer, I. (2012b). A patient reported outcome measure for spiritual care. *Spiritual care and health: Improving outcome and enhancing well being*. Clydebank, Scotland.

Snowden, A., & Telfer, I. (2015). CCL PROM: To Validity and Beyond. In *Spiritual Wellbeing at the Heart of Person-Centred Care: Co-creating Community Through Research and Innovation*. Glasgow, Scotland. Retrieved from www.events.nes.scot.nhs.uk/media/69361/register-now-spritual-wellbeing-flyer-october15.pdf.

Snowden, A., Telfer, I. J., Kelly, E. K., Bunniss, S., & Mowat, H. (2013). I was able to talk about what was on my mind. The operationalisation of person centred care. *The Scottish Journal of Healthcare Chaplaincy*, 16, 14–24.

Snowden, A., Telfer, I. J., Kelly, E. K., Bunniss, S., & Mowat, H. (2013a). The construction of the Lothian PROM. *The Scottish Journal of Healthcare Chaplaincy*, 16, 3–13.

Snowden, A., Telfer, I., Kelly, E., Mowat, H., Bunniss, S., & Howard, N. (2012). *Healthcare Chaplaincy/: The Lothian Chaplaincy patient reported outcome measure (PROM)*. Gourock. Retrieved from www.snowdenresearch.co.uk.

Snowden, A., Watson, R., Stenhouse, R., & Hale, C. (2015). Factor and Rasch analysis of the trait emotional intelligence questionnaire short form. *Journal of Advanced Nursing*, 71(12), 2936–2949.

Spiliotopoulou, G. (2009). Reliability reconsidered: Cronbach's alpha and paediatric assessment in occupational therapy. *Australian Occupational Therapy Journal*, 56(3), 150–155. doi:10.1111/j.1440-1630.2009.00785.x

Stewart-Brown, S. (2013). The Warwick-Edinburgh Mental Wellbeing Scale (WEMWBS): Performance in different cultural and geographical groups. In C. Keyes (Ed.), *Mental wellbeing: International contributions to the study of positive mental health* (pp.133–150). Dordrecht: Springer Science Business Media.

Stewart-Brown, S. (2014). Measuring wellbeing: What does the Warwick-Edinburgh Mental Wellbeing Scale have to offer integrated care? *European Journal of Integrative Medicine*, 7, 384–388. doi:10.1016/j.eujim.2014.08.004

Stewart-Brown, S., Tennant, A., Tennant, R., Platt, S., Parkinson, J., & Weich, S. (2009). Internal construct validity of the Warwick-Edinburgh Mental Wellbeing Scale (WEMWBS): A Rasch analysis using data from the Scottish Health Education Population Survey. *Health and Quality of Life Outcomes*, 7, 15. doi:10.1186/1477-7525-7-15

Swailes, S., & McIntyre-Bhatty, T. (2002). The "Belbin" team role inventory: Reinterpreting reliability estimates. *Journal of Managerial Psychology*, 17(6), 529–536. doi:10.1108/02683940210439432

Tennant, R., Hiller, L., Fishwick, R., Platt, S., Joseph, S., Weich, S., … Stewart-Brown, S. (2007). The Warwick-Edinburgh mental wellbeing scale (WEMWBS): Development and UK validation. *Health and Quality of Life Outcomes*, 5, 63. doi:10.1186/1477-7525-5-63

Van Gestel-Timmermans, H., Van Den Bogaard, J., Brouwers, E., Herth, K., & Van Nieuwenhuizen, C. (2010). Hope as a determinant of mental health recovery. *Scandinavian Journal of Caring Sciences*, 24 Suppl 1, 67–74. http://doi.org/10.1111/j.1471-6712.2009.00758.x

Visser, A., Garssen, B., & Vingerhoets, A. J. (2016). Existential wellbeing. *The Journal of Nervous and Mental Disease*.

Vlasblom, J. P., Walton, N. P., van der Steen, J. T., Doolaard, J. J., & Jochemsen, H. (2014). Developments in healthcare chaplaincy in the Netherlands and Scotland: A content analysis of professional journals. *Health and Social Care Chaplaincy*, 2(2), 235–254. doi:10.1558/hscc.v2i2.20409

Williams, B., Brown, T., & Onsman, A. (2012). Exploratory factor analysis: A five- step guide for novices. *Australasian Journal of Paramedicine*, 8(3), 1–13.

Wolpert, M. (2014). Uses and abuses of patient reported outcome measures (PROMs): Potential iatrogenic impact of PROMs implementation and how it can be mitigated. *Administration and Policy in Mental Health*, 41(2), 141–145. doi:10.1007/s10488-013-0509-1

Appendix

Source, summary, measure, and salience to chaplaincy PROM

Authors	Summary	Measures	Salience to PROM development
Ai and McCormick (2009)	Case studies are used to illustrate the actions of the chaplain at the bedside in end of life care. A new scale is presented for chaplains to assess diverse afterlife beliefs.	Connection of the soul (COS)	Recognition of importance of "being with," caring and compassion as unique contribution of chaplain. Within the health care team, the chaplain is often uniquely situated as one who is designated to take time to "be with" the patient and who by both personal virtue and professional training can embody a caring and compassionate presence to the vulnerable patient.
Pargament, Feuille, and Burdzy (2011)	Pargament was the original developer of the 14 item brief RCOPE, a measure of religious coping with life stressors. The items within the scale were developed from interviews with people suffering life stressors. Important distinction emerged between negative and positive religious coping. The negative religious coping subscale has been particularly useful as a predictor of health outcome.	Brief RCOPE	This article integrates discussion of psychometric quality with religious coping, a factor specifically associated with spiritual care. This may be particularly pertinent in light of discussions that suggest there is little unique to the chaplaincy role, given that other professions can claim to meet certain spiritual needs.

Authors	Summary	Measures	Salience to PROM development
Farber et al. (2010)	This study sought to quantify the degree to which personal meaning accounted for various differences amongst a cohort of 132 people with HIV. They found that "personal meaning" was associated with psychological wellbeing.	LRI-R, GWB, MOS, Social Support Survey, LOT-R, CHIP	Personal meaning is a pertinent construct to the work of chaplaincy, so this study illuminated some of the issues in trying to account for such a variable. The Life Regard Index seems promising in this regard, although this particular study could not identify any causality because of its design.
Gonzalez, Hartig, Patil, Martinsen, and Kirkevold (2011)	This small ($n = 46$) study measured the efficacy of therapeutic horticulture on depression and in particular existential issues. The intervention significantly correlated with a consistent improvement in depression but not existential issues. Existential issues were measured with the LRI-R.	LRI-R, BDI	This article is relevant because existential issues were postulated to be relevant to chaplaincy interventions. The findings suggested that depression in this case may not be directly correlated with existential issues as measured in this way. This could be a function of the measure, the sample size or genuine discord, although the authors imply the former because the participants claimed the intervention was meaningful and influential on their view of life. These all need to be considered in PROM development.
Hebert, Jenckes, Ford, O'Connor, and Cooper (2001)	Study designed to ascertain the preferences and concerns of seriously ill people when discussing religious and spiritual beliefs with clinicians. God, prayer, spiritual beliefs were all mentioned as sources of support and healing. Willingness to discuss these issues was closely related to the therapeutic relationship.	Thematic	Relevant in ascertaining the pertinent categories of discussion and also relevant that clinicians didn't always meet these needs. In general people didn't expect clinicians to fulfill these needs but if they disclosed them then they hoped the beliefs would be valued.

Kannan (2008)	The purpose of this study was to describe the relationships among symptom experience, symptom management, and symptom outcome based on spiritual wellbeing. Kannan found that greater spiritual existential wellbeing was significantly associated with improved physical function.	Revised Symptom Management Conceptual Model	Important because they found a relationship between self-reported spiritual wellbeing and physical function. This type of result supports chaplaincy from a clinical perspective. The self-report methodology makes it relevant to a potential spiritual PROM.
Van Gestel-Timmermans, Van Den Bogaard, Brouwers, Herth, and Van Nieuwenhuizen (2010)	Discusses the function of hope in recovery from mental ill-health. The study develops and validates a Dutch version of the Herth Hope Index to assess the degree to which hope may be construed and measured.	HHI, MANSA, RAND-36, CISS, MHCS	Although the authors conclude the tool is a valid measure of hope they warn against using subscales within it in isolation. This may be due to "interconnectedness" as being an historical factor of this index. Useful for showing how scales can and should be compared with each other in order to develop and clarify constructs like hope, loneliness and coping.
Bay, Beckman, Trippi, Gunderman, and Terry (2008)	RCT studied the efficacy of chaplaincy against patient outcomes of anxiety, depression, hope, positive and negative religious coping, and religious coping styles. They found chaplain visits increased positive religious coping and decreased negative religious coping.	Hamilton Anxiety and Depression Scale (HADS); Herth Hope Index; 14 item brief RCOPE	No significant differences were found between any of the major scales, suggesting it may be difficult to detect efficacy using this type of methodology. Nevertheless, some non-significant trends towards positive religious coping were encouraging. The measures used in this study were highly pertinent to our project.

ARTICLE 21

A National Study of Chaplaincy Services and End-of-Life Outcomes

Kevin J Flannelly[1], Linda L Emanuel[2,*], George F Handzo[3], Kathleen Galek[4], Nava R Silton[5] and Melissa Carlson[6]

1 The Spears Research Institute, HealthCare Chaplaincy, 307 East 60th Street, New York, NY 10022, USA.

2 Buehler Center on Aging, Health & Society, Northwestern University Feinberg School of Medicine, 750 N. Lake Shore Drive, Suite 601, Chicago, IL 60611, USA.

3 HealthCare Chaplaincy, 307 East 60th Street, New York, NY 10022, USA.

4 The Spears Research Institute, HealthCare Chaplaincy, 307 East 60th Street, New York, NY 10022, USA.

5 Department of Psychology, Marymount Manhattan College, 221 East 71st Street, New York, NY 10021, USA.

6 Mount Sinai School of Medicine, Annenberg Building Floor 10, 1468 Madison Avenue, New York, NY 10029, USA.

* Correspondence: l-emanuel@northwestern.edu

© 2012 Flannelly et al.; licensee BioMed Central Ltd. This is an Open Access article distributed under the terms of the Creative Commons Attribution License (http://creativecommons.org/licenses/by/2.0), which permits unrestricted use, distribution, and reproduction in any medium, provided the original work is properly cited.

Abstract

Background: Medicine has long acknowledged the role of chaplains in healthcare, but there is little research on the relationship between chaplaincy care and health outcomes. The present study examines the association between chaplaincy services and end-of-life care service choices.

Methods: HealthCare Chaplaincy purchased the AHA survey database from the American Hospital Association. The Dartmouth Atlas of Health Care database was provided to HealthCare Chaplaincy by The Dartmouth Institute for Health Policy & Clinical Practice, with the permission of Dartmouth Atlas Co-Principal Investigator Elliot S. Fisher, M.D., M.P.H. The Dartmouth Atlas of Health Care is available interactively online at www.dartmouthatlas.org. Patient data are aggregated at the hospital level in the Dartmouth Atlas of Health Care. IRB approval was not sought

---

Flannelly, K.J., Emanuel, L.L., Handzo, G.F., Galek, K., Silton, N.R., and Carlson, M. (2012) "A national study of chaplaincy services and end-of-life outcomes." *BMC Palliative Care*, 11, 10.

for the project because the data are available to the public through one means or another, and neither database contains data about individual patients, i.e. all the variables are measures of hospital characteristics. We combined and analyzed data from the American Hospital Association's Annual Survey and outcome data from The Dartmouth Atlas of Health Care in a cross-sectional study of 3,585 hospitals. Two outcomes were examined: the percent of patients who (1) died in the hospital, and (2) were enrolled in hospice. Ordinary least squares regression was used to measure the association between the provision of chaplaincy services and each of the outcomes, controlling for six factors associated with hospital death rates.

Results and discussion: The analyses found significantly lower rates of hospital deaths ($\beta = .04$, $p < .05$) and higher rates of hospice enrollment ($\beta = .06$, $p < .001$) for patients cared for in hospitals that provided chaplaincy services compared to hospitals that did not.

Conclusions: The findings suggest that chaplaincy services may play a role in increasing hospice enrollment. This may be attributable to chaplains' assistance to patients and families in making decisions about care at the end of life, perhaps by aligning their values and wishes with actual treatment plans. Additional research is warranted.

Key words: chaplaincy care, pastoral care, health outcomes, end-of-life care, hospice

Introduction

Most individuals in the United States (U.S.) who are seriously ill say they want to die at home.[1] Yet, research has consistently shown that the majority of older U.S. adults,[2,3,4] especially those with chronic diseases,[2,3,5] die in the hospital. This is the case in other countries, too, according to studies conducted in the 1990s.[6,7]

More recent research has found that high rates of hospital deaths among older adults and those with chronic illnesses exists in most of the countries in which it has been studied, including Australia,[8] Belgium,[9,10,11] Canada,[12] Korea,[13] Singapore,[14] the U.K.[11] and the U.S.[15] Exceptions to this observation are The Netherlands[11] and Sweden.[16]

A number of factors have been examined that contribute to the high rates of hospital deaths. U.S. studies consistently have found that hospital deaths are related to hospital bed availability and vary across states and regions of the country, with hospital death rates being lowest in the Western states.[3,4,5] This association between hospital bed availability and rate of hospital deaths has been found in Belgium and the United Kingdom, as well.[11]

Another geographically related variable that is associated with rates of hospital deaths is population density. Research in Belgium,[10] Germany,[17] and Taiwan[18] has shown that people living in urban areas are more likely to die in the hospital than those living in rural areas, although findings from other studies are inconsistent.[2, 7] The observed relationship between hospital deaths and population density, as well as the regional differences, may be partly attributable to the number of available hospital beds per capita, with areas that have a greater number of hospital beds per person having higher rates of hospital deaths.[3, 19]

Geographically based (e.g. census tracks) measures of socio-economic status have also been found to be associated with hospital death rates. For example, Belgian[9] and American researchers[19] have reported that individuals from poorer neighborhoods have higher rates of hospital deaths than those from wealthier neighborhoods.

Recent studies have begun to explore the degree to which different healthcare services are associated with different end-of-life outcomes. For instance, an Australian study reported that community nursing services, which included emotional support for patients and families, were associated with lower hospital death rates.[20] Other Australian studies reported that community-based palliative care services were associated with lower rates of hospital deaths.[8, 21] The lower rates of hospital deaths were associated with higher rates of institutional hospice deaths in one study[21] and higher rates of home deaths in the other.[8] A Belgian study also found that community-based palliative care services were associated with lower rates of hospital deaths and higher rates of home deaths.[22]

U.S. research suggests that hospital-based palliative care programs can affect hospice enrollment and hospital deaths. One study, for example, reported that in-patient palliative care produced higher rates of referrals to home-based hospice programs than usual acute care,[23] and another reported that palliative care teams successfully diverted patients into inpatient and home-based hospice programs.[24] In a randomized control trial, patients who received palliative care services had fewer admissions to intensive care units (ICU) and longer hospice stays.[25] Other research further indicates that palliative care teams may help to reduce hospital deaths, especially ICU deaths.[26]

Chaplains have long been considered to be an integral part of the palliative care team[27] and they have routinely provided emotional and spiritual support to patients and family members even when palliative care services were not available.[28, 29, 30, 31, 32] However, only two studies to date have examined the effectiveness of chaplaincy care, one of which found chaplaincy care reduced patient anxiety[33] and the other of which reported that it helped patients contend with spiritual distress.[34]

Although no previous research has examined the relationship between chaplaincy care and end-of-life outcomes, there is reason to believe that spiritual care, like that provided by chaplains, may affect end-of-life decision-making. Recent research has found that patients who say their spiritual needs were met by hospital staff were more likely to receive hospice care and less likely to receive aggressive treatment.[35, 36]

We have noticed that one of the things that chaplains do for patients is help them understand and feel comfortable with their core values and how these can be synthetic with their health care goals. Since people generally prefer to die at home, chaplains may help patients and families to resolve issues about end of life care, so that patients are less likely to die in the hospital.

Study aims

The present study was designed to test two hypotheses about the provision of chaplaincy services and end-of-life outcomes. First, hospitals that provide chaplaincy services will have lower rates of hospital deaths than hospitals that do not provide chaplaincy services. Second, hospitals that provide chaplaincy services will have higher rates of hospice enrollment than hospitals that do not provide chaplaincy services.

Methods

Study sample

The study combined datasets from the American Hospital Association (AHA) and The Dartmouth Atlas of Health Care. The AHA regularly conducts surveys of its member hospitals in which hospital administrators are asked to report the facilities and services the hospital provides, along with various other characteristics of the hospital. The present study used data from the 2005 fiscal-year survey. The Dartmouth Atlas of Health Care combined data from the Center for Medicare and Medicaid Services on traditional, fee-for-service medical claims to track patients who died between January 1, 2001 and December 31, 2005, and had one or more of nine chronic diseases: congestive heart failure, chronic lung disease, cancer, coronary artery disease, renal failure, peripheral vascular disease, diabetes, chronic liver disease, and dementia. The Dartmouth Atlas uses discharge claims to assign patients to the hospital in which they died, or were admitted most often during the last two years of life. Patients who only had surgical admissions were excluded from The Dartmouth Atlas database.

Of the 4,271 healthcare facilities in The Dartmouth Atlas, 4,180 (97.9%) were matched by name to hospitals in the AHA database. Of these, 3,603 completed the AHA annual survey for fiscal-year 2005. After excluding children's, orthopedic, and obstetrics/gynecology hospitals, and rehabilitation and long-term care facilities, the sample consisted of 3,585 hospitals: 3,566 general medical, one surgical, eight heart, and ten cancer hospitals.

Dependent variables

Two measures from The Dartmouth Atlas served as dependent variables: (1) the percent of patients who died in each hospital; and (2) the percent of patients who enrolled in home-based hospice.

Independent variable

The independent variable for the study was whether or not a hospital provided chaplaincy services by hospital staff or through a vendor. The AHA Survey's definition for "Chaplaincy/Pastoral Care Services" is: "A service ministering religious activities and providing pastoral counseling to patients, their families, and staff of a health care organization." Hospitals that had chaplaincy services were coded as 1 and those that did not were coded as 0.

Control variables

Six control variables were used in the analyses: (1) whether the hospital was located in a western state (Alaska, Arizona, California, Colorado, Hawaii, Idaho, Montana, Nevada, New Mexico, Oregon Utah, Washington, and Wyoming); (2) the population density of its catchment area; (3) number of hospital beds; (4) the proportion of Medicaid patients; (5) whether the hospital has a palliative care team; and (6) type of hospital. The three categorical variables (1, 5 and 6) were dummy coded as explained below.

It was essential to control for the region of the U.S. in which the hospital was located (i.e., western states), since several studies have found that hospital deaths are lower in the western states than in other states.[3, 4] This variable also controls for regional differences in palliative care and chaplaincy services.[37, 38, 39] Population density was included as a control variable in the analyses because it also has been found to be related to the rate of hospital deaths.[17, 18, 22] The AHA survey measures population density on a 0–6 scale, reflecting the size of the Metropolitan Statistical Area in which a hospital is located.

The next control variable, hospital beds, was included to control for bed availability, which is associated with hospital death rates,[3, 11, 19] and the fact that larger hospitals (as measured by beds) are more likely to provide palliative and chaplaincy services[37, 38, 39, 40]. This variable was measured by the AHA bed size code, which uses a 1–8 scale.

The proportion of each hospital's Medicaid patients was used as a proxy for socio-economic status of patients.[41] It was calculated by dividing the hospital's number of Medicaid discharges by its number of licensed beds. To control for the net effects of palliative care services, hospitals that had a palliative care program were dummy coded as 1 and those that did not have one were coded as 0. Similarly, we controlled for type of hospital by dummy coding the 19 specialty hospitals as 1 and the general hospitals as 0.

Regression models

The association between chaplaincy and each of the dependent variables was tested by using ordinary least-squares (OLS) regression, controlling for western states, population density, number of hospitals beds, socio-economic status, type of hospital, and whether a hospital had a palliative care program. Because 95 hospitals did not have data on hospice enrollment, only 3,490 hospitals were used in the analysis of this dependent variable. Other analyses are described in the results section.

Results

Table 1 presents the univariate statistics for the independent, dependent and control variables. Of the 3,585 hospitals in the sample, nearly 2,457 hospitals provided chaplaincy services (68.5%), and 1,092 hospitals provided palliative care services (30.5%). Just under 18% were located in the 13 western states. The average rates of hospital deaths and hospice enrollment were approximately, 35% and 29%, respectively.

Table 1: Univariate statistics for independent, dependent, and control variables

(N = 3,585 hospitals)	Number	Percent
Hospitals with Chaplaincy Services	2,457	68.5
Hospitals in Western States	630	17.6
Hospitals with Palliative Care	1,092	30.5
Specialty Hospitals	19	0.6
	Mean	S.D.
Rate of Hospital Deaths	34.9	7.6
Rate of Hospice Enrollment	29.2	12.2
Population Density	2.2	2.4
Number of Hospital Beds	3.9	1.8
Socio-Economic Status (Proportion of Medicaid Patients)	1.5	2.9

On a scale of 0–6, the mean population density of 2.2 indicates that the average hospital in the sample was located in a geographical area with a population of over 250,000 residents. The average size of hospitals in the study was between 100 and 200 beds, based on the AHA bed size code.

Table 2 presents the results of the OLS regression models predicting rates of hospital deaths and hospice enrollment. The values given in the table are standardized betas (βs), which show the unique association of chaplaincy services and each of the control variables with the two dependent variables: hospital deaths and hospice enrollment.

Table 2: Estimated net association of chaplaincy services variables with the rate of hospital deaths and rate of hospice enrollment, controlling for the six other variables in the model

Variables	Hospital deaths	Hospice enrollment
Western States	-0.12***	0.02
Population Density	0.02	0.29***
Number of Hospital Beds	0.27***	0.06**
Socio-Economic Status	0.02	-0.08***
Palliative Care	-0.07***	-0.02
Specialty Hospitals	0.03	0.01
Chaplaincy Services	-0.04*	0.06***
Adjusted R^2	0.08	0.12

* $p < .05$ ** $p < .01$ *** $p < .001$ Values in the table are standardized betas.

As hypothesized, chaplaincy services were associated with significantly lower rates of hospital deaths ($\beta = -.04$, $p < .01$) compared to hospitals that did not provide chaplaincy services, controlling for region of the country, population density, hospital beds, socio-economic status, palliative care and type of hospital (see Table 2). As expected, hospitals located in western states and those with palliative care teams had significantly lower rates of hospital deaths.

Number of hospital beds was positively and significantly related to hospital deaths, but population was not. However, these two variables were positively correlated, and the association between hospital deaths and population density ($\beta = 0.14$) was statistically significant ($p < .001$) when the model was re-run without number of beds. This supports previous findings that population density is positively related to hospital deaths and shows that the inclusion of number of beds in the model captured a substantial portion of the variation in hospital deaths that would otherwise have been attributable to population density.

As hypothesized, chaplaincy services also were associated with significantly higher rates of hospice enrollment ($\beta = .06$, $p < .001$). Population density and number of beds were positively related to hospice enrollment, while socio-economic status was negatively related to enrollment.

Discussion

The findings support both hypotheses: that chaplaincy services are significantly associated with (1) lower rates of hospital deaths and (2) higher rates of hospice enrollment. Although these associations are relatively small, they can have profound consequences for patients and families. One would not expect appreciably larger net effects of specific services, since many unknown variables also contribute to the outcomes being examined. Nevertheless, the fact that the regression model for rates of hospital deaths replicated the effects of variables known to be related to hospital death rates from previous research lends credence to the generalizability of the findings. While palliative care exhibited the expected negative association with hospital deaths, it is not apparent why it did not have a significant positive association with hospice enrollment.

Chaplains often help patients and family members to feel comfortable with their core values and to see how these can be congruent with their healthcare goals. Since most people prefer to die at home,[1,42,43] discussions of values and goals with chaplains might partially account for the observed association of chaplaincy services with decreased hospital deaths and increased hospice enrollment.

The present results are consistent with recent research that patients who said their spiritual needs were met by hospital staff were more likely to receive hospice care and less likely to receive aggressive treatment.[35, 36] Related research has found that families of dying patients who felt supported,[44] and were able to discuss spiritual issues when making end-of-life decisions were more satisfied with those decisions.[44]

Other research has found that meeting the spiritual needs of patients is associated with higher levels of patient[45] and family[46, 47] satisfaction with the quality of overall care. Meeting spiritual needs is particularly important at the end of life in order to achieve spiritual and psychological healing when physical healing is no longer possible, and palliation is the goal.[48, 49] At this time of life, it is essential to align treatment with the patient's goals,[50] which are often influenced by spirituality and religion.[51]

A recent study of patients in a palliative care unit with end-stage cancer found that 88% of patients expressed the desire to work with a chaplain.[52] Roughly half of the patients indicated they would like the chaplain to provide a sense of "presence," listen to them, visit with them, or accompany them on their journey. The more religious patients also desired various spiritual interventions from the hospital chaplain.

Surveys of hospital administrators in the U.S. have found that professional chaplains are expected to play a number of roles.[53, 54] In addition to providing spiritual and emotional support to patients and families, generally, chaplains are also expected to help patients and family members address end-of-life issues and deal with difficult decisions. Related U.S. research indicates that hospital staff refer patients and families to chaplains for such reasons,[32] and that chaplains spend a considerable amount of time dealing with these kinds of issues.[55, 56] Moreover, Australian studies have found that the majority of hospital chaplains helped patients and families make treatment decisions,[57] and that many chaplains assisted families and staff dealing with pain control and life support issues.[58, 59, 60]

This study has a number of limitations, including the fact that the AHA survey only indicated whether or not a hospital provided chaplaincy services. It did not provide information about the specific nature, scope, and quality of the services. Another limitation is that the patient outcome data are aggregated across a 5-year period (2001–2005), and there is evidence that the provision of chaplaincy services increased somewhat during this time.[37] This introduces some degree of error to the models, which are based on the hospital services that existed in fiscal year 2005 (2004–2005).

Although the analyses controlled for a number of variables that have been shown to be associated with end-of-life outcomes, the presence of chaplaincy services could still be a proxy for some other variable or variables. It could, for example, be an indication that a hospital is committed to providing patient-centered and family-focused care in which all members of the team are dedicated to listening to the patient and aligning care with patient and family wishes. Since the evidence indicates that this stance generally leads to less use of hospital resources at the end of life, these hospitals might have fewer hospital deaths even if they did not have chaplains. Nonetheless, this type of care, whether provided by a chaplain or another discipline, appears to have an impact.

Its limitations notwithstanding, we believe the present study provides support for the possible role of chaplains in reducing hospital deaths and increasing hospice enrollment. This could be attributable to the fact that chaplains assist patients and families in making decisions about care at the end of life and aligning their values and wishes with actual treatment plans.

Conclusions

The findings suggest that chaplaincy services may play a role in decreasing hospital deaths and increasing hospice enrollment. This may be attributable to chaplains' assistance to patients and families in making decisions about care at the end of life, perhaps by aligning their values and wishes with actual treatment plans. Additional research is warranted.

Competing interests

The authors declare that they have no competing interests.

Acknowledgements

This study was funded in part by a grant from the Fannie E. Rippel Foundation.

Authors' contributions

KJF designed the study with KG, NRS and MC, all of whom wrote the initial draft. KJF, LLE and GFH were the primary authors. KJF conducted the statistical analyses. All the authors reviewed drafts and approved the final content.

Received: 26 January 2012

Accepted: 2 July 2012

Published: 2 July 2012

References
1. Fried TR, Bradley EH, Towle VR, Allore H: Understanding the treatment preferences of seriously ill patients. *N Engl J Med* 2002, 346:1061–1066.
2. Gruneir A, Mor V, Weitzen S, Truchil R, Teno J, Roy J: Where people die: a multilevel approach to understanding influences on site of death in America. *Med Care Res Rev* 2007, 64:351–378.
3. Hansen SM, Tolle SW, Martin DP: Factors associated with lower rates of in-hospital death. *J Palliat Med* 2002, 5:677–685.
4. Mitchell SL, Teno JM, Miller SC, Mor V: A national study of the location of death for older persons with dementia. *J Am Geriatr Soc* 2005, 53:299–305.
5. Weitzen S, Teno JM, Fennell M, Mor V: Factors associated with site of death: a national study of where people die. *Med Care* 2003, 41:323–335.
6. Tang ST, McCorkle R: Determinants of place of death for terminal cancer patients. *Cancer Invest* 2001, 19:165–180.
7. Burge F, Lawson B, Johnston G: Trends in the place of death of cancer patients, 1992–1997. *CMAJ* 2003, 168:265–270.
8. McNamara B, Rosenwax L: Factors affecting place of death in Western Australia. *Health Place* 2007, 13:356–367.
9. Houttekier D, Cohen J, Bilsen J, Deboosere P, Verduyckt P, Deliens L: Determinants of the place of death in the Brussels metropolitan region. *J Pain Symptom Manage* 2009, 37:996–1005.
10. Cohen J, Bilsen J, Hooft P, Deboosere P, van der Wal G, Deliens L: Dying at home or in an institution using death certificates to explore the factors associated with place of death. *Health Policy* 2006, 78:319–329.
11. Houttekier D, Cohen J, Bilsen J, Addington-Hall J, Onwuteaka-Philipsen B, Deliens L: Place of death in metropolitan regions: metropolitan versus non-metropolitan variation in place of death in Belgium, The Netherlands and England. *Health Place* 2010, 16:132–139.
12. Motiwala SS, Croxford R, Guerriere DN, Coyte PC: Predictors of place of death for seniors in Ontario: a population-based cohort analysis. *Can J Aging* 2006, 25:363–371.
13. Yun YH, Lim MK, Choi KS, Rhee YS: Predictors associated with the place of death in a country with increasing hospital deaths. *Palliat Med* 2006, 20:455–461.
14. Beng AK, Fong CW, Shum E, Goh CR, Goh KT, Chew SK: Where the elderly die: the influence of socio-demographic factors and cause of death on people dying at home. *Ann Acad Med Singapore* 2009, 38:676–683.
15. Muramatsu N, Hoyem RL, Yin H, Campbell RT: Place of death among older Americans: does state spending on home- and community-based services promote home death? *Med Care* 2008, 46:829–838.
16. Hanratty B, Burstrom B, Walander A, Whitehead M: Hospital deaths in Sweden: are individual socioeconomic factors relevant? *J Pain Symptom Manage* 2007, 33:317–323.
17. Pinzon LC, Weber M, Claus M, et al.: Factors influencing place of death in Germany. *J Pain Symptom Manage* 2011, 41:893–903.
18. Lin HC, Lin YJ, Liu TC, Chen CS, Lin CC: Urbanization and place of death for the elderly: a 10-year population-based study. *Palliat Med* 2007, 21:705–711.

19. Lackan NA, Eschbach K, Stimpson JP, Freeman JL, Goodwin JS: Ethnic differences in in-hospital place of death among older adults in California: effects of individual and contextual characteristics and medical resource supply. *Med Care* 2009, 47:138–145.
20. Howat A, Veitch C, Cairns W: A retrospective review of place of death of palliative care patients in regional north Queensland. *Palliat Med* 2007, 21:41–47.
21. Currow DC, Burns CM, Abernethy AP: Place of death for people with noncancer and cancer illness in South Australia: a population-based survey. *J Palliat Care* 2008, 24:144–150.
22. Cohen J, Houttekier D, Chambaere K, Bilsen J, Deliens L: The use of palliative care services associated with better dying circumstances. Results from an epidemiological population-based study in the Brussels metropolitan region. *J Pain Symptom Manage* 2011, 42:839–851.
23. Reville B, Miller MN, Toner RW, Reifsnyder J: End-of-life care for hospitalized patients with lung cancer: utilization of a palliative care service. *J Palliat Med* 2010, 13:1261–1266.
24. Fromme EK, Bascom PB, Smith MD, et al.: Survival, mortality, and location of death for patients seen by a hospital-based palliative care team. *J Palliat Med* 2006, 9:903–911.
25. Gade G, Venohr I, Conner D, et al.: Impact of an inpatient palliative care team: A randomized control trial. *J Palliat Med* 2008, 11:180–190.
26. Elsayem A, Smith ML, Parmley L, et al.: Impact of a palliative care service on in-hospital mortality in a comprehensive cancer center. *J Palliat Med* 2006, 9:894–902.
27. Weissman DE, Meier DE: Center to advance palliative care inpatient unit operational metrics: consensus recommendations. *J Palliat Med* 2009, 12:21–25.
28. Vanderwerker LC, Flannelly KJ, Galek K, et al.: What do chaplains really do? III. Referrals in the New York Chaplaincy Study. *J Health Care Chaplain* 2008, 14:57–73.
29. Handzo GF, Flannelly KJ, Kudler T, et al.: What do chaplains really do? II. Interventions in the New York Chaplaincy Study. *J Health Care Chaplain* 2008, 14:39–56.
30. Flannelly K, Weaver A, Handzo G: A three-year study of chaplains' professional activities at Memorial Sloan-Kettering Cancer Center in New York City. *Psycho-Oncology* 2003, 12:760–768.
31. Fogg SL, Weaver AJ, Flannelly KJ, Handzo GF: An analysis of referrals to chaplains in a community hospital in New York over a seven year period. *J Pastoral Care Counsel* 2004, 58:225–235.
32. Galek K, Vanderwerker LC, Flannelly KJ, et al.: Topography of referrals to chaplains in the Metropolitan Chaplaincy Study. *J Pastoral Care Counsel* 2009, 63(6):1–13.
33. Iler WL, Obenshain D, Camac N: The impact of daily visits from chaplains on patients with chronic obstructive pulmonary disease (COPD): A pilot study. *Chaplaincy Today* 2001, 17:5–11.
34. Bay PS, Beckman D, Trippi J, Gunderman R, Terry C: The effect of pastoral care services on anxiety, depression, hope, religious coping, and religious problem solving styles: a randomized controlled study. *J Relig Health* 2008, 47:57–69.
35. Balboni TA, Paulk ME, Balboni MJ, et al.: Provision of spiritual care to patients with advanced cancer: associations with medical care and quality of life near death. *J Clin Oncol* 2010, 28:445–452.
36. Balboni T, Balboni M, Paulk ME, et al: Support of cancer patients' spiritual needs and associations with medical care costs at the end of life. *Cancer* 2011, 117:5383–5391.
37. Cadge W, Freese J, Christakis NA: The provision of hospital chaplaincy in the United States: A national overview. *South Med J* 2008, 101:626–630.
38. Flannelly KJ, Handzo GF, Weaver AJ: Factors affecting healthcare chaplaincy and the provision of pastoral care in the United States. *J Pastoral Care Counsel* 2004, 58:127–130.
39. Goldsmith B, Dietrich J, Du Q, Morrison RS: Variability in access to hospital palliative care in the United States. *J Palliat Med* 2008, 11:1094–1102.
40. Morrison RS, Maroney-Galin C, Kralovec PD, Meier DE: The growth of palliative care programs in United States hospitals. J Palliat Med 2005, 8:1127–1134.

41. Gelfman LP, Meier DE, Morrison RS: Does palliative care improve quality? A survey of bereaved family members. *J Pain Symptom Manage* 2008, 36:22–28.
42. Flory J, Yinong Y-X, Gurol I, Levinsky N, Ash A, Emanuel E: Place of death: US trends since 1980. *Health Affairs (Project Hope)* 2004, 23:194–200.
43. Pritchard RS, Fisher ES, Teno JM, et al.: Influence of patient preferences and local health system characteristics on the place of death. SUPPORT Investigators. Study to Understand Prognoses and Preferences for Risks and Outcomes of Treatment. *J Am Geriatr Soc* 1998, 46:1242–1250.
44. Gries CJ, Curtis JR, Wall RJ, Engelberg RA: Family member satisfaction with end-of-life decision making in the ICU. *Chest* 2008, 133:704–712.
45. Astrow AB, Wexler A, Texeira K, He MK, Sulmasy DP: Is failure to meet spiritual needs associated with cancer patients' perceptions of quality of care and their satisfaction with care? *J Clin Oncol* 2007, 25:5753–5757.
46. Daaleman TP, Williams CS, Hamilton VL, Zimmerman S: Spiritual care at the end of life in long-term care. *Med Care* 2008, 46:85–91.
47. Wall RJ, Engelberg RA, Gries CJ, Glavan B, Curtis JR: Spiritual care of families in the intensive care unit. *Crit Care Med* 2007, 35:1084–1090.
48. Billings JA, Pantilat S: Survey of palliative care programs in United States teaching hospitals. *J Palliat Med* 2001, 4:309–314.
49. Sulmasy DP: Spiritual issues in the care of dying patients: "...it's okay between me and god". *J Am Med Assoc* 2006, 296:1385–1392.
50. Meier DE, Casarett DJ, von Gunten CF, Smith WJ, Storey CP: Palliative medicine: politics and policy. *J Palliat Med* 2010, 13:141–146.
51. Balboni TA, Vanderwerker LC, Block SD, et al.: Religiousness and spiritual support among advanced cancer patients and associations with end-of-life treatment preferences and quality of life. *J Clin Oncol* 2007, 25:555–560.
52. Mako C, Galek K, Poppito SR: Spiritual pain among patients with advanced cancer in palliative care. *J Palliat Med* 2006, 9:1106–1113.
53. Flannelly KJ, Galek K, Bucchino J, Handzo GF, Tannenbaum HP: Department directors' perceptions of the roles and functions of hospital chaplains: A national survey. *Hosp Top* 2005, 83:19–27.
54. Flannelly K, Handzo G, Weaver A, Smith W: A national survey of health care administrators' views on the importance of various chaplain roles. *J Pastoral Care Counsel* 2005, 59:87–96.
55. Handzo GF, Flannelly KJ, Murphy KM, et al.: What do chaplains really do? I. Visitation in the New York Chaplaincy Study. *J Health Care Chaplain* 2008, 14:20–38.
56. Vanderwerker LC, Handzo GF, Fogg SL, Overvold JA: Selected findings from the "New York" and the "Metropolitan" chaplaincy studies: A 10-year comparison of chaplaincy in the New York City area. *J Health Care Chaplain* 2008, 15:13–24.
57. Carey LB, Cohen J: Religion, spirituality and health care treatment decisions: the role of chaplains in the Australian clinical context. *J Health Care Chaplain* 2008, 15:25–39.
58. Carey LB, Newell CJ: Chaplaincy and resuscitation. *Resuscitation* 2007, 75:12–22.
59. Carey LB, Newell CJ, Rumbold B: Pain control and chaplaincy in Australia. *J Pain Symptom Manage* 2006, 32:589–601.
60. Carey LB, Newell CJ: Withdrawal of life support and chaplaincy in Australia. *Crit Care Resusc* 2007, 9:34–39.

Full citations of the 21 articles

Bay, P.S., Beckman, D., Trippi, J., and Gunderman, C.T. (2008) 'The effect of pastoral care services on anxiety, depression, hope, religious coping, and religious problem solving styles: a randomized controlled study.' *Journal of Religion & Health, 47,* 57-69.

Berning, J.N., Poor, A.D., Buckley, S.M., Patel, K.R., Lederer, D.J., Goldstein, N.E., Brodie, D., and Baldwin, M.R. (2016) 'A Novel picture guide improve spiritual care and reduce anxiety in mechanically ventilated adults in the intensive care unit.' *Annals of the American Thoracic Society, 13,* 8, 1333-42.

Cadge, W., Freese, J., and Christakis, N.A. (2008) 'The provision of hospital chaplaincy in the United States: a national overview.' *Southern Medical Journal, 101,* 6, 626-630.

Donohue, P.K., Norvell, M., Boss, R., Shepard, J., Frank, K., Patron, C., and Crowe, T. (2017) 'Hospital chaplains: through the eyes of parents of hospitalized children.' *Journal of Palliative Medicine 20,* 2, 1352-1358.

Flannelly, K.J., Emanuel, L.L., Handzo, G.F., Galek, K., Silton, N.R., and Carlson, M. (2012) 'A national study of chaplaincy services and end-of-life outcomes.' *BMC Palliative Care, 11,* 10.

Grossoehme, D.H., Szczesniak, R.D., Mrug, S., Dimitriou, S.M., Marshall, A.L., and McPhail, G.L. (2016) 'Adolescents' spirituality and cystic fibrosis airway clearance treatment adherence: examining mediators.' *Journal of Pediatric Psychology 41,* 19, 1022-1032.

Hui, D., de la Cruz, M., Thorney, S., Parsons, H.A., Delgado-Guay, M., and Bruera, E. (2011) 'The frequency and correlates of spiritual distress among patients with advanced cancer admitted to an acute palliative care unit.' *American Journal of Hospice and Palliative Medicine, 28,* 4, 264-270.

Johnson, J.R., Engelberg, R.A., Nielsen, E.L., Kross, E.K., Smith, N.L., Hanada, J.C., Doll O'Mahoney, S.K., and Curtis, J.R. (2014) 'The association of spiritual care providers' activities with family members' satisfaction with care after a death in the ICU.' *Critical Care Medicine, 42,* 9, 1991-2000.

Johnson, R.M., Wirpsa, M.J., Boyken, L., Sakumoto, M., Handzo, G., Kho, A., and Emanuel, L. (2016) 'Communicating chaplains' care: narrative documentation in a neuroscience-spine intensive care unit.' *Journal of Health Care Chaplaincy, 22,* 4, 133-50.

Kestenbaum, A., Shields, M., James, J., Hocker, W., Morgan, S., Karve, S., Rabow, MW, and Dunn, L.B. (2017) 'What impact do chaplains have? A pilot study of spiritual AIM for advanced cancer patients in outpatient palliative care.' *Journal of Pain and Symptom Management, 54,* 5, 707-714.

King, S.D., Fitchett, G., Murphy, P., Pargament, K.I., Harrison, D.A., and Loggers, E.T. (2017) 'Determining best methods to screen for religious/spiritual distress.' *Supportive Care in Cancer, 25,* 471-79.

Marin, D.B., Sharma, V., Sosunov, E., Egorova, N., Goldstein, R., and Handzo, G.F. (2015) 'Relationship between chaplain visits and patient satisfaction.' *Journal of Health Care Chaplaincy, 21,* 14-24.

Massey, K., Barnes, M.J.D., Villines, D., Goldstein, J.D., Hisey Pierson, A.L., Scherer, C., Vander Laan, B., and Summerfelt, W.T. (2015) 'What do I do? Developing a taxonomy of chaplaincy activities and interventions for spiritual care in intensive care unit palliative care.' *BMC Palliative Care, 14,* 10, 1-8.

Monod, S.M., Rochat, E., Büla, C.J., Jobin, G., Martin, E., and Spencer, B. (2010) 'The spiritual distress assessment tool: an instrument to assess spiritual distress in hospitalized elderly persons.' *BMC Geriatrics, 10*, 88-96.

Nolan, S. (2016) '"He needs to talk!": a chaplain's case study of nonreligious spiritual care.' *Journal of Health Care Chaplaincy, 22*, 1, 1-16.

Nuzum, D., Meaney, S., and O'Donoghue, K. (2017) 'The spiritual and theological challenges of stillbirth by bereaved parents.' *The Journal of Religion & Health 56*, 1081-1095.

Piderman, K.M., Radecki, B.C., Jenkins, S.M., Lapid, M.I., Kwete, G.M., Sytsma, T.T., Lovejoy, L.A., Yoder, T.J., and Jatoi, A. (2017a) 'The impact of a spiritual legacy intervention in patients with brain cancer and other neurologic illnesses and their support persons.' *Psychooncology, 26*, 3, 346-353.

Raffay, J., Wood, E., and Todd, A. (2016) 'Service user views of spiritual and pastoral (chaplaincy) in NHS mental health services: a co-produced constructivist grounded theory investigation.' *BMC Psychiatry, 16*, 200.

Ragsdale, J.R., Hegner, M.A., Mueller, M., and Davies, S. (2014) 'Identifying religious and/or spiritual perspectives of adolescents and young adults receiving blood and marrow transplants: a prospective qualitative study.' *Biological Blood Marrow Transplantation 20*, 8, 1242-1257.

Schultz, M., Lulav-Grinwald, D., and Bar-Sela, G. (2014) 'Cultural differences in spiritual care: findings of an Israeli oncologic questionnaire examining patient interest in spiritual care.' *BMC Palliative Care, 13*, 1, 19-29.

Snowden, A. and Telfer, I. (2017) 'Patient reported outcome measure of spiritual care as delivered by chaplains.' *Journal of Health Care Chaplaincy, 23*, 4, 131-155.